New Insights into Pediatric Pulmonology

New Insights into Pediatric Pulmonology

Editors

Lea Bentur
Ronen Bar-Yoseph

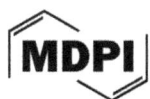

Basel • Beijing • Wuhan • Barcelona • Belgrade • Novi Sad • Cluj • Manchester

Editors
Lea Bentur
Pediatric Pulmonary Institute
and CF Center
Ruth Rappaport Children's
Hospital
Haifa, Israel

Ronen Bar-Yoseph
Pediatric Pulmonary Institute
and CF Center
Ruth Rappaport Children's
Hospital
Haifa, Israel

Editorial Office
MDPI
St. Alban-Anlage 66
4052 Basel, Switzerland

This is a reprint of articles from the Special Issue published online in the open access journal *Journal of Clinical Medicine* (ISSN 2077-0383) (available at: https://www.mdpi.com/journal/jcm/special_issues/Pediatric_Pulmonology).

For citation purposes, cite each article independently as indicated on the article page online and as indicated below:

Lastname, A.A.; Lastname, B.B. Article Title. *Journal Name* **Year**, *Volume Number*, Page Range.

ISBN 978-3-0365-9362-3 (Hbk)
ISBN 978-3-0365-9363-0 (PDF)
doi.org/10.3390/books978-3-0365-9363-0

© 2023 by the authors. Articles in this book are Open Access and distributed under the Creative Commons Attribution (CC BY) license. The book as a whole is distributed by MDPI under the terms and conditions of the Creative Commons Attribution-NonCommercial-NoDerivs (CC BY-NC-ND) license.

Contents

About the Editors vii

Liron Borenstein-Levin, Noa Avishay, Orit Soffer, Shmuel Arnon, Arieh Riskin, Gil Dinur, et al.
Transcutaneous CO_2 Monitoring in Extremely Low Birth Weight Premature Infants
Reprinted from: *J. Clin. Med.* **2023**, *12*, 5757, doi:10.3390/jcm12175757 1

Yakov Sivan, Yael Bezalel, Avital Adato, Navit Levy and Ori Efrati
Congenital Central Hypoventilation Syndrome in Israel—Novel Findings from a New National Center
Reprinted from: *J. Clin. Med.* **2023**, *12*, 3971, doi:10.3390/jcm12123971 11

Noga Arwas, Sharon Uzan Shvartzman, Aviv Goldbart, Romi Bari, Itai Hazan, Amir Horev and Inbal Golan Tripto
Elevated Neutrophil-to-Lymphocyte Ratio Is Associated with Severe Asthma Exacerbation in Children
Reprinted from: *J. Clin. Med.* **2023**, *12*, 3312, doi:10.3390/jcm12093312 23

Jolanta Tomczonek-Moruś, Natalia Krysiak, Agnieszka Blomberg, Marta Depczyk-Bukała, Marcin Tkaczyk and Krzysztof Zeman
Role of Lung Ultrasonography (LUS) as a Tool for Evaluating Children with Pediatric Inflammatory Multisystem Syndrome Temporally Associated with SARS-CoV-2 (PIMS-TS)
Reprinted from: *J. Clin. Med.* **2023**, *12*, 2850, doi:10.3390/jcm12082850 35

Richard De Vuyst, Elizabeth Jalazo, Tamy Moraes Tsujimoto, Feng-Chang Lin, Joseph Muenzer and Marianne S. Muhlebach
Airway Findings in Patients with Hunter Syndrome Treated with Intravenous Idursulfase
Reprinted from: *J. Clin. Med.* **2023**, *12*, 480, doi:10.3390/jcm12020480 43

Ophir Bar-On, Hagit Levine, Patrick Stafler, Einat Shmueli, Eyal Jacobi, Ori Goldberg, et al.
Lactose-Containing Dry-Powder Inhalers for Patients with Cow's Milk Protein Allergy—The Conundrum; A National Survey of Pediatric Pulmonologists and Allergologists
Reprinted from: *J. Clin. Med.* **2022**, *11*, 7346, doi:10.3390/jcm11247346 55

Hagit Levine, Ophir Bar-On, Vered Nir, Nicole West, Yotam Dizitzer, Huda Mussaffi and Dario Prais
Reversible Bronchial Obstruction in Primary Ciliary Dyskinesia
Reprinted from: *J. Clin. Med.* **2022**, *11*, 6791, doi:10.3390/jcm11226791 63

Roberto Grandinetti, Valentina Fainardi, Carlo Caffarelli, Gaia Capoferri, Angela Lazzara, Marco Tornesello, et al.
Risk Factors Affecting Development and Persistence of Preschool Wheezing: Consensus Document of the Emilia-Romagna Asthma (ERA) Study Group
Reprinted from: *J. Clin. Med.* **2022**, *11*, 6558, doi:10.3390/jcm11216558 71

Kamal Masarweh, Oz Mordechai, Michal Gur, Ronen Bar-Yoseph, Lea Bentur and Anat Ilivitzki
Challenges in DICER1-Associated Lung Disease
Reprinted from: *J. Clin. Med.* **2023**, *12*, 1918, doi:10.3390/jcm12051918 103

Michal Gur, Mordechai Pollak, Ronen Bar-Yoseph and Lea Bentur
Pregnancy in Cystic Fibrosis—Past, Present, and Future
Reprinted from: *J. Clin. Med.* **2023**, *12*, 1468, doi:10.3390/jcm12041468 115

Miles Weinberger, Dennis Buettner and Ran D. Anbar
A Review, Update, and Commentary for the Cough without a Cause: Facts and Factoids of the Habit Cough
Reprinted from: *J. Clin. Med.* **2023**, *12*, 1970, doi:10.3390/jcm12051970 . . . . **129**

About the Editors

Lea Bentur

Professor Lea Bentur is the former head of the Pediatric Pulmonary Institute at Ruth Rappaport Children's Hospital, Rambam Health Care Campus, Israel. She is also the former head of the Israeli Pediatric Pulmonary Association and Israeli CF Association. Her main research interests include asthma, cystic fibrosis, childhood congenital lung disease, preschool pulmonary function tests, and the effects of smoking on pulmonary function.

Ronen Bar-Yoseph

Dr. Ronen Bar-Yoseph is the head of the Pediatric Pulmonology Institute and head of the Children's Physical Activity and Exercise Clinic and Lab at Ruth Rappaport Children's Hospital, Rambam Health Care Campus, Israel. His main research interest are pediatric pulmonology, cardiopulmonary exercise testing, exercise physiology, the pediatric origin of adult diseases.

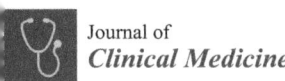

Article

Transcutaneous CO_2 Monitoring in Extremely Low Birth Weight Premature Infants

Liron Borenstein-Levin [1,2,*], Noa Avishay [2], Orit Soffer [1], Shmuel Arnon [3,4], Arieh Riskin [2,5], Gil Dinur [1,2], Karen Lavie-Nevo [2,6], Ayala Gover [2,6], Amir Kugelman [1,2] and Ori Hochwald [1,2]

[1] Department of Neonatology, Rambam Health Care Campus, Haifa 3109601, Israel; oritsof@gmail.com (O.S.); gil.dinur@gmail.com (G.D.); amirkug@gmail.com (A.K.); o_hochwald@rambam.health.gov.il (O.H.)
[2] Rappaport Faculty of Medicine, Technion-Israel Institute of Technology, Haifa 3200003, Israel; noa.avishai@gmail.com (N.A.); arik.riskin@gmail.com (A.R.); klavie@gmail.com (K.L.-N.); ayalagover@gmail.com (A.G.)
[3] Department of Neonatology, Meir Medical Center, Kfar-Saba 4428164b, Israel; shmuelar@clalit.org.il
[4] Faculty of Medicine, Tel Aviv University, Tel Aviv 69978, Israel
[5] Department of Neonatology, Bnai Zion Medical Center, Haifa 32000, Israel
[6] Department of Neonatology, Carmel Medical Center, Haifa 3436212, Israel
* Correspondence: liron.boren@gmail.com; Tel.: +972-54-2243556

Abstract: Extremely low birth weight (ELBW) premature infants are particularly susceptible to hypocarbia and hypercarbia, which are associated with brain and lung morbidities. Transcutaneous CO_2 ($TcCO_2$) monitoring allows for continuous non-invasive CO_2 monitoring during invasive and non-invasive ventilation and is becoming more popular in the NICU. We aimed to evaluate the correlation and agreement between CO_2 levels measured by a $TcCO_2$ monitor and blood gas CO_2 ($bgCO_2$) among ELBW infants. This was a prospective observational multicenter study. All infants < 1000 g admitted to the participating NICUs during the study period were monitored by a $TcCO_2$ monitor, if available. For each $bgCO_2$ measured, a simultaneous $TcCO_2$ measurement was documented. In total, 1828 pairs of $TcCO_2$–$bgCO_2$ values of 94 infants were collected, with a median (IQR) gestational age of 26.4 (26.0, 28.3) weeks and birth weight of 800 (702, 900) g. A moderate correlation (Pearson: r = 0.64) and good agreement (bias (95% limits of agreement)):(2.9 [−11.8, 17.6] mmHg) were found between the $TcCO_2$ and $bgCO_2$ values in the 25–70 mmHg $TcCO_2$ range. The correlation between the $TcCO_2$ and $bgCO_2$ trends was moderate. CO_2 measurements by $TcCO_2$ are in good agreement (bias < 5 mmHg) with $bgCO_2$ among premature infants < 1000 g during the first week of life, regardless of day of life, ventilation mode (invasive/non-invasive), and sampling method (arterial/capillary/venous). However, wide limits of agreement and moderate correlation dictate the use of $TcCO_2$ as a complementary tool to blood gas sampling, to assess CO_2 levels and trends in individual patients.

Keywords: non-invasive CO_2 monitoring; premature infant; transcutaneous CO_2 monitoring

1. Introduction

Extremely premature infants are susceptible to hyper- or hypocapnia and rapid fluctuations in $PaCO_2$, especially during the first week of life [1]. While monitoring $PaCO_2$ in a blood sample is the "gold standard", it only allows for interval monitoring and not continuous monitoring. Thus, periods of abnormally high or low $PaCO_2$ may be missed, and corrective ventilation measurements may be delayed.

Two methods that allow for non-invasive, continuous CO_2 monitoring in the NICU are End-tidal CO_2 ($EtCO_2$) monitoring and Transcutaneous CO_2 ($TcCO_2$) monitoring. In $EtCO_2$ monitoring, the capnograph sensor is connected to the endotracheal tube and allows for mainstream or side-stream measurements of $EtCO_2$ [2]. $EtCO_2$ monitoring was found to have a good correlation with $bgCO_2$ among ventilated term and preterm infants [3,4],

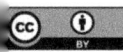

though the agreement was only moderate during the first day of life [5], and was negatively influenced by the severity of lung disease [4,6,7]. Among infants receiving mechanical ventilation in the NICU, the use of continuous $EtCO_2$ monitoring was found to improve the control of CO_2 levels within a safe range. In a subgroup analysis of extremely low birth weight premature infants (ELBW), the prevalence of intraventricular hemorrhage and periventricular leukomalacia was lower in the $EtCO_2$-monitored group; however, this group was too small to draw firm conclusions [8]. The main clinical limitation of $EtCO_2$ monitoring in the neonatal intensive care unit (NICU) is that it cannot be used in infants supported by high-frequency oscillatory ventilation (HFOV) or non-invasive ventilation, which are ventilation modes that are commonly used in this population [2].

$TcCO_2$ is based on the ability of CO_2 to diffuse through body tissues and skin and be detected by a sensor on the surface of the skin. By warming the sensor, local hyperemia is induced, which increases the supply of arterial blood to the dermal capillary bed below the sensor [9]. $TcCO_2$ monitors are currently widely used in the NICU [10,11]. Historically, neonatal studies have shown that $TcCO_2$ correlates better with $PaCO_2$ compared to $EtCO_2$ [12–14], though more recent studies revealed inconclusive results [5,15–17].

Given the importance of avoiding extreme CO_2 values and fluctuations during the first week of life among ELBW premature infants, the growing popularity of $TcCO_2$ monitoring in the NICU, and the inconclusive data regarding their accuracy in this population, we conducted this study. Our aim was to evaluate the correlation and agreement between CO_2 levels measured by the $TcCO_2$ monitor and blood gas CO_2 ($bgCO_2$) among ELBW infants during their first days of life. We hypothesized that $TcCO_2$ monitoring will be in good correlation and agreement with $bgCO_2$ measurements as well as CO_2 trends

2. Materials and Methods

These data were part of a prospective, observational, multicenter study studying the impact of $TcCO_2$ monitoring on neurologic and respiratory complications among ELBW infants (under submission). This study was approved by the research ethics board of all centers participating in the study. Written informed consent was obtained from the parents of all infants prior to study entry.

2.1. Study Population

All premature infants < 1000 g admitted to the participating NICUs during the study period and needing respiratory support during the first day of life were monitored by $TcCO_2$ monitor (Sentec AG, Therwil, Switzerland), if available, during the first week of life or longer as clinically indicated. Respiratory support included invasive support (Conventional mechanical ventilation (CMV) and HFOV) and non-invasive support including nasal intermittent positive pressure ventilation (NIPPV), continuous positive airway pressure (CPAP), and heated humidified high flow nasal cannula (HHHNC).

Infants with severe congenital malformation, birth asphyxia, known intraventricular hemorrhage stage III–IV in the first 24 h of life, or if active treatment was not initiated were excluded from the study.

2.2. Study Design

$TcCO_2$ monitoring was started during the first 12 h of life. Probe placement was in predefined areas as per manufacturer instructions. The sensor temperature was set to 41 °C in accordance with the manufacturer's instructions [18]. Calibration of the $TcCO_2$ was automatically performed every 4 h and following any reposition of the probe. Sensor membranes were changed every 28 days or sooner in case of any visible damage or repeated calibration errors. Skin fixation adhesives and contact gel were used in accordance with manufacturer guidelines.

Blood samples were taken at the discretion of the bedside care team, following meticulous placement of the probe and allowing for an adequate time period to achieve equilibrium. For each blood sample drawn for blood gas monitoring, a simultaneous TcCO$_2$ measure was recorded, as well as other clinical and respiratory support data.

2.3. Statistical Analysis

Data are presented as mean ± standard deviation (SD) for normally distributed variables, or median with interquartile range (IQR) for variables with non-parametric distribution. The correlation between TcCO$_2$ and bgCO$_2$ was measured using Pearson correlation. To determine the agreement between the two CO$_2$ measuring methods, a Bland–Altman analysis was performed on all matched TcCO$_2$–bgCO$_2$ samples, correcting for multiple measurements per patient [19]. Data are presented as bias (mean difference) and 95% limits of agreement (LoA) (i.e., 1.96 times the SD of the bias). The correlation of measurement trends was assessed for all consecutive pairs of TcCO$_2$ and bgCO$_2$ using Pearson correlation.

Logistic regression analysis was used to examine the relationship between different variables examined and the likelihood that the TcCO$_2$–bgCO$_2$ difference will be <|5|, which we consider clinically acceptable [3]. We incorporated into the model risk factors with p value < 0.05.

Statistical analyses were performed with SPSS version 25 (IBM SPSS, Chicago, IL, USA). Bland–Altman plot according to multiple measurements per subject was performed by MedCalc® Statistical Software version 20.218 (MedCalc Software Ltd., Ostend, Belgium).

3. Results

The study was conducted between March 2018 and September 2021 in the NICU's in Rambam, Bnai Zion, Meir, and Carmel medical centers. A total of 1828 pairs of TcCO$_2$ and bgCO$_2$ of 94 ELBW premature infants were collected, with a median (IQR) GA of 26.4 (26.0, 28.3) weeks and birth weight of 800 (702, 900) g. Demographic data are presented in Table 1.

Table 1. Demographics.

	Premature Neonates n = 94
Gestational Age, weeks	26.4 (26.0, 28.3)
Birth weight, g	800 (702, 900)
Small for gestational age	8 (8)
Prenatal steroids	65 (69)
Preeclampsia	25 (27)
Multiple births	26 (28)
Male gender	40 (43)
Delivery mode—Cesarean section	72 (77)
Apgar 5'	8 (6, 9)
Intubation at delivery room	41 (44)
Umbilical cord pH	7.27 (7.19, 7.33)
RDS requiring surfactant treatment	56 (60)
Ionotropic support during first week	5 (6)
Sepsis during the first week	5 (6)
Deceased during first week	2 (2)
Deceased during NICU stay	6 (6)
Number of samples per infant	19 (14, 23)

Values are presented as median (IQR) or n (%). IQR—interquartile range, NICU—neonatal intensive care unit, RDS—respiratory distress syndrome.

The Bland–Altman analysis showed a mean bias of 3.6 mmHg with a 95% confidence LoA from −14.3 to +21.4 mmHg (Figure 1A). Pearson's correlation coefficient between TcCO$_2$ and bgCO$_2$ was r = 0.64 (Figure 1B). The corrected Bland–Altman analysis according to multiple measurements per subject showed similar results (mean bias of 3.6 mmHg with a 95% confidence LoA from −14.1 to +21.2 mmHg).

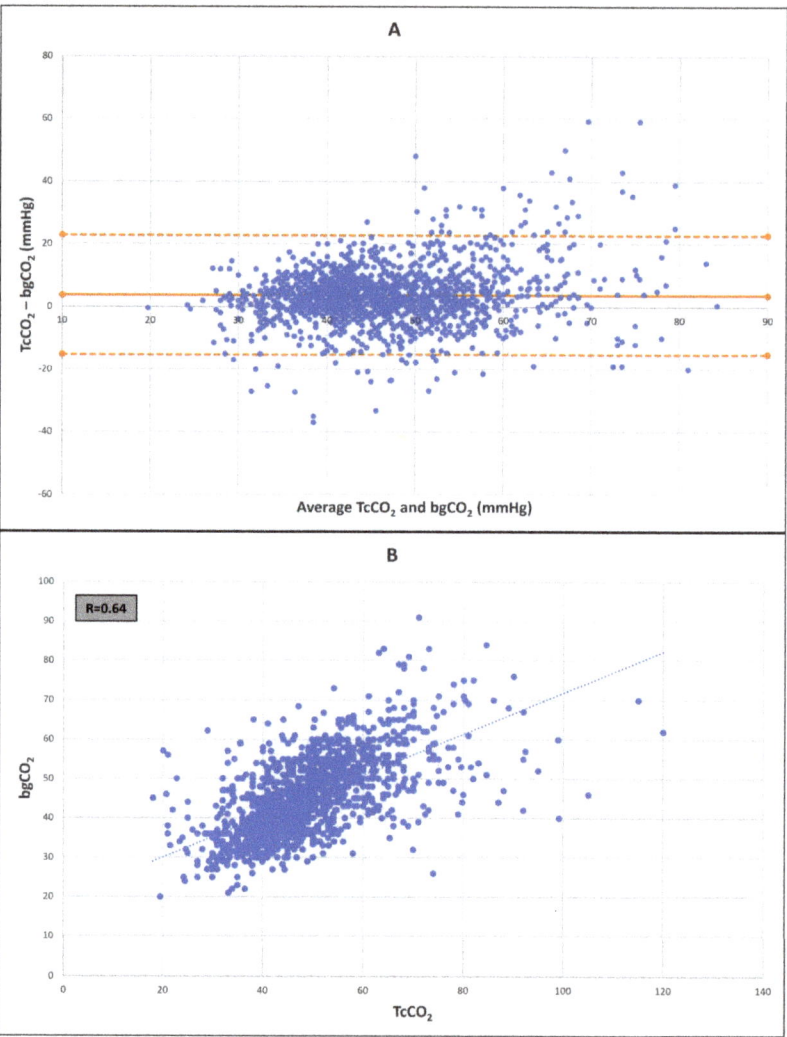

Figure 1. (**A**) Bland–Altman plot of the differences between $TcCO_2$ and $bgCO_2$. Orange lines represent the bias (solid line) and 2SD (dotted lines). (**B**) Pearson correlation between $TcCO_2$ and $bgCO_2$. $bgCO_2$—blood gas CO_2; $TcCO_2$—transcutaneous CO_2.

Similarly, moderate correlation and good agreement were demonstrated in $TcCO_2$ values ranges of 30–60 mmHg and 25–70 mmHg (the ranges that are most frequently seen at the bedside) (Table 2). For $TcCO_2$ below 25 and above 70 mmHg the correlation was poor (r = −0.41 and 0.14, respectively) as was the agreement (bias (LoA) −16.3 [−40.0, 7.4] and 20.1 [−9, 49.1] mmHg, respectively). However, the number of samples at these extremes was small.

Table 2. Subgroup analysis of correlation and agreement.

Parameter	No. of Samples	R	Bias (SD)	Lower LoA, Upper LoA
Per TcCO$_2$ measurements range				
All (20–115 mmHg)	1828	0.64	3.6 (9.1)	−14.3, 21.4
30–60 mmHg	1576	0.60	2.3 (6.8)	−11.1, 15.7
25–70 mmHg	1724	0.65	2.9 (7.4)	−11.8, 17.6
Per age (days) at sampling *				
Day of life 1	286	0.75	1 (6.8)	−12.3, 14.4
Day of life 1–3	887	0.71	2.0 (6.7)	−11.1, 15.1
Day of life 4+	851	0.59	3.8 (8.1)	−12.0, 19.6
Per sampling mode *				
Capillary	454	0.67	3.2 (8.1)	−12.6, 19.1
Arterial	1019	0.67	2.9 (7.4)	−11.6, 17.6
Venous	88	0.72	1.8 (6.2)	−10.3, 13.9
Per mode of ventilation *				
Non-invasive ventilation ˆ	900	0.65	3.1 (7.1)	−10.8, 17.1
Invasive ventilation	684	0.61	2.52 (8.1)	−13.6, 18.3
HFOV	243	0.6	2.28 (9.3)	−16.1, 20.6
CMV	442	0.62	2.6 (7.9)	−12.7, 18.1

* Data are presented for TcCO$_2$ measurements between 25 and 70 mmHg. ˆ Non-invasive ventilation includes nasal intermittent positive pressure ventilation (NIPPV), continuous positive airway pressure (CPAP), and heated humidified high-flow nasal cannula (HHHNC). CMV—Conventional mechanical ventilation; HFOV—High-frequency oscillatory ventilation; LoA—Limit of agreement.

The CO$_2$ range for TcCO$_2$ was 18–120 mmHg and for bgCO$_2$ was 20–91 mmHg.

Ninety-six percent of the samples were taken during the first week of life. Samples taken during the first 3 days of life had a stronger correlation and lower bias but still a wide LoA. Similar results are seen for venous samples as compared to arterial or capillary. Samples taken during non-invasive ventilation had a similar correlation and agreement as samples taken during the different invasive ventilation modes (HFOV and CMV) (Table 2).

In 950 out of 1724 of the samples (55%), the TcCO$_2$ reading was within the ±5 mmHg range as compared to bgCO$_2$. A total of 491/1724 (29%) were within the 6–10 absolute difference range, and in 283/1724 samples (16%), the difference was >10.

Multivariable logistic regression showed that sampling during the first 3 days of life and venous sampling significantly increase the likelihood that the TcCO$_2$–bgCO$_2$ difference will be less than or equal to five (95% CI for first 3 days of life—1.52 [1.24–1.87], $p < 0.001$, and for venous sampling—1.87 [1.16–3.01], $p = 0.01$), while HFOV increases the likelihood of absolute difference greater than five (95% CI 0.78 [0.59–0.97], $p = 0.037$).

To evaluate the trending accuracy of TcCO$_2$, we studied samples taken during the first 3 days of life. We chose this time period because, in the first days of life, blood gas sampling is usually more frequent and therefore we avoided, as much as possible, studying samples taken more than 12 h apart. A moderate correlation was found between the trending of each two successive measurements of TcCO$_2$ vs. bgCO$_2$- r = 0.52 (Figure 2A). However, studying individual infants, we observed a good correlation in CO$_2$ trends in some infants while a poor trend in others (Figure 2B,C).

We did not observe any burns or skin breakdowns among the participating infants.

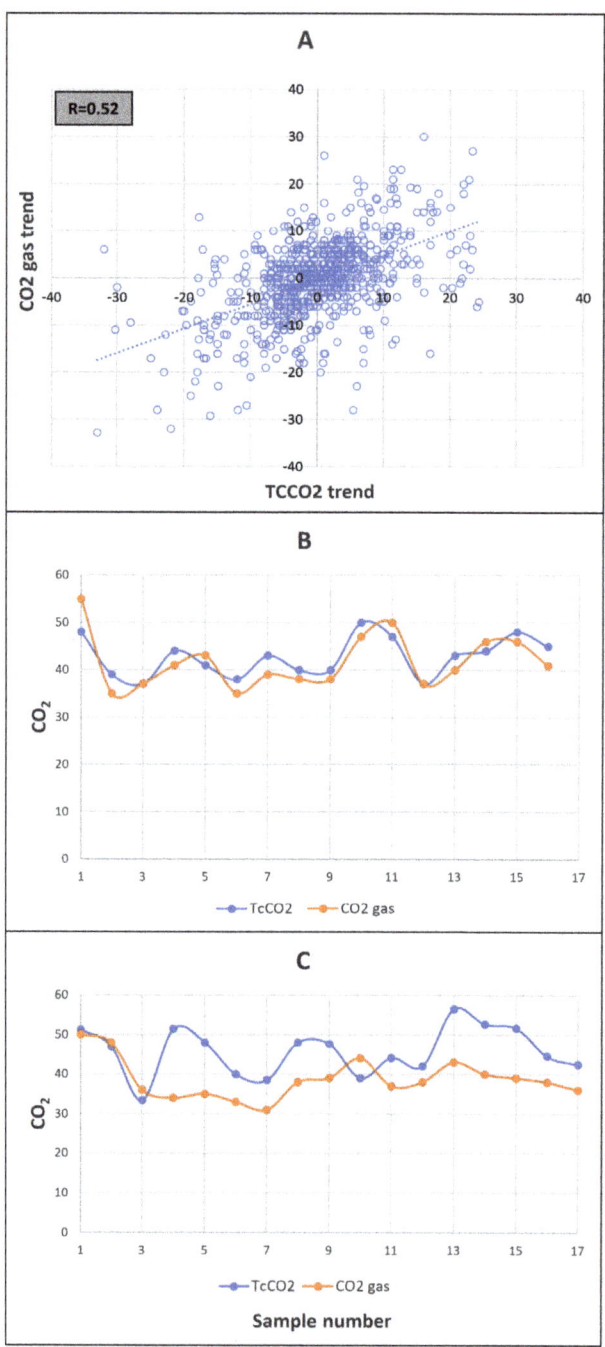

Figure 2. Comparison of the trending of $TcCO_2$ and $bgCO_2$: (**A**) Scatter plot of the change in the measured value between 2 consecutive measurements in $bgCO_2$ vs. $TcCO_2$ during the first 3 days of life (n = 657). (**B**,**C**) Examples of the trends in individual infants. Example B demonstrates a good agreement and trending between $TcCO_2$ and $bgCO_2$ measurements, while in example C, the agreement as well as trending is changing.

4. Discussion

In this large, prospective, multicenter study, we found a moderate correlation between transcutaneously measured CO_2 values and blood gas CO_2, among ELBW premature infants during their first week of life; a period when they are especially vulnerable to the harms of both hypocarbia and hypercarbia. The agreement between the two measuring methods was good; however, a wide limit of agreement exists.

The accuracy of $TcCO_2$ monitoring among premature infants was previously studied in the NICU in various clinical situations. Mukhopadhyay et al. [20] analyzed 1338 paired samples of $TcCO_2$ and $bgCO_2$, of mostly premature infants (mean ± SD GA 28.6 ± 4.3), in two different time periods, and found a bias ± SD of 5.2 ± 8.6 mmHg. Aliwalas et al. [5] studied 81 pairs of samples of intubated preterm infants ≤ 28 weeks gestation with RDS at 4, 12, and 24 h of age and showed bias ± SD of 2.2 ± 2.3, 4.4 ± 1.2, and 2.6 ± 1.8 mmHg, respectively. Van Weteringen reported a bias of 4.7 mmHg (95% LoA −7.8 to 17.1 mmHg) in 216 paired samples of premature infants (median (IQR) GA 26.4 [25.3–27.5]) with a similar agreement in subgroup analysis based on birth weight (below or above 1000 g), week of life (during or after the first week of life), and sepsis status (no sepsis, suspected and proven sepsis) [21]. A good correlation and agreement were also demonstrated when using a reduced temperature probe [18,22]. A poor correlation was found by Janaillac et al. [23]; however, these results should be addressed with caution as the average time lag between the pairs of samples was 4 min.

In our study, we focused on a homogenous group of ELBW premature infants during their first week of life, when they are most vulnerable to both hypocarbia and hypercarbia [24]. Studying 1828 paired samples, we found a bias of 3.6 mmHg, which is considered acceptable (<5 mmHg), with LoA from −14.3 to +21.4 mmHg. These results are comparable to previous studies and highlight the advantages of this CO_2 monitoring method—it is reliable, and it allows the continuous non-invasive monitoring of CO_2 in ELBW infants supported by all modes of invasive or non-invasive ventilation. Our study also demonstrates the disadvantage of this method, which is the wide LoA, also reported by others who have studied $TcCO_2$ monitoring [18,20,21]. A wide LoA was found also for $EtCO_2$ monitoring [3,4,6,7]. This emphasizes the importance of combining these methods with blood gas sampling, as these two non-invasive methods, $TcCO_2$ and $EtCO_2$, cannot be used as independent indicators of CO_2 levels.

Studying the impact of hemodynamic stability including blood pressure, oxygenation, arterial pH, and medications on $TcCO_2$, Bhat et al. found that the major factors affecting the $TcCO_2$ to $bgCO_2$ agreement were hypoxia and acidosis [25]. We were able to demonstrate similar agreement during the first days of life when the hemodynamic stability and oxygenation of ELBW infants are a concern, and it is reassuring that $TcCO_2$ is indeed a reliable method for CO_2 monitoring in this population.

In our study, we chose to focus on measurements between 25 and 70 mmHg as measurements above 70 mmHg and below 25 mmHg were found to have poor correlation and agreement. Poor correlation in the hypercarbia range was also demonstrated by Uslu et al. [26] and is suggested to result from impaired capillary blood flow and gas diffusion to the skin when the pH decreases. Interestingly, in the hypocapnia range, the bias was inverted, showing $TcCO_2$ measurements lower than $bgCO_2$ measurements. Low $TcCO_2$ readings that fall below the $bgCO_2$ value may indicate a technical problem as $TcCO_2$ values are generally higher than $PaCO_2$ values due to a local increase in CO_2 by the elevated temperature and by CO_2 production of epidermal cells [9]. This is also demonstrated by a mean bias > 0 mmHg. It is possible that the small number of measurements in the extreme values of CO_2 is the reason for the poor correlation and agreement in these ranges. We suggest, in any case, to exercise caution when interpreting $TcCO_2$ measurements in the extreme ranges.

Other studies found that the sampling method or mode of ventilation could affect the accuracy of $TcCO_2$ measurements. For example, Mukhopadhyay et al. found that HFOV support significantly increases the odds of increased bias [20], and others found that $tcCO_2$

was more accurate for capillary blood samples than for arterial blood samples [16,20,27]. In our study, 84% of the samples were within an absolute range of ±10 mmHg. We found a slight improvement in correlation and reduced bias in venous samples, and samples taken during the first 3 days of life. No statistical differences were found in samples collected while infants were on CMV or HFOV (Table 2). In multivariate analysis, venous sampling was associated with bias < 5 mmHg and HFOV with bias > 5 mmHg. However, these small differences are purely statistical and have no clinical significance.

As expected, TcCO$_2$ was also accurate during non-invasive ventilation. These results are reassuring as one of the main advantages of monitoring CO$_2$ transcutaneously is the ability to use it during non-invasive ventilation and during HFOV, which is technically challenging with other modes of non-invasive CO$_2$ monitoring [2].

TcCO$_2$ monitoring is suggested to be used as a complementary tool to blood gas sampling to allow trending of CO$_2$ levels. TcCO$_2$ trends have been successfully used to identify optimal lung volume during HFOV in neonates [28] and are proposed to allow early diagnosis of pneumothorax [29]. During the first 3 days of life, we found a moderate correlation between the TcCO$_2$ trends and bgCO$_2$ trends. We noticed excellent trending in some infants while poor trending in others. This observation reinforces the need to ascertain the trending in each individual patient, and a high index of suspicion whenever the TcCO$_2$ measurement does not fit the clinical scenario.

The main limitation of our study is that the samples were taken according to clinical need and not at a predetermined interval, which could have better delineated the trend-monitoring ability of this monitoring method. Another limitation is that the number of measurements per infant varies, but this was corrected by Bland–Altman analysis according to multiple measurements per subject. Furthermore, we did not record the sensor location and time from the last calibration. This prevented us from further studying the sensor location effect on the accuracy of the measurements as well as assessing the technical challenges associated with sensor positioning in the high-humidity environment required for ELBW during the first weeks of life. However, sensor location and calibration were performed as per the manufacturer's instructions; therefore, it represents the standard practice. The large number of samples most probably compensates for any false samples, if any. Due to the small number of infants with active sepsis or ionotropic support, we could not perform a multifactorial analysis to isolate parameters that could affect perfusion, as reported by others [30]. The advantages of our study are the large number of samples, the prospective nature of the study, and the focus on ELBW infants during their first week of life; the most vulnerable population during the most critical time period for CO$_2$ fluctuations.

5. Conclusions

CO$_2$ measurements by TcCO$_2$ have a moderate correlation with bgCO$_2$ among premature infants < 1000 g during the first week of life. While agreement between the TcCO$_2$ and bgCO$_2$ measurements is good, the wide LoA, as well as the moderate correlation of trends, dictate the use of this continuous non-invasive method as a complementary tool along with blood gas sampling to assess CO$_2$ levels and trending.

Author Contributions: Conceptualization L.B.-L. and A.K.; methodology L.B.-L., A.R., A.K. and O.H.; formal analysis A.R. and O.H.; investigation L.B.-L., S.A., A.R., K.L.-N. and A.G.; resources A.K. data curation N.A., O.S., S.A., G.D., K.L.-N. and A.G.; writing—original draft preparation, L.B.-L.; writing—review and editing A.R., A.K., O.H., N.A., O.S., S.A., G.D., K.L.-N. and A.G.; supervision, O.H. All authors have read and agreed to the published version of the manuscript.

Funding: No grant was received to support this study. Consumables and two monitors used to measure TcCO$_2$ at the Rambam Medical Center were provided by Sentec.

Institutional Review Board Statement: The study was conducted in accordance with the Declaration of Helsinki, and approved by the Institutional Review Board of all centers participating in the study the Institutional Review Board of Rambam Medical Center, Haifa, Israel (protocol code 0269-17-RMB approved on 15 August 2017), the Institutional Review Board of Bnai Zion Medical Center, Haifa

Israel (protocol code BNZ-17-0099, approved on 25 October 2017), the Institutional Review Board of Carmel Medical Center, Haifa, Israel (protocol code 0144-17-CMC, approved on 8 April 2018), and the Institutional Review Board of Meir Medical Center, Kfar-Saba, Israel (protocol code 0053-18-MMC, approved on 26 January 2018).

Informed Consent Statement: Informed consent was obtained from the parents of all infants involved in the study.

Data Availability Statement: Data are available upon reasonable request from the corresponding author.

Conflicts of Interest: The authors declare no conflict of interest. Sentec had no role in the design of the study; in the collection, analyses, or interpretation of data; in the writing of the manuscript; or in the decision to publish the results.

References

1. Wong, S.K.; Chim, M.; Allen, J.; Butler, A.; Tyrrell, J.; Hurley, T.; McGovern, M.; Omer, M.; Lagan, N.; Meehan, J.; et al. Carbon dioxide levels in neonates: What are safe parameters? *Pediatr. Res.* **2022**, *91*, 1049–1056. [CrossRef] [PubMed]
2. Hochwald, O.; Borenstein-Levin, L.; Dinur, G.; Jubran, H.; Ben-David, S.; Kugelman, A. Continuous Noninvasive Carbon Dioxide Monitoring in Neonates: From Theory to Standard of Care. *Pediatrics* **2019**, *144*, e20183640. [CrossRef] [PubMed]
3. Rozycki, H.J.; Sysyn, G.D.; Marshall, M.K.; Malloy, R.; Wiswell, T.E. Mainstream end-tidal carbon dioxide monitoring in the neonatal intensive care unit. *Pediatrics* **1998**, *101 Pt 1*, 648–653. [CrossRef] [PubMed]
4. Kugelman, A.; Zeiger-Aginsky, D.; Bader, D.; Shoris, I.; Riskin, A. A novel method of distal end-tidal CO_2 capnography in intubated infants: Comparison with arterial CO_2 and with proximal mainstream end-tidal CO_2. *Pediatrics* **2008**, *122*, e1219–e1224. [CrossRef] [PubMed]
5. Aliwalas, L.L.D.; Noble, L.; Nesbitt, K.; Fallah, S.; Shah, V.; Shah, P.S. Agreement of carbon dioxide levels measured by arterial, transcutaneous and end tidal methods in preterm infants < or = 28 weeks gestation. *J. Perinatol.* **2005**, *25*, 26–29. [CrossRef]
6. Singh, B.S.; Gilbert, U.; Singh, S.; Govindaswami, B. Sidestream microstream end tidal carbon dioxide measurements and blood gas correlations in neonatal intensive care unit. *Pediatr. Pulmonol.* **2013**, *48*, 250–256. [CrossRef] [PubMed]
7. Trevisanuto, D.; Giuliotto, S.; Cavallin, F.; Doglioni, N.; Toniazzo, S.; Zanardo, V. End-tidal carbon dioxide monitoring in very low birth weight infants: Correlation and agreement with arterial carbon dioxide. *Pediatr. Pulmonol.* **2012**, *47*, 367–372. [CrossRef]
8. Kugelman, A.; Golan, A.; Riskin, A.; Shoris, I.; Ronen, M.; Qumqam, N.; Bader, D.; Bromiker, R. Impact of Continuous Capnography in Ventilated Neonates: A Randomized, Multicenter Study. *J. Pediatr.* **2016**, *168*, 56–61.e2. [CrossRef]
9. Eberhard, P. The design, use, and results of transcutaneous carbon dioxide analysis: Current and future directions. *Anesth. Analg.* **2007**, *105*, S48–S52. [CrossRef]
10. Ochiai, M.; Kurata, H.; Inoue, H.; Ichiyama, M.; Fujiyoshi, J.; Watabe, S.; Hiroma, T.; Nakamura, T.; Ohga, S. Transcutaneous blood gas monitoring among neonatal intensive care units in Japan. *Pediatr. Int.* **2020**, *62*, 169–174. [CrossRef]
11. Rüdiger, M.; Töpfer, K.; Hammer, H.; Schmalisch, G.; Wauer, R.R. A survey of transcutaneous blood gas monitoring among European neonatal intensive care units. *BMC Pediatr.* **2005**, *5*, 30. [CrossRef] [PubMed]
12. Hand, I.L.; Shepard, E.K.; Krauss, A.N.; Auld, P.A. Discrepancies between transcutaneous and end-tidal carbon dioxide monitoring in the critically ill neonate with respiratory distress syndrome. *Crit. Care Med.* **1989**, *17*, 556–559. [CrossRef] [PubMed]
13. Geven, W.B.; Nagler, E.; de Boo, T.; Lemmens, W. Combined transcutaneous oxygen, carbon dioxide tensions and end-expired CO_2 levels in severely ill newborns. *Adv. Exp. Med. Biol.* **1987**, *220*, 115–120. [CrossRef] [PubMed]
14. Epstein, M.F.; Cohen, A.R.; Feldman, H.A.; Raemer, D.B. Estimation of $PaCO_2$ by two noninvasive methods in the critically ill newborn infant. *J. Pediatr.* **1985**, *106*, 282–286. [CrossRef] [PubMed]
15. Tingay, D.G.; Stewart, M.J.; Morley, C.J. Monitoring of end tidal carbon dioxide and transcutaneous carbon dioxide during neonatal transport. *Arch. Dis. Child. Fetal Neonatal Ed.* **2005**, *90*, F523–F526. [CrossRef] [PubMed]
16. Werther, T.; Aichhorn, L.; Stellberg, S.; Cardona, F.S.; Klebermass-Schrehof, K.; Berger, A.; Schmölzer, G.M.; Wagner, M. Monitoring of carbon dioxide in ventilated neonates: A prospective observational study. *Arch. Dis. Child. Fetal Neonatal Ed.* **2022**, *107*, 293–298. [CrossRef] [PubMed]
17. Tingay, D.G.; Mun, K.S.; Perkins, E.J. End tidal carbon dioxide is as reliable as transcutaneous monitoring in ventilated postsurgical neonates. *Arch. Dis. Child. Fetal Neonatal Ed.* **2013**, *98*, F161–F164. [CrossRef] [PubMed]
18. Aly, S.; El-Dib, M.; Mohamed, M.; Aly, H. Transcutaneous Carbon Dioxide Monitoring with Reduced-Temperature Probes in Very Low Birth Weight Infants. *Am. J. Perinatol.* **2017**, *34*, 480–485. [CrossRef]
19. Bland, J.M.; Altman, D.G. Agreement between methods of measurement with multiple observations per individual. *J. Biopharm. Stat.* **2007**, *17*, 571–582. [CrossRef]
20. Mukhopadhyay, S.; Maurer, R.; Puopolo, K.M. Neonatal Transcutaneous Carbon Dioxide Monitoring—Effect on Clinical Management and Outcomes. *Respir. Care* **2016**, *61*, 90–97. [CrossRef]
21. van Weteringen, W.; van Essen, T.; Gangaram-Panday, N.H.; Goos, T.G.; de Jonge, R.C.J.; Reiss, I.K.M. Validation of a New Transcutaneous $tcPO_2$/$tcPCO_2$ Sensor with an Optical Oxygen Measurement in Preterm Neonates. *Neonatology* **2020**, *117*, 628–636. [CrossRef] [PubMed]

22. Sullivan, K.P.; White, H.O.; Grover, L.E.; Negron, J.J.; Lee, A.F.; Rhein, L.M. Transcutaneous carbon dioxide pattern and trend over time in preterm infants. *Pediatr. Res.* **2021**, *90*, 840–846. [CrossRef] [PubMed]
23. Janaillac, M.; Labarinas, S.; Pfister, R.E.; Karam, O. Accuracy of Transcutaneous Carbon Dioxide Measurement in Premature Infants. *Crit. Care Res. Pract.* **2016**, *2016*, 8041967. [CrossRef] [PubMed]
24. Fabres, J.; Carlo, W.A.; Phillips, V.; Howard, G.; Ambalavanan, N. Both extremes of arterial carbon dioxide pressure and the magnitude of fluctuations in arterial carbon dioxide pressure are associated with severe intraventricular hemorrhage in preterm infants. *Pediatrics* **2007**, *119*, 299–305. [CrossRef] [PubMed]
25. Bhat, R.; Kim, W.D.; Shukla, A.; Vidyasagar, D. Simultaneous tissue pH and transcutaneous carbon dioxide monitoring in critically ill neonates. *Crit. Care Med.* **1981**, *9*, 744–749. [CrossRef] [PubMed]
26. Uslu, S.; Bulbul, A.; Dursun, M.; Zubarioglu, U.; Turkoglu, E.; Guran, O. Agreement of Mixed Venous Carbon Dioxide Tension ($PvCO_2$) and Transcutaneous Carbon Dioxide ($PtCO_2$) Measurements in Ventilated Infants. *Iran. J. Pediatr.* **2015**, *25*, e184. [CrossRef] [PubMed]
27. Baumann, P.; Gotta, V.; Adzikah, S.; Bernet, V. Accuracy of a Novel Transcutaneous PCO_2 and PO_2 Sensor with Optical PO_2 Measurement in Neonatal Intensive Care: A Single-Centre Prospective Clinical Trial. *Neonatology* **2022**, *119*, 230–237. [CrossRef] [PubMed]
28. Tingay, D.G.; Mills, J.F.; Morley, C.J.; Pellicano, A.; Dargaville, P.A. Indicators of optimal lung volume during high-frequency oscillatory ventilation in infants. *Crit. Care Med.* **2013**, *41*, 237–244. [CrossRef]
29. McIntosh, N.; Becher, J.C.; Cunningham, S.; Stenson, B.; Laing, I.A.; Lyon, A.J.; Badger, P. Clinical diagnosis of pneumothorax is late: Use of trend data and decision support might allow preclinical detection. *Pediatr. Res.* **2000**, *48*, 408–415. [CrossRef]
30. Sivan, Y.; Eldadah, M.K.; Cheah, T.E.; Newth, C.J. Estimation of arterial carbon dioxide by end-tidal and transcutaneous P_{CO_2} measurements in ventilated children. *Pediatr. Pulmonol.* **1992**, *12*, 153–157. [CrossRef]

Disclaimer/Publisher's Note: The statements, opinions and data contained in all publications are solely those of the individual author(s) and contributor(s) and not of MDPI and/or the editor(s). MDPI and/or the editor(s) disclaim responsibility for any injury to people or property resulting from any ideas, methods, instructions or products referred to in the content.

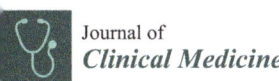

Journal of Clinical Medicine

Article

Congenital Central Hypoventilation Syndrome in Israel—Novel Findings from a New National Center

Yakov Sivan [1,2,3,*], Yael Bezalel [1], Avital Adato [4,5], Navit Levy [1] and Ori Efrati [1,3]

1. National CCHS Center & Department of Pediatric Pulmonology, Edmond and Lily Safra Children's Hospital, Sheba Medical Center, Tel Aviv 5262000, Israel
2. Adelson School of Medicine, Ariel University, Ariel 4070000, Israel
3. Faculty of Medicine, Tel Aviv University, Tel Aviv 6997801, Israel
4. Yad LaNeshima, The Israeli CCHS Patients' Foundation, Tel Aviv 6927728, Israel
5. Department of Natural and Life Sciences, The Open University of Israel, Ra'anana 4353701, Israel
* Correspondence: sivan@tauex.tau.ac.il; Tel.: +972-524262020

Abstract: Background. Congenital central hypoventilation syndrome (CCHS) is a rare autosomal-dominant disorder of the autonomic nervous system that results from mutations in the *PHOX2B* gene. A national CCHS center was founded in Israel in 2018. Unique new findings were observed. Methods. All 27 CCHS patients in Israel were contacted and followed. Novel findings were observed. Results. The prevalence of new CCHS cases was almost twice higher compared to other countries. The most common mutations in our cohort were polyalanine repeat mutations (PARM) 20/25, 20/26, 20/27 (combined = 85% of cases). Two patients showed unique recessive inheritance while their heterozygotes family members were asymptomatic. A right-sided cardio-neuromodulation was performed on an eight-year-old boy for recurrent asystoles by ablating the parasympathetic ganglionated plexi using radiofrequency (RF) energy. Over 36 months' follow-up with an implantable loop-recorder, no bradycardias/pauses events were observed. A cardiac pacemaker was avoided. Conclusions. A significant benefit and new information arise from a nationwide expert CCHS center for both clinical and basic purposes. The incidence of CCHS in some populations may be increased. Asymptomatic NPARM mutations may be much more common in the general population, leading to an autosomal recessive presentation of CCHS. RF cardio-neuromodulation offers a novel approach to children avoiding the need for permanent pacemaker implantation.

Keywords: congenital central hypoventilation syndrome (CCHS); polyalanine repeat mutations (PARM); non-polyalanine repeat mutations (NPARM); asystole; radiofrequency cardio-neuromodulation

1. Introduction

Congenital central hypoventilation syndrome (CCHS) is a rare disorder of the autonomic nervous system (ANS) that results from mutations in the paired-like homeobox 2b (*PHOX2B*) gene located on chromosome 4p12. *PHOX2B* encodes a transcription factor that is important for the development of the ANS. CCHS characteristically manifests after birth with hypoventilation and respiratory insufficiency with hypoxemia and hypercarbia due to chemoreceptor insensitivity [1–3]. Additionally, features may include Hirschsprung's disease (HSCR), cardiac sinus pauses, ocular involvement, temperature sensation and control and increased risk for neural crest tumors. It is estimated that more than 3000 cases have been diagnosed worldwide since 1970, with increased prevalence since 2003 when *PHOX2B* genetic testing became available [4–6]; however, this is likely an underestimate [2,4]. Data on disease prevalence have been reported from only a few populations, suggesting an incidence of 1:148,000–1:200,000 live births [7,8].

CCHS is inherited in an autosomal dominant pattern [1,2,6], where about 90% of *PHOX2B* mutations are represented by expansions of a polyalanine tract, encoded by exon 3, of the normal (wild-type) allele from 20 repeats to 24–33 repeats on the mutated alleles.

This is collectively defined as polyalanine repeat mutations (PARM) [2,3]. About 10% of CCHS cases result from frameshift, missense and nonsense mutations in one *PHOX2B* allele, while the polyalanine expansion is normal (20 on both alleles), and are defined as non-PARM (NPARM) [2]. PHOX2B is a transcription factor encoded by a three-exons gene, which is a member of the paired family of homeobox proteins localized to the nucleus. It is involved in neural crest cell migration and plays a critical role in early embryonic neuronal formation and differentiation, especially in the ANS from the neural crest cell derivative, and in the development of several major noradrenergic neuron populations and the determination of the neurotransmitter phenotype. Normal function of the *PHOX2B* gene is also required for central nervous chemo-sensitivity (mainly to hypercarbia) postnatally throughout the life span. The physiologic ventilatory control abnormality in CCHS appears to be in the integration of chemoreceptor input to central ventilatory controllers, rather than abnormalities in the chemoreceptors themselves [9].

Most CCHS cases occur de novo [2,3]; hence, parents have normal phenotype and genotype. Cases where one of the parents is a mosaic also occur. The PARMs show a genotype–phenotype relationship [2,9,10]. In CCHS, the central drive is decreased, more during sleep than during wakefulness. Hence, all CCHS patients exhibit hypoventilation and decreased response to hypercarbia during sleep. While milder cases with 24–26 PARM require assisted ventilation only while asleep and during intercurrent infections or after general anesthesia, patients with 27 PARM and higher usually require ventilator support 24 h/day. However, unlike PARM, due to the rarity of CCHS, the fact that NPARMs comprise only about 10% of all CCHS cases, and since each specific NPARM results from a different point mutation, not enough data have accumulated to correlate specific NPARMs with clinical presentation. Recently, an international collaboration looking for genotype–phenotype relationships from 302 NPARM cases showed immense genotypic and phenotypic variability associated with CCHS *PHOX2B* NPARM cases [11]. Patients with *PHOX2B* NPARMs can have highly variable phenotypes, ranging from severe respiratory conditions to mild and even subclinical manifestations that may become evident with an additional internal or external stressor [12,13].

Due to the rarity of CCHS, patients with multi-organ involvement are followed and treated by professionals of various specialties, and different countries and regions implement different strategies. Fortunately, specialized CCHS centers and clinics have evolved, contributing significantly to knowledge and experience that improved and optimized CCHS patient management. Moreover, the clinical and research experience accumulated in these specialized centers has been shared and circulated around the world, allowing small countries and communities to follow and implement large centers' experience with their designated protocols. This is of main virtue also since CCHS is a multi-organ systems disease that may require the involvement of cardiologists, neurologists, geneticists, neurologists, gastroenterologists, ENT, speech therapists, ophthalmologists, sleep specialists and more. Despite the complexity of the phenotypic manifestations, with good medical multidisciplinary support, CCHS patients reach "normal life milestones", including attending schools, maintaining employment, marrying and having families [2]. A crucial prerequisite is early diagnosis and devoted management by specialized professionals before hypoxic brain damage occurs.

In Israel, over the years, CCHS patients have been managed mainly for their ventilatory support by pediatric pulmonologists around the country. In January 2018, a national CCHS center was founded in the Edmond and Lily Safra Children's Hospital, Sheba Medical Center, and organized evaluation, follow-up, treatment, family support and genetic consultation for CCHS patients and their families was initiated, applying US leading centers protocols (mainly CAMP in Chicago).

The purpose of this report is to share our experience and present some unique and novel findings that accumulated over a relatively short period of four years.

2. Patients and Methods

This study was approved by the local IRB (Helsinki Committee). There was no need for patient consent. We were able to reach and contact all CCHS patients in Israel. This was achieved in several ways:

(a) From the Israeli pediatric pulmonologists ($n = 60$) who follow and manage all CCHS cases. Being a small country, all pediatric pulmonologists join the Israeli Pediatric Pulmonology Society and network and meet five times yearly.
(b) From the database of the Israeli CCHS Foundation ("Yad LaNeshima", www.cchsisrael.org).
(c) Information on CCHS and the new national center was distributed officially to all four insurance agencies, hospitals and community clinics by a formal statement from the chief manager of the Ministry of Health. Israel employs a free-of-charge national health service and by law, all residents are automatically enrolled in and entitled for medical services.
(d) The information was circulated to all pediatricians (including all sub-specialties and neonatologists) via the Israeli Society of Pediatrics.
(e) Information on CCHS and the new national center was circulated both in a television program and daily newspapers.

All CCHS patients and families were invited for evaluation and treatment in the new national CCHS center. Data collected included demographic information, ethnic origin, genetic results, and the full medical history of patient and family. The patients underwent an initial clinical and laboratory evaluation by specialists of the following disciplines:

Cardiology: cardiac echocardiogram, ECG and 72 h Holter recording; radiology: chest radiography and abdominal ultrasound; ENT: tracheoscopy for those who had a tracheostomy; respiratory: pediatric pulmonologist and pediatric intensivist, gas exchange measurement and ventilator adjustment. Other disciplines were involved according to patients' clinical presentation. These disciplines are services in the Safra Children's Hospital, which is a part of the general Sheba Medical Center. Each of these disciplines agreed to consult, follow and treat all patients whenever a problem in their field needed their assistance. All these services have received a detailed explanation and talks on CCHS with specific relation to their field and also increased their knowledge from the literature whenever needed. Additionally, consultation with experienced centers overseas (mainly CAMP) took place when needed. Polysomnography was performed in patients who did not have recent sleep evaluation. Follow-up included 6–12 months of scheduled visits that included repeat assessment as detailed above.

All patients under 18 years old are followed in the community by a dedicated physician experienced in home ventilation who in addition to scheduled home visits is available for phone consultations and home visits as needed.

The staff of the new CCHS center includes one doctor and one coordinator nurse both at 30% of their time (1.5 days/week). The staff of the CCHS center is available to the patients 24/7 for assistance by phone and patients are seen, in addition, whenever a medical problem arises that requires in-house assessment. Being recognized as a national center, all relevant hospital services for CCHS are available to all patients and insurance coverage is guaranteed by law.

3. Results

Twenty patients were located at the time of the national CCHS center foundation (January 2018). Age ranged between 1 and 33 years. Over the following four years, seven new patients were diagnosed at birth and joined the center (male: 16 of 27). Patients' distribution by year of birth is presented in Figure 1.

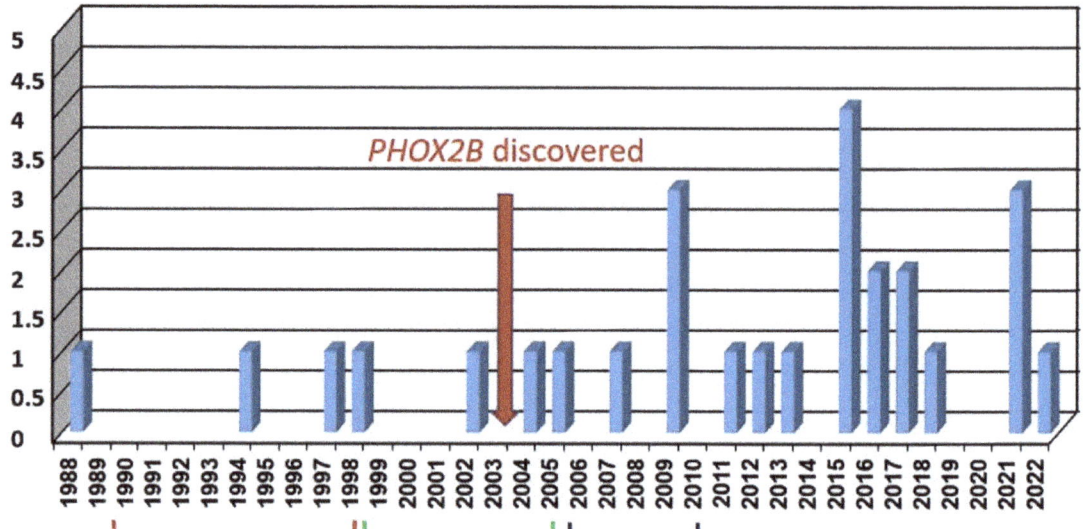

Figure 1. CCHS—new cases by year of birth.

Several novel and unique findings were observed.

3.1. Incidence

The overall rate of new CCHS cases over the last 20 years (since gene discovery) is 1:166,000 live-births with a rate of 1:127,000 for the Jewish population—almost twice the reported rate from other countries [4]. Interestingly, and with adjustment to the natural increase in number of births per year, the rate for the years 2003–2006 was 1:240,000 and increased to 1:165,000 for 2007–2014 and to 1:148,000 for 2015–2022. The rate for the Jewish population was 1:166,000, 1:149,000 and 1:109,000 for the three periods, respectively. Three patients were from Arabic Islamic ethnic origin: one Israeli, one from the Palestinian Authority, one from the city of Gaza. The latter two were not included in the rate calculation. 9 patients out of 27 (33%) were ultra-orthodox Jews, which accounts for 9 of 24 (39%) Jewish ultra-orthodox patients out all Jewish cases, while the average prevalence of that population over the last 20 years is only 11% of the general society and 14% of the Jewish population.

3.2. Genotype

Overall, the distribution of mutations was similar to the distribution reported from countries with large populations [14]. A total of 25 patients out of 27 (93%) had an autosomal dominant genotype, where 23 of 27 (85%) patients had a PARM on a single *PHOX2B* allele with the most common mutations being 20/25, 20/26 and 20/27 PARM, and 2 patients (7%) had an NPARM on one allele. An additional two patients (7%) had an unusual novel recessive genotype with a full respiratory phenotype (Figure 2). One of these carries a co-occurrence of 20/24 *PHOX2B* PARM on one allele and a new NPARM missense variant on the other allele (NM_003924.4:c.785G>T, p.Gly262Val). The two parents and 50% of their siblings as well as both grandfathers of both sides carry these PARM or NPARM mutations, respectively, being completely asymptomatic (Figure 3). This case has been reported in detail previously [15]. The other case was homozygote for two identical NPARMs on both *PHOX2B* alleles. This mutation is the same as the missense variants found in the previous recessive genotype patient (NM_003924.4:c.785G>T, p.Gly262Val). Both parents were found to carry this NPARM on one allele only and are completely asymptomatic. Hence, in both cases CCHS follows an autosomal recessive inheritance pattern.

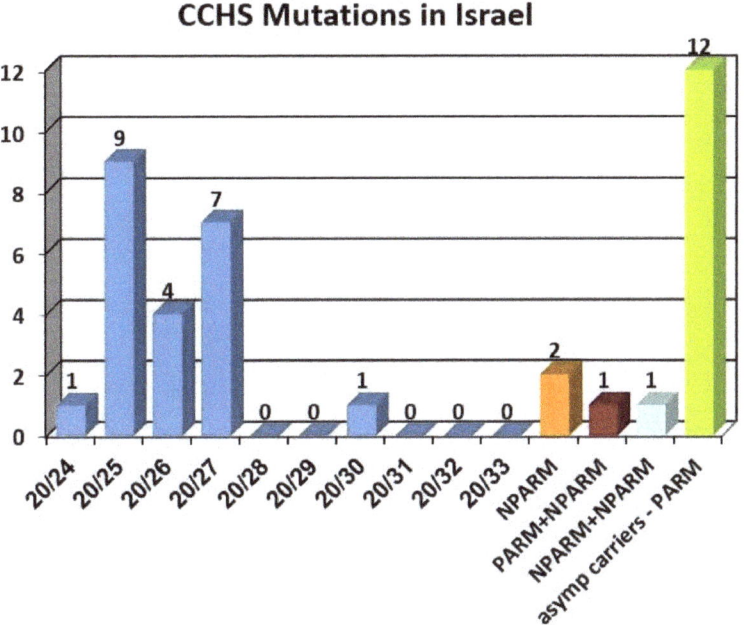

Figure 2. Distribution CCHS mutations.

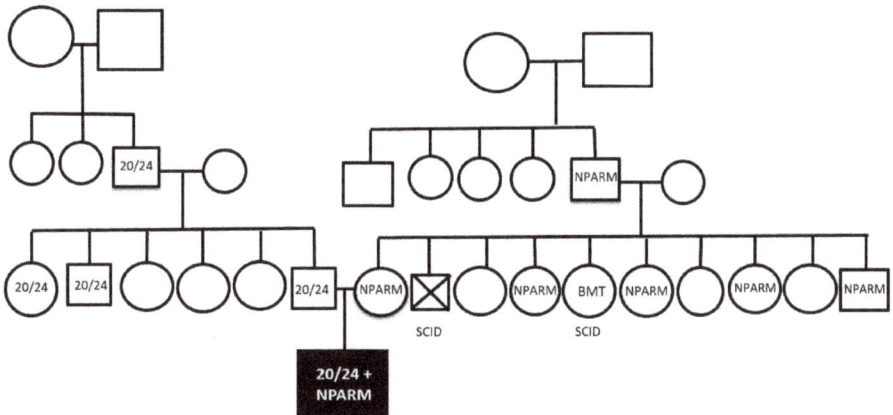

Figure 3. Pedigree of the family. Squares indicate males and circles indicate females. The proband is indicated by the black square. SCID—severe combined immune deficiency. BMT—bone marrow transplantation. The marked square with X indicates an uncle (mother's brother) who died of SCID. Adapted with permission from reference [15].

3.3. Genotype–Phenotype Relationship

While patients with PARM followed the previously described genotype–phenotype relationship, patients with NPARM and the homozygote patients with the autosomal recessive genotype had unpredictable and unique clinical presentation and course. The patient with the NPARM/24 mutation requires assisted ventilation when asleep, but no other clinical or laboratory manifestations have been observed over seven years. The patient with the recessive homozygote NPARM CCHS had a difficult course since birth, including 24/7 respiratory support and gastrointestinal and cardiac involvement.

The two NPARM patients with a "classical" autosomal dominant (heterozygote) NPARM genotype presented unique clinical manifestations. One was a seven-year-old boy, born in Gaza. His parents are second- degree cousins. At the age of three months, he was transferred to our pediatric oncology department due to chest and abdominal masses, which were diagnosed as neuroblastoma. Further evaluation due to suspected color change verified CCHS due to a novel heterozygous *PHOX2B* NPARM (c.369delC p.Pro123fs) in exon 2 of the *PHOX2B* gene, within the region encoding the homeobox domain of the protein. Initial respiratory evaluation during sleep showed no desaturations below 91% and CO_2 levels up to 45 mmHg. Due to the lack of facilities and experts in his neighborhood, the parents decided not to consider assisted respiratory support but to monitor nocturnal oxygen saturation. He responded to his hemato-oncologic treatment. However, over the years, respiratory assessment showed gradual worsening with recent evaluation showing desaturations down to 85% and hypercapnia up to 54 mmHg during sleep. Assisted ventilator support during sleep was started. Repeat examinations showed no cardiac, GI or other clinical manifestations.

The other NPARM patient was an eight-year-old girl that carried another novel *PHOX2B* mutation, a c.314T>C transition that causes a phenylalanine to serine missense, at position 105 within the homeobox domain of the PHOX2B protein (c.314T>C, F105S). This mutation was also detected in other family members with no disease manifestation (Figure 4). This patient has Hirschsprung's disease. Repeated polysomnography showed transient hypercapnia up to 50 mmHg with oxygen saturations of mostly 95–97% and no desaturations below 91%. Hence, the parents decided to continue with saturation monitoring during sleep alone.

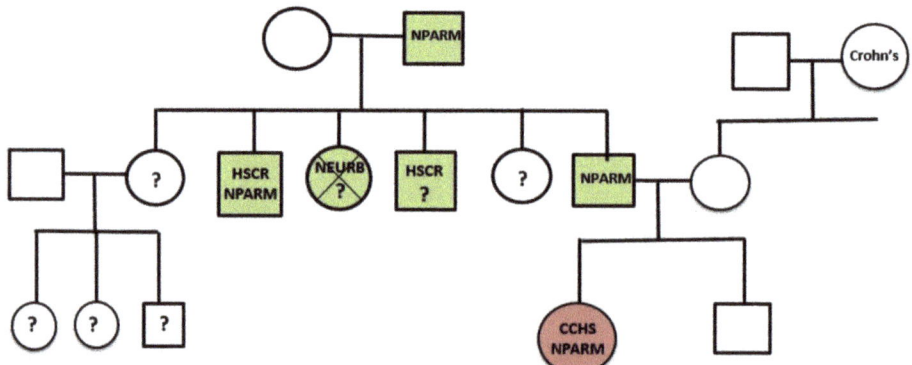

Figure 4. Pedigree of family. Squares indicate males and circles indicate females. HSCR—Hirschsprung's disease, Neurb—neuroblastoma.

3.4. Cardio-Neuromodulation by Radiofrequency Ablation for Cardiac Asystoles

A nine-year old boy with 20/27 PARM CCHS had recurrent asymptomatic episodes of sinus pause documented in a yearly routine of 72-hour Holter monitor recording There were overall 23 pauses of 3–4 s during both sleep and awake time. Three repeat Holter recordings showed similar findings. The patient is appropriately ventilated during sleep through a tracheostomy since birth. Of note, the parents reported two recent seizure episodes.

A permanent pacemaker (PPM) implantation was considered. However, given the relatively high rate of complications and the effects on quality of life associated with cardiac pacing, we applied a novel approach based on the idea that the sinus pauses resulted from increased vagal tone. A cardio-neuromodulation of the sinus node using radio-frequency (RF) ablation of the anterior right-ganglionated plexi was performed using a technique that has previously been reported only in adults [16]. The procedure was performed using a retrograde-arterial and a right-atrial-venous approach, guided by the merged image of an electro-anatomical mapping (CARTO® mapping system; BIOSENSEWEBSTER) and of a pre-procedural cardiac computed tomography. Baseline intravenous injection of 1 mg (0.04 mg/kg) atropine resulted in a 40 beats per minute (bpm) increase in heart rate. RF ablations of the high postero-septal right atrial (RA) region opposite to the right superior pulmonary vein and the high anterior septum part opposite the aorta were performed. Post-ablation intravenous atropine had no effect on heart rate, consistent with a successful endpoint. In addition, following the ablation procedure an implantable loop recorder (ILR) was inserted and programmed to record any R-R interval longer than 3 s.

Over 36 months of follow-up with an ILR and repeated Holter monitor recordings, the patient has been asymptomatic with no documented bradycardic episodes. His documented average heart rate is 104 bpm and the minimum heart rate was 73 bpm. Of note, no further seizure episodes occurred, suggesting that these events were indeed syncope episodes. A cardiac pacemaker was avoided.

4. Discussion

Our data provide several new findings that may add to clinical practice and basic understandings in CCHS. We nevertheless believe that the main message of our experience is that a significant additional benefit arises from a nationwide or regional expert-based CCHS center that covers the entire country or region, depending on the population size, for both clinical and basic purposes. Our findings show that data from even a small country with a small cohort may provide new important information on CCHS over a relatively short period. This may be of major importance due to the rarity of the disease and the benefit of a designated professional center. The recognition that rare diseases, and specifically CCHS, need to be consolidated to maximally learn from the children and to optimally improve the care of the affected children, and that the ability to study cohorts of children with CCHS at these centers leads to the major advances that follow has been highlighted by Weese-Mayer et al. in 2009 [14]. Our findings strongly support this conclusion. Additionally, our experience shows that a center with minimal manpower may cope with a population of 8–9 million people when all the services of the various relevant disciplines are available, cooperative and covered by law.

While only five patients were diagnosed over the 15 years 1988–2003 (0.33 cases/year), 27 patients were diagnosed over the 18 years 2004–2022. This is obviously the result of increased awareness and especially the discovery of the *PHOX2B* gene and the capability for laboratory diagnosis that started in 2003 [5,6].

The distribution of the PARMs and the incidence of NPARM in our population is similar to the distribution described from 640 cases from several populations and countries [14], suggesting that this is indeed the spread of CCHS worldwide. More information from other countries is, therefore, very valuable.

We faced a significant practical problem to persuade some of our patients and family members to cooperate and follow the recommended clinical practices and to agree to evaluate their asymptomatic family members. This was apparent in two groups: ultra-orthodox Jewish families, and older patients. Interestingly, the occurrence of ultra-orthodox Jewish patients in our cohort is much higher than their occurrence in the general population (33% of the cohort and 39% of Jewish CCHS cases compared to 11% and 14%, respectively). We have no explanation for this observation and CCHS has not been found to be more frequent in ultra-orthodox Jewish people from other countries with a large Jewish population.

Some ultra-orthodox Jewish patients and their family members only partially followed our clinical recommendations and were not interested in genetic consultation, stating that they will never stop or hold pregnancy anyway, and hence amniocentesis in following pregnancies was unacceptable. This was due to religious beliefs and the instructions of their rabbis. Fortunately, some of these families agreed to preconception diagnosis. Nevertheless, some ultra-orthodox families were reluctant to perform any family screening for *PHOX2B* tests. This emphasizes the need to adjust practices to specific populations and receive help from religious authorities, such as Jewish rabbis whom ultra-orthodox Jewish follow and obey much more than their cooperation with medical experts. Indeed, collaborating with some rabbis was partially successful in convincing family members to agree to *PHOX2B* testing, albeit limited to the parents and only some of the patients' and parents' siblings.

The other challenging group was older patients who had not received designated care, explanation and comprehensive clinical support before the start of our program. For example, it was difficult to convince patients 20 years old and older to start periodic 72-h Holter recordings after this had not been performed before; consequently, some did not follow the recommendations. This highlights the need to establish authorized and recognized national or regional CCHS centers early, in addition to investing in increasing the awareness of the relevant colleagues nationwide.

Some new interesting understandings may be derived from the two cases with a recessive CCHS genotype, whose multiple heterozygous family members do not manifest any CCHS symptoms. Hence, the c.785G>T variant on *PHOX2B* exon 3 results in a glycine to valine substitution at position 262, which is the second amino acid right after the polyalanine repeat. Although glycine is a neutral and non-polar amino acid and valine has a hydrophobic side chain, in-silico analyses suggest that this variant is likely to be tolerated. However, segregation of this variant among members of two Israeli families indicates that one allele of this variant may be insufficient to cause clinically apparent disease, thus presenting a true autosomal recessive pattern of CCHS, which is unusual for this syndrome, although it has been described for the 20/24 PARM when present in homozygosity [17]. It is speculated that the specific c.785G>T NPARM causes subthreshold decrements in *PHOX2B* functioning and when present on both alleles there is sufficient impairment of the PHOX2B protein function to cause clinical expression of the CCHS phenotype.

This c.785G>T variant is present in population databases (rs768420488, ExAC 0.003%). The finding of the same mutation in the two patients reported here and the observation of several asymptomatic carriers in both families suggests that this NPARM may be much more common in the population and probably in a specific population. This homozygote NPARM was not observed in a recent large study of 302 CCHS cases with NPARM [11]. At present, the rarity of the cases does not seem to justify preconception screening; nevertheless, this position may change if additional unrelated cases are reported, especially in a specific population, since asymptomatic heterozygotes have been found. Additionally, the fact that previous cases carrying this NPARM have not been reported suggests that unlike most NPARMs this specific mutation in one allele does not cause clinical disease unless the other *PHOX2B* allele also harbors a PARM or an NPARM.

The fact that heterozygote family members with the novel missense NPARM are completely asymptomatic while when this NPARM combines with a 24-polyalanine expansion or with the same NPARM on the other allele, it presents as a CCHS phenotype, may suggest that with this specific NPARM the amount of undamaged protein from one allele is enough for normal life, and that this specific NPARM does not have a toxic gain of function. This presents a true autosomal recessive pattern. Obviously, we do not know the prevalence of this NPARM in the general population. The finding of asymptomatic family members with 20/24 PARM is not surprising, since this PARM has been reported to present with either clinically CCHS from birth, late-onset CCHS or as asymptomatic carriers [2,15,18–20]. It is speculated that the 20/24 PARM may also cause a non-clinically important decrease in the PHOX2B protein that decreases further to impair function when the other allele is also mutated.

Although most CCHS cases occur de novo, phenotypic variability when the mutation was inherited from an asymptomatic or a mild phenotypic parent has been reported especially with NPARMs and the 20/24 PARM [3,15,21,22].

The two heterozygote (autosomal dominant) NPARM cases are also unique in that both do not receive assisted ventilation. These patients were introduced to us when they already were three and four years old and the parents were reluctant to consider assisted ventilator support with or without tracheostomy that will significantly affect their quality of life. Interestingly, although CCHS patients due to NPARM are usually considered to have a worse clinical course, and most require assisted ventilator support also when awake, at present, these two patients grow and develop well without assisted ventilation. However, the patient from Gaza, who at the beginning showed reasonable gas exchange including during sleep, progressed to hypoventilation over time and assisted ventilation during sleep has been recently applied.

The other heterozygote NPARM case showed variable penetrance in several family members carrying the same NPARM. Variable penetrance was previously reported in a family with three generations carrying a novel NPARM with both severely affected and asymptomatic members having the NPARM [21]. This variable penetrance in our and the abovementioned families supports the hypothesis that the CCHS phenotypic manifestations may be influenced by environmental or genetic modifiers that presently are unknown.

Our approach to performing a right-sided cardio-neuromodulation by ablating the parasympathetic ganglionated plexi area using radiofrequency energy in a CCHS patient with sinus pauses is novel. Prolonged sinus pauses were documented in this population and are associated with an increased risk of sudden cardiac death, where 83% of the carriers of the *PHOX2B* 20/27 PARM mutation will suffer from sinus pauses longer than 3 s at some point. Hence, in order to detect sinus pauses before they present clinically, an annual 72-hour Holter recording is recommended [23]. Given their increased risk of sudden death, the common practice in this population is to insert a cardiac pacemaker when prolonged pauses (>3 s) are observed, even when symptoms have not yet occurred [4,23].

Radiofrequency (RF) ablation of right-sided parasympathetic ganglionated plexi (PGPs) is a novel approach to treat neurally-mediated syncope and functional sinus node dysfunction [16]. This method has been implemented merely in the adult population. Targeting the anatomically known locations of the PGPs affecting the sinus and AV nodes causes a vagolytic effect, with a subsequent increase in sinus rhythm and enhancement of AV conduction, respectively.

Only two pediatric cases of RF ablation for vagal denervation were reported thus far from Brazil and the US [24,25]. Both were 15–16-year-old adolescents with recurrent syncope episodes. There were no previous reports of such a therapeutic approach in a CCHS patient. The latter population displays a variety of associated cardiovascular symptoms, namely attenuated heart rate variability, increased incidence of atrial and ventricular ectopy, sinus bradycardia and prolonged sinus pauses [22,26,27]. Since the chances of future sinus pauses in CCHS cases increases with age, their only therapeutic option until now was a permanent pacemaker implantation. The observation that continuous monitoring for 36 months following the procedure did not document bradycardic events (no R-R interval longer than two seconds) is reassuring and supports that the mechanism behind the episodes is vagally-mediated rather than intrinsic degenerative disease of the conduction system.

Avoiding permanent pacemaker implantation in children and young adults with CCHS is of paramount importance, since these patients also suffer from many other major problems. In addition to avoiding the insertion procedure, RF ablation for vagal denervation may prevent lifelong pace-maker complications such as infection, reverse ventricular remodeling, ventricular dysfunction and the need for hardware exchange. Obviously, there is a need for additional experience and controlled studies to assess this therapeutic option, especially in CCHS patients. Interestingly, this patient did not have any further seizure episode. We speculate that the two seizure events he had prior to the procedure might have been syncope-related rather than of primary neurologic origin.

5. Summary and Conclusions

A significant additional benefit arises from a nationwide or regional expert CCHS center both for clinical and basic purposes. Data from a small center with limited resources may provide new important information on CCHS. The rate of CCHS in some populations may be higher than reported. Asymptomatic NPARM mutations may be much more common in the general population than previously known, leading to an autosomal recessive presentation of CCHS. Whether such mutations, and specifically the c.785G>T, p.Gly262Val NPARM, should be screened in population where it has been found waits for additional findings. RF cardio-neuromodulation offers a novel approach to children and may be specifically beneficial to CCHS patients with cardiac pauses, avoiding the need for permanent pacemaker implantation.

Author Contributions: Conceptualization, Y.S., Y.B. and O.E.; Methodology, Y.S. and N.L.; Formal analysis, Y.S., N.L., A.A; Investigation, Y.S., Y.B., A.A., N.L.; Resources, Y.S., Y.B., A.A., N.L. and O.E.; Data curation, Y.S., Y.B., A.A. and N.L.; Writing—original draft, Y.S. and A.A.; Writing—review and editing, Y.S., Y.B., A.A., N.L. and O.E.; Supervision, Y.S. All authors have read and agreed to the published version of the manuscript.

Funding: This research received no external funding.

Institutional Review Board Statement: The Sheba Medical Center Research Ethics Committees not required.

Informed Consent Statement: Not applicable.

Data Availability Statement: Not applicable.

Acknowledgments: The authors thank our colleagues from the Department of Cardiology for permitting to include in brief the case who underwent RF cardio-neuromodulation: Yoav Bolkier, Roy Beinart, Uriel Katz, Shai Tejman-Yarden and Eyal Nof. This case may be reported in the future in detail.

Conflicts of Interest: The authors declare no conflict of interest.

References

1. Trang, H.; Brunet, J.F.; Rohrer, H.; Gallego, J.; Amiel, J.; Bachetti, T.; Fischbeck, K.H.; Similowski, T.; Straus, C.; Ceccherini, I.; et al. European Central Hypoventilation Syndrome Consortium. Proceedings of the fourth international conference on central hypoventilation. *Orphanet. J. Rare. Dis.* **2014**, *9*, 194–218. [CrossRef] [PubMed]
2. Weese-Mayer, D.E.; Berry-Kravis, E.M.; Ceccherini, I.; Keens, T.G.; Loghmanee, D.A.; Trang, H. An official ATS clinical policy statement: Congenital central hypoventilation syndrome: Genetic basis, diagnosis, and management. *Am. J. Respir. Crit. Care Med.* **2010**, *181*, 626–644. [CrossRef] [PubMed]
3. Trang, H.; Samuels, M.; Ceccherini, I.; Frerick, M.; Garcia-Teresa, M.A.; Peters, J.; Schoeber, J.; Migdal, M.; Markstrom, A.; Ottonello, G.; et al. Guidelines for diagnosis and management of congenital central hypoventilation syndrome. *Orphanet. J. Rare Dis.* **2020**, *15*, 252. [CrossRef] [PubMed]
4. Slattery, S.M.; Perez, I.A.; Ceccherini, I.; Chen, M.L.; Kurek, K.C.; Yap, K.L.; Keens, T.G.; Khaytin, I.; Ballard, H.A.; Sokol, E.A.; et al. Transitional care and clinical management of adolescents, young adults, and suspected new adult patients with congenital central hypoventilation syndrome. *Clin. Auton. Res.* **2022**. [CrossRef] [PubMed]
5. Weese-Mayer, D.E.; Berry-Kravis, E.M.; Zhou, L.; Maher, B.S.; Silvestri, J.M.; Curran, M.E.; Marazita, M.L. Idiopathic congenital central hypoventilation syndrome: Analysis of genes pertinent to early autonomic nervous system embryologic development and identification of mutations in *PHOX2B*. *Am. J. Med. Genet.* **2003**, *123A*, 267–278. [CrossRef]
6. Amiel, J.; Laudier, B.; Attié-Bitach, T.; Trang, H.; de Pontual, L.; Gener, B.; Trochet, D.; Etchevers, H.; Ray, P.; Simonneau, M.; et al Polyalanine expansion and frameshift mutations of the paired-like homeobox gene *PHOX2B* in congenital central hypoventilation syndrome. *Nat. Genet.* **2003**, *33*, 459–461. [CrossRef]
7. Trang, H.; Dehan, M.; Beaufils, F.; Zaccaria, I.; Amiel, J.; Gaultier, C. French CCHS, Working Group: The French Congenital Central Hypoventilation Syndrome Registry: General data, phenotype, and genotype. *Chest* **2005**, *127*, 72–79. [CrossRef]
8. Shimokaze, T.; Sasaki, A.; Meguro, T.; Hasegawa, H.; Hiraku, Y.; Yoshikawa, T.; Kishikawa, Y.; Hayasaka, K. Genotype-phenotype relationship in Japanese patients with congenital central hypoventilation syndrome. *J. Hum. Genet.* **2015**, *60*, 473–477. [CrossRef]

9. Spengler, C.M.; Gozal, D.; Shea, S.A. Chemoreceptive mechanisms elucidated by studies of congenital central hypoventilation syndrome. *Respir. Physiol.* **2001**, *129*, 247–255. [CrossRef]
10. Matera, I.; Bachetti, T.; Puppo, F.; Di Duca, M.; Morandi, F.; Casiraghi, G.M.; Cilio, M.R.; Hennekam, R.; Hofstra, R.; Schöber, J.G.; et al. PHOX2B mutations and polyalanine expansions correlate with the severity of the respiratory phenotype and associated symptoms in both congenital and late onset central hypoventilation syndrome. *J. Med. Genet.* **2004**, *41*, 373–380. [CrossRef]
11. Berry-Kravis, E.M.; Zhou, L.; Rand, C.M.; Weese-Mayer, D.E. Congenital central hypoventilation syndrome: *PHOX2B* mutations and phenotype. *Am. J. Respir. Crit. Care Med.* **2006**, *174*, 1139–1144. [CrossRef]
12. Zhou, A.; Rand, C.M.; Hockney, S.M.; Niewijk, G.; Reineke, P.; Speare, V.; Berry-Kravis, E.M.; Zhou, L.; Jennings, L.J.; Yu, M.; et al. Paired-like homeobox gene (*PHOX2B*) nonpolyalanine repeat expansion mutations (NPARMs): Genotype–phenotype correlation in congenital central hypoventilation syndrome (CCHS). *Genet. Med.* **2021**, *23*, 1656–1663. [CrossRef]
13. Kasi, A.S.; Li, H.; Jurgensen, T.J.; Guglani, L.; Keens, T.G.; Perez, I.A. Variable phenotypes in congenital central hypoventilation syndrome with *PHOX2B* nonpolyalanine repeat mutations. *J. Clin. Sleep Med.* **2021**, *17*, 2049–2055. [CrossRef]
14. Weese-Mayer, D.E.; Rand, C.M.; Berry-Kravis, E.; Jennings, L.J.; Loghmanee, D.A.; Patwari, P.P.; Ceccherini, I. Congenital central hypoventilation syndrome from past to future: Model for translational and transitional autonomic medicine. *Pediatr. Pulmonol.* **2009**, *44*, 521–535. [CrossRef]
15. Sivan, Y.; Zhou, A.; Jennings, L.J.; Berry-Kravis, E.M.; Yu, M.; Zhou, L.; Rand, C.M.; Weese-Mayer, D.E. Congenital central hypoventilation syndrome: Severe disease caused by co-occurrence of two *PHOX2B* variants inherited separately from asymptomatic family members. *Am. J. Med. Genet. A* **2019**, *179*, 503–506. [CrossRef]
16. Debruyne, P.; Rossenbacker, T.; Collienne, C.; Roosen, J.; Ector, B.; Janssens, L.; Charlier, F.; Vankelecom, B.; Dewilde, W.; Wijns, W. Unifocal Right-Sided Ablation Treatment for Neurally Mediated Syncope and Functional Sinus Node Dysfunction Under Computed Tomographic Guidance. *Circ. Arrhythm. Electrophysiol.* **2018**, *11*, e006604. [CrossRef]
17. Trochet, D.; de Pontual, L.; Straus, C.; Feingold, J.; Goridis, C.; Lyonnet, S.; Amiel, J. *PHOX2B* germline and somatic mutations in late-onset central hypoventilation syndrome. *Am. J. Respir. Crit. Care Med.* **2008**, *177*, 906–911. [CrossRef]
18. Repetto, G.M.; Corrales, R.J.; Abara, S.G.; Zhou, L.; Berry-Kravis, E.M.; Rand, C.M.; Weese-Mayer, D.E. Later-onset congenital central hypoventilation syndrome due to a heterozygous 24-polyalanine repeat expansion mutation in the *PHOX2B* gene. *Acta Paediatr.* **2009**, *98*, 192–195. [CrossRef]
19. Cohen-Cymberknoh, M.; Shoseyov, D.; Goldberg, S.; Gross, E.; Amiel, J.; Kerem, E. Late-onset central hypoventilation presenting as extubation failure. *Isr. Med. Assoc. J.* **2010**, *12*, 249–250.
20. Sivan, Y. Ondine's curse--never too late. *Isr. Med. Assoc. J.* **2010**, *12*, 234–236.
21. Kasi, A.S.; Jurgensen, T.J.; Yen, S.; Kun, S.S.; Keens, T.G.; Perez, I.A. Three-generation family with congenital central hypoventilation syndrome and novel *PHOX2B* gene non-polyalanine repeat mutation. *J. Clin. Sleep Med.* **2017**, *13*, 925–927. [CrossRef] [PubMed]
22. Pace, N.P.; Pace Bardon, M.; Borg, I. A respiratory/Hirschsprung phenotype in a three-generation family associated with a novel pathogenic *PHOX2B* splice donor mutation. *Mol. Genet. Genom. Med.* **2020**, *8*, e1528. [CrossRef] [PubMed]
23. Gronli, J.O.; Santucci, B.A.; Leurgans, S.E.; Berry-Kravis, E.M.; Weese-Mayer, D.E. Congenital Central Hypoventilation Syndrome: *PHOX2B* Genotype Determines Risk for Sudden Death. *Pediatric. Pulmonol.* **2008**, *43*, 77–86. [CrossRef] [PubMed]
24. Scanavacca, M.; Hachul, D.; Pisani, C.; Sosa, E. Selective vagal denervation of the sinus and atrioventricular nodes, guided by vagal reflexes induced by high frequency stimulation, to treat refractory neurally mediated syncope. *J. Cardiovasc. Electrophysiol.* **2009**, *20*, 558–563. [CrossRef]
25. Kumthekar, R.N.; Sumihara, K.; Moak, J.P. Pediatric Radiofrequency Ablation of cardiac parasympathetic ganglia to achieve vagal denervation. *HeartRhythm Case Rep.* **2020**, *6*, 879–883. [CrossRef]
26. Laifman, E.; Keens, T.G.; Bar Cohen, Y.; Perez, I.A. Life-threatening cardiac arrhythmias in congenital central hypoventilation syndrome. *Eur. J. Pediatr.* **2020**, *179*, 821–825. [CrossRef]
27. Silvestri, J.M.; Hanna, B.D.; Volgman, A.S.; Jones, P.J.; Barnes, S.D.; Weese-Mayer, D.E. Cardiac rhythm disturbances among children with idiopathic congenital central hypoventilation syndrome. *Pediatr. Pulmonol.* **2000**, *29*, 351–358. [CrossRef]

Disclaimer/Publisher's Note: The statements, opinions and data contained in all publications are solely those of the individual author(s) and contributor(s) and not of MDPI and/or the editor(s). MDPI and/or the editor(s) disclaim responsibility for any injury to people or property resulting from any ideas, methods, instructions or products referred to in the content.

Elevated Neutrophil-to-Lymphocyte Ratio Is Associated with Severe Asthma Exacerbation in Children

Noga Arwas [1,2,†], Sharon Uzan Shvartzman [2,†], Aviv Goldbart [1,2,3], Romi Bari [2,4], Itai Hazan [2,4], Amir Horev [2,5,†] and Inbal Golan Tripto [1,2,3,*,†]

1. Department of Pediatrics, Soroka University Medical Center, Beer-Sheva 8410101, Israel; noga.arwas@gmail.com (N.A.)
2. Faculty of Health Sciences, Ben-Gurion University of the Negev, Beer-Sheva 8410101, Israel; uzansharon1@gmail.com (S.U.S.); romiba6@gmail.com (R.B.); itaihazan@gmail.com (I.H.); horev8@gmail.com (A.H.)
3. Pediatric Pulmonary Unit, Soroka University Medical Center, Beer-Sheva 8410101, Israel
4. Clinical Research Center, Soroka University Medical Center, Beer-Sheva 8410101, Israel
5. Pediatric Dermatology Service, Soroka University Medical Center, Beer-Sheva 8410101, Israel
* Correspondence: inbalgt@clalit.org.il; Tel.: +972-8-6403064; Fax: +972-8-6287163
† These authors contributed equally to this work.

Abstract: Asthma is the most common chronic respiratory disease in children. The neutrophil-to-lymphocyte ratio (NLR) is a marker of a chronic inflammatory state; however, data on the association of NLR with acute asthma exacerbations in children is lacking. In this cross-sectional study, between 2016 and 2021, children aged 2–18 years who were referred to the emergency department (ED) due to asthma exacerbation, were included. NLR, calculated from complete blood count upon arrival, was assessed as a continuous variable and was classified into four groups according to quartiles. The association between severity parameters and NLR quartiles was examined. A total of 831 ED visits for asthma exacerbation were included in the study. The median NLR was 1.6, 3.8, 6.7, and 12.9 in quartiles 1–4, respectively ($p < 0.001$). Demographic parameters, background diseases, and chronic medications were similar between the quartiles. Higher heart rate, body temperature, systolic blood pressure, and respiratory rate were observed in the higher NLR quartiles, as well as lower oxygen saturation. Higher urgency scale and higher rates of intravenous magnesium sulfate were observed in the higher NLR quartiles, with higher admission rates and prolonged hospitalizations. In summary, NLR upon admission is associated with the severity of asthma exacerbation and higher chances of hospitalization among children in the ED.

Keywords: neutrophil-to-lymphocyte ratio; asthma; asthma exacerbation; emergency department; children; chronic inflammation

1. Introduction

Asthma is the most common chronic respiratory disease in children. It is characterized by chronic airway inflammation and hyper-responsiveness. Asthma exacerbations are well-known complications, impairing patients' quality of life and causing substantial healthcare costs [1,2]. In a US study conducted between 2010 and 2015, asthma exacerbations accounted for 3% of emergency department (ED) visits and 6% of hospitalizations among children aged 5–17 years [3]. Among the common triggers for acute exacerbations in the pediatric population are respiratory viral infections and exposure to allergens [4].

Assessing the risk for a severe exacerbation at the initial evaluation in an asthma patient may be challenging. Some of the predictors previously reported include spirometry measurements, such as forced expiratory volume in the first second (FEV1), number of exacerbations in the previous year, and patients' self-report on asthma control [5,6]. Several pediatric asthma scores are available to help classify the severity of exacerbation, including the Preschool Respiratory Assessment Measure (PRAM), the Pediatric Asthma Severity Score (PASS), and the Pediatric Asthma Score (PAS). Most scores assess different clinical-based parameters such as signs of increased work of breathing and accessory muscle use, air entry, and wheezing. Some include respiratory rate and oxygen saturation in addition to clinical observation [7]. In the acute ED setting, there is high variability among different centers in the management of acute exacerbation and admission criteria. The proportion admitted to the hospital ranges from 1.2–53%, according to different reports [8], and there is a non-negligible rate of relapse among discharged patients [9]. To date, there is no single validated model in determining the need for hospitalization in acute asthma exacerbation. Gorelick et al. suggested a model that can distinguish the patients that can be discharged from the ED from those needing further care, based on a clinical score, and the number of albuterol treatments given in the ED. Nevertheless, their model did not determine the need for a short stay versus more intensive inpatient-level care [8].

In the pathogenesis of asthma, airway inflammation is assumed to include two main subtypes, either induced by interleukin (IL)-5-mediated eosinophilic inflammation or an IL-8-mediated neutrophilic inflammation [10,11]. The role of systemic inflammation in asthma has not been well understood. An elevated level of circulating pro-inflammatory factors may be found in asthmatic patients. These include an increase in immune cells such as neutrophils and IL-6 and tumor necrosis factor (TNF)-α, which stimulates the production of acute-phase proteins [12,13]. Based on sputum eosinophil and neutrophil proportions [14], airway inflammatory patterns may represent different asthma phenotypes, with varying risks for exacerbations and response to treatment [15]. An increased neutrophil count in the sputum has been associated with steroid-refractory asthma and was negatively correlated with airflow obstruction parameters [14,16,17]. Peripheral blood counts may be of value in distinguishing between asthma phenotypes through correlation with sputum cell counts. Blood eosinophils, eosinophil-to-lymphocyte ratio (ELR), eosinophil-to-neutrophil ratio (ENR), and eosinophil-to-monocyte ratio (EMR) can predict eosinophilic asthma in adult patients [18].

The neutrophil-to-lymphocyte ratio (NLR) is a marker of a chronic inflammatory state. Previous data suggest its use as a prognostic factor indicating an accelerated inflammatory response in several diseases [19]. NLR was described in evaluating obstructive sleep apnea, allergic rhinitis, and chronic obstructive pulmonary disease (COPD) [20,21]. Moosman et al. reported age- and sex-specific pediatric reference values for the NLR and other blood count-derived biomarkers from 60,682 patients, from birth to 18 years of age. They found that the major changes in laboratory analysis from the neonatal period to adolescence were characterized by higher values directly after birth, which gradually decreased during the first two years of life. Another peak was observed in adolescence, with little change in most of the childhood years. No significant differences were found between boys and girls. It was also concluded that NLR was significantly increased in several diseases with inflammatory components, such as appendicitis; 65.7% of patients with appendicitis showed a higher NLR than the calculated upper reference limit. Regarding the respiratory system, they found that 22.7% of patients suffering from cystic fibrosis had pathological NLR values. In patients with asthma, NLR was also significantly increased; 20.6% of asthmatic patients presented with NLR > 97.5th percentile [22].

Measuring NLR is widely available, fast, and inexpensive, suiting both hospital and outpatient settings [23], though the clinical use of NLR in asthma patients is still debated. Imtiaz et al. did not find a relationship between asthma and NLR [24]. However, Zhang et al. reported an elevated NLR in adult patients with neutrophilic asthma [18]. In a study assessing the association of blood cell count parameters with severe asthma exacerbations, NLR was correlated with an increased risk for a severe exacerbation within the next year, with a predictor cutoff of 2.1 [23]. Multiple studies describe NLR in adult asthma exacerbation; however, there are only a few studies on children. Several previous studies evaluated NLR in correlation to a single parameter of hospitalized versus non-hospitalized pediatric patients [25]. Dogru et al. reported that NLR was higher by 17% in asthmatic children than in non-asthmatic controls [26]. Zhu et al. reported a combined score of C-Reactive-Protein and NLR levels, serving as a marker for differentiation between children with exacerbated asthma and healthy children [27]. In another recent study that included 89 children with asthma, the combination of NLR, alanine aminotransferase ratio, and NLR–albumin ratio was suggested as a clinical biomarker for asthma exacerbation in children [28].

To date, NLR is not routinely used to evaluate acute asthma exacerbation in children. Therefore, we aim to investigate the association of NLR with severity assessment and management of acute asthma exacerbation in children.

2. Materials and Methods

This is a cross-sectional study examining the NLR and its association with acute asthma exacerbation in the Soroka University Medical Center, a single tertiary center in southern Israel. We identified children who were diagnosed with asthma as a background disease and were referred to the ED due to asthma exacerbation. We collected data on their medical history, laboratory results, and vital signs during their ED visit and hospitalization.

2.1. Patients

A total of 715 pediatric patients aged 2–18 who presented during 813 ED visits for asthma exacerbation, between 2016 and 2021, were included in the study. All patients were presented with asthma-related symptoms (e.g., shortness of breath, wheezing, tachypnea), and underwent a complete blood count (CBC) upon arrival. In order to enhance precision, we included only the patients treated during the visit with anti-asthmatic medications. Children with respiratory symptoms that could be explained by factors other than asthma (e.g., suspected bacterial infection, chronic inflammatory diseases) were excluded from the cohort. We collected clinical, radiological, and laboratory data on each patient using electronic health record data. Data collected included: demographic data, chronic diagnoses, chronic medication purchases, vital signs on admission, radiological findings on chest X-ray (interpreted by either a pediatric radiologist or a pediatric pulmonologist), treatment at the ED, steroid use up to seven days prior to the ED visit, ED urgency scale based on the Canadian Triage Assessment Score (a clinical scale between 1–5, given at triage, according to initial patient assessment, with 1 being the most urgent and 5 the least urgent) [29], physical examination findings, CBC parameters, ED treatment, the decision of admission or discharge, treatment at the pediatric ward, pediatric intensive care unit (PICU) admissions, and length of hospitalization stay (LOS). Chronic diagnoses were extracted from the medical records, according to the ICD-9. The chronic diseases were categorized according to the involved system: endocrine disorders such as hypothyroidism and diabetes mellitus, cardiac diseases such as atrial septal defect and ventricular septal defect, metabolic diseases such as Niemann–Pick and mucopolysaccharidoses, developmental diseases such as cerebral palsy and autistic spectrum disorders, neuromuscular diseases such as Duchenne muscular dystrophy and myasthenia gravis, and gastrointestinal diseases such as inguinal hernia and short bowel syndrome. Pulmonary hypertension (PHT) was defined by echocardiographic diagnosis, that is, based on the task force of the European Society of Cardiology and the European Respiratory Society definitions of estimated systolic PAP ≥ 40 mmHg by Echo [30]. Bronchopulmonary dysplasia (BPD) was defined as a chronic lung disease of premature infants (<32 weeks gestational age), characterized by persistent parenchymal lung disease with radiographic confirmation, that requires oxygen or other respiratory support for ≥ 3 consecutive days, at 36 weeks postmenstrual age [31–33]. The study received the approval of the local institutional ethics committee (No. 184-20).

2.2. NLR

NLR was calculated by dividing the absolute neutrophil count by the absolute lymphocyte count in the blood count measured during the ED visit. Subsequently, the NLR was assessed as a continuous variable and was classified into four groups according to quartiles.

In this manner, the cohort was divided into four quartiles [34,35], with NLR quartiles 1, 2, 3, and 4 representing 0–24.99%, 25–49.99%, 50–74.99%, and 75–100%, respectively.

2.3. Statistical Analysis

Comparisons of demographic, clinical, and radiological parameters, as well as admissions outcomes, were made using appropriate univariate analyses. Continuous variables are reported as mean ± standard deviation (SD), median and interquartile range (IQR) for both normal and abnormal distribution. Categorical variables are presented as percentages. Comparisons were made with the appropriate statistical test. Continuous variables were compared with an ANOVA test, ordinal variables were compared with the Kruskal–Wallis test, and nominal variables were compared using chi-square analysis.

Given 117 repeated visits, we conducted several generalized estimating equations (GEE), with a logistic distribution. We chose the following variables as dependent variables: hospital admissions, the need for a resuscitation room, intravenous magnesium sulfate, admission $\geq$ two days, room air saturation < 92% [36], and tachypnea according to age. NLR quartiles were defined as primary independent variables. All regressions were adjusted for age. The results of the GEE models are shown schematically in Figure 1. The results are also shown in Supplementary Table S1 as an odds ratio (OR), 95% confidence interval (CI), and *p*-value.

A two-sided *p* value < 0.05 was considered statistically significant for all statistical tests. Reported *p*-values were rounded to two decimal places. All statistical analyses were performed using R statistical software version 4.05.

3. Results

A total of 831 ED visits for asthma exacerbation were included in the study during 2016–2021. Of all visits during the study period (5 years): 638, 59, 8, 5, 3, and 2 children visited 1, 2, 3, 4, 5, and 8 times, respectively. The median NLR was 1.6, 3.8, 6.7, and 12.9 in quartiles 1, 2, 3, and 4, respectively (*p* < 0.001). Similar demographic parameters were observed between the quartiles except for age, which was older in the higher quartiles (median age of 3.4, 4.6, 4.4, and 6.2 years in quartiles 1, 2, 3, and 4, respectively (*p* < 0.001)). The majority of patients were males of Bedouin-Arab descent in all quartiles. Table 1 summarizes the background diseases with similar rates of prior steroid use, atopy, and different comorbidities between the quartiles.

Table 1. Demographic and background diseases, according to NLR [a] quartiles.

Characteristic	Quartile 1 N-207	Quartile 2 N-208	Quartile 3 N-208	Quartile 4 N-208	*p*-Value
NLR [a] Mean ± SD [b]	1.6 ± 0.6	3.8 ± 0.7	6.8 ± 1.1	14.5 ± 5.5	**<0.001**
Age (years) Mean ± SD [b]	5.3 ± 3.9	6.2 ± 4.1	6.1 ± 3.8	7.1 ± 3.8	**<0.001**
Male gender, n/N (%)	120/207 (58%)	129/208 (62%)	129/207 (62%)	114/208 (55%)	0.3
Bedouin ethnicity, n/N (%)	114/178 (64%)	123/181 (68%)	120/183 (66%)	129/171 (75%)	0.11
Steroid use before admission, n/N (%)	38/207 (18%)	37/208 (18%)	53/208 (25%)	48/208 (23%)	0.2
Prematurity (<36 + 6 weeks), n/N (%)	9/207 (4.3%)	2/208 (1.0%)	2/208 (1.0%)	1/208 (0.5%)	**0.013**
Bronchopulmonary dysplasia, n/N (%)	5/207 (2.4%)	2/208 (1.0%)	3/208 (1.4%)	0/208 (0%)	0.10
Pulmonary hypertension, n/N (%)	2/207 (1.0%)	0/208 (0%)	7/208 (3.4%)	5/208 (2.4%)	**0.023**
Developmental disease, n/N (%)	11/207 (5.3%)	7/208 (3.4%)	9/208 (4.3%)	4/208 (1.9%)	0.3
Neuromuscular disease, n/N (%)	9/207 (4.3%)	1/208 (0.5%)	2/208 (1.0%)	3/208 (1.4%)	**0.025**
Cardiac disease, n/N (%)	11/207 (5.3%)	7/208 (3.4%)	13/208 (6.2%)	6/208 (2.9%)	0.3
Metabolic disease, n/N (%)	4/207 (1.9%)	1/208 (0.5%)	0/208 (0%)	0/208 (0%)	**0.018**
Atopic dermatitis, n/N (%)	80/207 (39%)	95/208 (46%)	76/208 (37%)	81/208 (39%)	0.3
Allergic rhinitis, n/N (%)	5/207 (2.4%)	8/208 (3.8%)	3/208 (1.4%)	10/208 (4.8%)	0.2
Atopic diseases (combined), n/N (%)	81/207 (39%)	98/208 (47%)	77/208 (37%)	85/208 (41%)	0.2

[a] Neutrophil-to-Lymphocyte ratio. [b] SD—standard deviation. Bold values denote statistical significance at the $p \leq 0.05$ level.

Prematurity, neuromuscular disease, and metabolic disease were more common in the lower quartiles, while pulmonary hypertension was more common in the higher quartiles. Regarding chronic medical treatment, no significant difference was observed in the chronic anti-asthmatic treatment, indicating similar asthma control between the quartiles. Antiepileptic medications were used more commonly in the lower quartiles (Table 2).

Table 2. Chronic medication treatment, according to the quartiles.

Characteristic	Quartile 1 N-207	Quartile 2 N-208	Quartile 3 N-208	Quartile 4 N-208	p-Value
Inhaled corticosteroids, n/N (%)	75/207 (36%)	91/208 (44%)	79/208 (38%)	82/208 (39%)	0.4
Inhaled corticosteroids and long-acting beta-agonist, n/N (%)	16/207 (7.7%)	25/208 (12%)	22/208 (11%)	22/208 (11%)	0.5
Short-acting beta-agonist, n/N (%)	17/207 (8.2%)	14/208 (6.7%)	21/208 (10%)	17/208 (8.2%)	0.7
Leukotriene receptor antagonists, n/N (%)	31/207 (15%)	32/208 (15%)	22/208 (11%)	18/208 (8.7%)	0.10
Anticholinergics, n/N (%)	0/207 (0%)	1/208 (0.5%)	1/208 (0.5%)	0/208 (0%)	1
Antiepileptic medications, n/N (%)	22/207 (11%)	13/208 (6.2%)	10/208 (4.8%)	6/208 (2.9%)	**0.008**
Cardiovascular medications, n/N (%)	16/207 (7.7%)	7/208 (3.4%)	10/208 (4.8%)	5/208 (2.4%)	0.053
Antibiotics (chronic use), n/N (%)	6/207 (2.9%)	7/208 (3.4%)	13/208 (6.2%)	5/208 (2.4%)	0.2

Bold values denote statistical significance at the $p \leq 0.05$ level.

Table 3 summarizes the mean vital signs in the ED, with an elevated heart rate (131, 134, 154, and 137 beats per minute in quartiles 1, 2, 3 and 4, respectively, $p = 0.01$), higher temperature (37.71, 37.74, 39.55, and 37.4 Celsius in quartiles 1, 2, 3 and 4, respectively, $p = 0.004$), and higher respiratory rate (39, 43, 44 and 42 breaths per minute in the quartiles 1, 2, 3 and 4, respectively, $p = 0.002$) in the higher quartiles. The rate of tachypnea (adjusted to normal values for age), was correlated with higher quartiles with 85%, 89%, 94%, and 97% in quartiles 1, 2, 3, and 4, respectively ($p < 0.001$). Room air oxygen saturation was lower in the higher quartiles (93.5%, 93%, 92.1%, 92.5%, $p < 0.001$).

Table 3. Measurements in the emergency department, according to quartiles.

Characteristic	Quartile 1 N-207	Quartile 2 N-208	Quartile 3 N-208	Quartile 4 N-208	p-Value
Heart rate (beats/minute) Mean ± SD [a] (N)	131 ± 21 (109)	135 ± 21 (107)	154 ± 146 (106)	137 ± 17 (99)	**0.010**
Temperature (°C) Mean ± SD [a] (N)	37.71 ± 0.95 (192)	37.74 ± 0.95 (176)	39.55 ± 24.99 (172)	37.40 ± 0.72 (165)	**0.004**
Oxygen saturation (room air) Mean ± SD [a] (N)	93.5 ± 7.1 (185)	93.0 ± 5.6 (179)	92.1 ± 5.5 (173)	92.5 ± 4.6 (176)	**<0.001**
Room air oxygen saturation < 92%	60/185 (32%)	75/179 (42%)	79/173 (46%)	75/176 (43%)	0.061
Systolic blood pressure (mm Hg) Mean ± SD [a] (N)	107 ± 11 (178)	108 ± 11 (162)	109 ± 11 (160)	111 ± 11 (171)	**0.002**
Diastolic blood pressure (mm Hg) Mean ± SD [a] (N)	66 ± 10 (178)	66 ± 9 (162)	66 ± 10 (160)	66 ± 9 (171)	1
Respiratory rate (breaths/minute) Mean ± SD [a] (N)	39 ± 13 (196)	43 ± 15 (185)	44 ± 13 (179)	42 ± 12 (183)	**0.002**
Tachypnea (respiratory rate according to age) [b] n/N (%)	167/196 (85%)	165/185 (89%)	169/179 (94%)	178/183 (97%)	**<0.001**

[a] SD—standard deviation. [b] Respiratory rate above the normal respiratory rate according to the American Heart Association. Bold values denote statistical significance at the $p \leq 0.05$ level.

ED intervention characteristics are summarized in Table 4. ED urgency scale showed a decline across the quartiles, which correlated with higher mean clinical urgency (3.17, 2.72, 2.52, and 2.49 in quartiles 1, 2, 3, and 4, respectively, $p < 0.001$). Rates of supplemental oxygen, inhalation of anticholinergic agents, and intravenous magnesium sulfate were significantly higher in the higher quartiles. No significant difference was observed in chest X-ray findings among the quartiles.

Table 4. Treatment and interventions in the emergency department, according to the quartiles.

Characteristic	Quartile 1 N-207	Quartile 2 N-208	Quartile 3 N-208	Quartile 4 N-208	p-Value
ED [a] Urgency [1], Median (IQR [b])	3.00 (3.00, 4.00)	3.00 (2.00, 3.25)	2.50 (1.00, 3.00)	3.00 (1.00, 3.00)	**<0.001**
Oxygen, n/N (%)	69/207 (33%)	98/208 (47%)	92/208 (44%)	101/208 (49%)	**0.007**
Inhalation of Beta-agonists, n/N (%)	125/207 (60%)	137/208 (66%)	134/208 (64%)	139/208 (67%)	0.5
Inhalation of Anticholinergic, n/N (%)	91/207 (44%)	104/208 (50%)	109/208 (52%)	124/208 (60%)	**0.015**
Inhaled corticosteroids, n/N (%)	9/207 (4.3%)	12/208 (5.8%)	15/208 (7.2%)	13/208 (6.2%)	0.7
Systemic Steroids PO, n/N (%)	82/207 (40%)	71/208 (34%)	62/208 (30%)	57/208 (27%)	**0.043**
Systemic Steroids IV, n/N (%)	18/207 (8.7%)	25/208 (12%)	23/208 (11%)	27/208 (13%)	0.5
Antihistamines, n/N (%)	1/207 (0.5%)	0/208 (0%)	0/208 (0%)	0/208 (0%)	0.2
Antibiotics, n/N (%)	10/207 (4.8%)	9/208 (4.3%)	6/208 (2.9%)	10/208 (4.8%)	0.7
Sodium chloride Inhalation, n/N (%)	113/207 (55%)	121/208 (58%)	127/208 (61%)	132/208 (63%)	0.3
Intravenous Magnesium Sulphate, n/N (%)	6/207 (2.9%)	20/208 (9.6%)	26/208 (12%)	32/208 (15%)	**<0.001**
Findings on chest X-ray, n/N (%)					
Normal	37/63 (59%)	43/82 (52%)	45/91 (49%)	54/95 (57%)	
Hyperinflation	8/63 (13%)	13/82 (16%)	19/91 (21%)	13/95 (14%)	0.8
Infiltrate	12/63 (19%)	16/82 (20%)	12/91 (13%)	17/95 (18%)	
Atelectasis	6/63 (9.5%)	10/82 (12%)	15/91 (16%)	11/95 (12%)	

[a] ED—Emergency department. [b] IQR—interquartile range. [1] Allon et al. [29]. Bold values denote statistical significance at the $p \leq 0.05$ level.

Data on admissions to the pediatric ward and PICU are presented in Table 5. Admission rate and length of stay (above 2 days) were significantly higher in the higher quartiles, with 66%, 76%, 79%, and 84% rates of admission in quartiles 1, 2, 3, and 4, respectively, ($p < 0.001$) and 35%, 36%, 42% and 48% for prolonged admission in quartiles 1, 2, 3 and 4, respectively ($p = 0.034$). The rate of PICU admissions was not statistically significant across the quartiles.

Table 5. Admissions and hospitalizations data, according to quartiles.

Characteristic	Quartile 1 N-207	Quartile 2 N-208	Quartile 3 N-208	Quartile 4 N-208	p-Value
Hospitalization, n/N (%)	137/207 (66%)	158/208 (76%)	165/208 (79%)	175/208 (84%)	**<0.001**
LOS *, Median (IQR)	2.00 (1.00, 3.00)	1.00 (1.00, 2.00)	2.00 (1.00, 2.00)	2.00 (1.00, 3.00)	0.2
LOS * $\geq$ 2, n/N (%)	73/207 (35%)	75/208 (36%)	88/208 (42%)	99/208 (48%)	**0.034**
PICU **, n/N (%)	5/207 (2.4%)	10/208 (4.8%)	12/208 (5.8%)	12/208 (5.8%)	0.3

* LOS—length of stay in the hospital, ** PICU—pediatric intensive care unit. Bold values denote statistical significance at the $p \leq 0.05$ level.

Figure 1 present a multivariate analysis via generalized estimating equations (GEE) with a logistic distribution. Hospital admissions, a treatment in the resuscitation room (reflecting high urgency scale) in the ED, treatment with intravenous magnesium sulfate, prolonged hospitalization ($\geq$two days), room air saturation < 92%, and tachypnea (normalized to age) showed an odds ratio of 2.9 (95% CI 1.79, 4.69, $p = 0.001$) for admission, 2.86 (95% CI 1.64, 5.0, $p < 0.001$) for treatment in the resuscitation room, 6.62 (95% CI 2.7, 16.2, $p < 0.001$) for intravenous magnesium sulfate treatment, 1.64 (95% CI 1.1, 2.45, $p = 0.015$) for prolonged hospitalization, 1.74 (95% CI 1.12, 2.7, $p = 0.014$) for room air saturation < 92% and 8 (95% CI 2.98, 21.5, $p < 0.001$) for tachypnea adjusted to age, in the higher quartile.

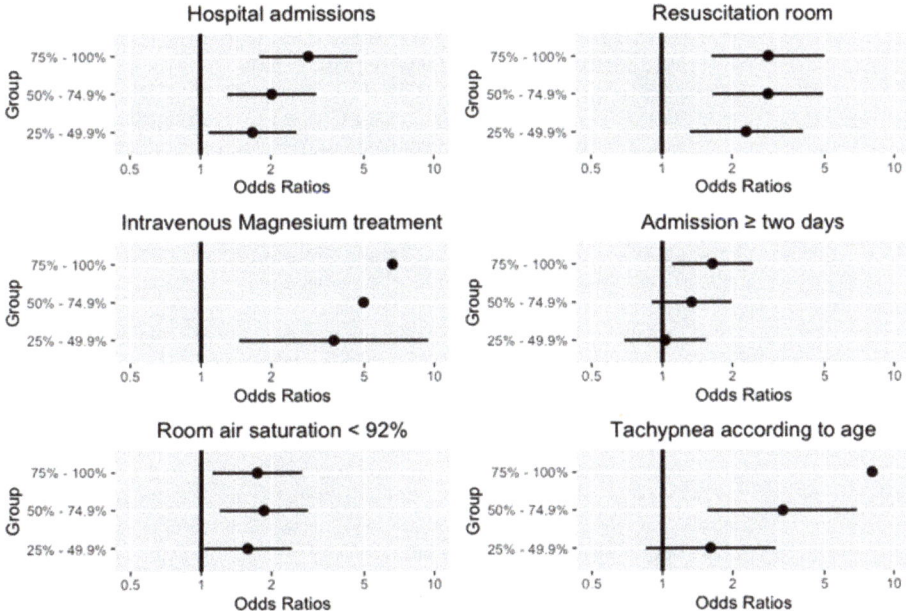

Figure 1. Multivariate GEE* logistic regressions for multiple independent variables, adjusted for age.

4. Discussion

The NLR, a blood count-derived parameter, is a marker of systemic inflammation, combining innate and allergic inflammation markers. It was previously suggested to be correlated with neutrophilic asthma [18], though its role in predicting the clinical outcome of asthmatic patients has not been elucidated yet. This study examined the correlation of the NLR with the clinical course of children who were presented with acute asthma exacerbation to the ED. Our results indicate that higher NLR is associated with a severe clinical course in children with acute exacerbations. Patients throughout the different quartiles had similar background diseases, chronic medical treatment, and asthma control.

Patients in the higher NLR quartiles were presented with more severe respiratory distress than in the lower quartiles, as reflected by higher heart rate, respiratory rate, and lower room air oxygen saturation. This finding was not attributable to fever or age, as this group had a slightly higher mean age and lower body temperature. A significant correlation was found between the NLR and the need for treatment in the resuscitation room, based on the ED urgency scale. This correlation suggested once more that patients with higher NLR appeared more clinically deteriorated than others and required more intensive treatment. Treatment with oxygen and intra-venous magnesium sulfate was also correlated with increased NLR.

Our results also demonstrated a higher hospitalization rate and length of stay with higher NLR. The risk for hospitalization for children within the highest NLR quartile was three times higher than in the lowest quartile, and the risk for prolonged hospitalization over two days equally increased. The PICU admission rate was twice as high among the higher quartiles, but this increase was not significant, possibly due to the small sample of children admitted to the PICU.

Our findings support previous data regarding the inferior prognosis of neutrophilic asthma. Neutrophilic asthma is characterized by at least 65% neutrophils in the sputum of, or above, 5×10^6 cells/mL [37]. Pathophysiologically, it is associated with activation of the Th17 pathway, IL-8 IL-1β, and TNFα. Recent data suggests it is correlated with decreasing FEV1 and resistance to steroid therapy [38]. To date, there are no specific therapeutical approaches to this asthma phenotype. Airway inflammation with dominant neutrophils can also be induced by respiratory tract infections, tobacco smoke exposure, and obesity.

Our study results are in congruence with previous data regarding the association of NLR with the severity of exacerbation among asthmatic children. In a recent study from China, that examined 81 pediatric patients with asthma exacerbation, the severe exacerbation group (n = 10) had the highest levels of NLR (7.19), compared with the mild or moderate exacerbation groups, though the specific criteria for subgroup division are unclear. The optimal NLR cutoff level suggested was 1.723, with a sensitivity of 0.73 and specificity of 0.906 [28].

A possible confounder influencing our results is a concurring bacterial infection which may elevate the neutrophil count. However, this seems unlikely in our cohort, due to the relatively lower body temperatures that characterized the highest NLR group and the similar use of antibiotics between the different groups as a surrogate marker for bacterial respiratory infection. Another possible influencing factor is previous steroid use, which was similar between the different groups in the week prior to their ED visit.

Another possible confounder is the physiologic distribution of NLR according to age and sex. All our groups presented similar sex distribution with a majority of male patients, and a slightly heterogenous age distribution. If we examine previous data on age-specific reference values, the pattern of change in the NLR values from birth to adolescence is mostly influenced by the highest peak in the neonatal and infancy period, which was not included in our study. Most of the childhood years are not characterized by substantial changes in the NLR [22].

Our study has a few limitations. First, is its retrospective nature. Our data was based on the documentation from the patient's electronic files. All patients were diagnosed and treated in a single tertiary center, with a potentially excessive influence of the unique demographics in our region. Bedouin Arabs consist of up to 75% of our cohort. The combination of several characteristic factors, such as low socioeconomic status, poor sanitation, crowded houses, high rates of malnutrition, and smoking, all contribute to the previously described data on higher morbidity, specifically, respiratory infections, among the Bedouin pediatric population [39,40]. Another limitation is that we did not capture data regarding viral PCR in nasal swabs, which are common triggers for asthma exacerbation in children and could differ in blood count parameters and clinical presentations. NLR from blood samples prior to the current ED visits was out of the scope of this study, but it could be interesting to investigate the association of NLR as a chronic marker for asthma control and exacerbations.

The strengths of our study are the relatively large population of children with a definition of asthma who were treated at the ED with anti-asthmatic treatments. In our study, we showed a significantly larger patient sample size. In addition, we examine multiple parameters of severity in order to demonstrate the potential clinical use of NLR in ED as an assessment tool for asthma exacerbation. We captured comprehensive ambulatory data on the patients, their blood tests, medication regimens, and radiology findings (that were interpreted by either a pediatric radiologist or a pulmonologist). Since the data was harvested from a single medical center, there is limited variability regarding admissions strategies and treatments, which strengthens the association between NLR and the severity measurements studied.

In conclusion, the NLR is an objective tool that may have a role in assessing pediatric asthma exacerbation severity and the need for hospitalization. It is a feasible and safe measure, suited for the pediatric ED setting. NLR could potentially supply an additional decision tool that could assist the clinician in the identification of severe asthma cases that require admission and further inpatient care. However, further studies are warranted for its implementation in the clinical setting, providing validated range and cutoff values in which a high probability of severe asthma is likely.

Supplementary Materials: The following supporting information can be downloaded at: https://www.mdpi.com/article/10.3390/jcm12093312/s1, Table S1: Several generalized estimating equations (GEE), with a logistic distribution, for the following variables: hospital admissions, the need for a resuscitation room, intravenous magnesium sulfate, admission ≥ two days, room air saturation < 92%, and tachypnea according to age.

Author Contributions: Conceptualization, I.G.T. and A.H.; methodology, I.G.T., A.G. and A.H.; software N.A., S.U.S., R.B. and I.H.; validation, R.B. and I.H.; formal analysis, R.B. and I.H.; investigation, R.B. and I.H.; resources, N.A. and S.U.S.; data curation, N.A. and S.U.S.; writing—original draft preparation, N.A. and S.U.S.; writing—review and editing, I.G.T., A.G. and A.H.; visualization, editing, I.G.T., A.G. and A.H.; supervision, I.G.T. and A.H.; project administration, I.G.T. and A.G. All authors have read and agreed to the published version of the manuscript.

Funding: This research received no external funding.

Institutional Review Board Statement: The study was conducted according to the guidelines of the Declaration of Helsinki and approved by the Institutional Review Board (or Ethics Committee) of Soroka University Medical Center (Number SOR 184-20).

Informed Consent Statement: Was not required since it was a retrospective cohort study.

Data Availability Statement: The database used and/or analyzed during the current study are available from the corresponding author on reasonable request.

Conflicts of Interest: The authors declare no conflict of interest.

Abbreviations

NLR	neutrophil-to-lymphocyte ratio
ED	emergency department
IQR	interquartile range
LOS	length of stay in the hospital
PICU	pediatric intensive care unit

References

1. Ivanova, J.I.; Bergman, R.; Birnbaum, H.G.; Colice, G.L.; Silverman, R.A.; McLaurin, K. Effect of asthma exacerbations on health care costs among asthmatic patients with moderate and severe persistent asthma. *J. Allergy Clin. Immunol.* **2012**, *129*, 1229–1235. [CrossRef] [PubMed]
2. Luskin, A.T.; Chipps, B.E.; Rasouliyan, L.; Miller, D.P.; Haselkorn, T.; Dorenbaum, A. Impact of asthma exacerbations and asthma triggers on asthma-related quality of life in patients with severe or difficult-to-treat asthma. *J. Allergy Clin. Immunol. Pract.* **2014**, *2*, 544–552.e1-2. [CrossRef] [PubMed]
3. Qin, X.; Zahran, H.S.; Malilay, J. Asthma-related emergency department (ED) visits and post-ED visit hospital and critical care admissions, National Hospital Ambulatory Medical Care Survey, 2010–2015. *J. Asthma* **2020**, *58*, 565–572. [CrossRef] [PubMed]
4. Fu, L.S.; Tsai, M.C. Asthma Exacerbation in Children: A Practical Review. *Pediatr. Neonatol.* **2014**, *55*, 83–91. [CrossRef] [PubMed]
5. Bateman, E.D.; Buhl, R.; O'Byrne, P.M.; Humbert, M.; Reddel, H.; Sears, M.R.; Jenkins, C.; Harrison, T.W.; Quirce, S.; Peterson, S.; et al. Development and validation of a novel risk score for asthma exacerbations: The risk score for exacerbations. *J. Allergy Clin. Immunol.* **2015**, *135*, 1457–1464.e4. [CrossRef]
6. Greenberg, S.; Liu, N.; Kaur, A.; Lakshminarayanan, M.; Zhou, Y.; Nelsen, L.; Gates, D.F.; Kuo, W.-L.; Smugar, S.S.; Reiss, T.F.; et al. The asthma disease activity score: A discriminating, responsive measure predicts future asthma attacks. *J. Allergy Clin. Immunol.* **2012**, *130*, 1071–1077.e10. [CrossRef]
7. Kline-Krammes, S.; Patel, N.H.; Robinson, S. Childhood asthma: A guide for pediatric emergency medicine providers. *Emerg. Med. Clin. N. Am.* **2013**, *31*, 705–732. [CrossRef] [PubMed]
8. Gorelick, M.; Scribano, P.V.; Stevens, M.W.; Schultz, T.; Shults, J. Predicting Need for Hospitalization in Acute Pediatric Asthma. *Pediatr. Emerg. Care* **2008**, *24*, 735–744. [CrossRef]

9. Emerman, C.L.; Cydulka, R.K.; Crain, E.F.; Rowe, B.H.; Radeos, M.S.; Camargo, C.A., Jr.; MARC Investigators. Prospective multicenter study of relapse after treatment for acute asthma among children presenting to the emergency department. *J. Pediatr.* **2001**, *138*, 318–324. [CrossRef] [PubMed]
10. Baines, K.J.; Simpson, J.L.; Bowden, N.A.; Scott, R.J.; Gibson, P.G. Differential gene expression and cytokine production from neutrophils in asthma phenotypes. *Eur. Respir. J.* **2010**, *35*, 522–531. [CrossRef]
11. Simpson, J.L.; Grissell, T.V.; Douwes, J.; Scott, R.J.; Boyle, M.J.; Gibson, P.G. Innate immune activation in neutrophilic asthma and bronchiectasis. *Thorax* **2007**, *62*, 211–218. [CrossRef] [PubMed]
12. Gabay, C.; Kushner, I. Acute-phase proteins and other systemic responses to inflammation. *N. Engl. J. Med.* **1999**, *340*, 448–454. [CrossRef] [PubMed]
13. Bruunsgaard, H.; Pedersen, B.K. Age-related inflammatory cytokines and disease. *Immunol. Allergy Clin. N. Am.* **2003**, *23*, 15–39. [CrossRef] [PubMed]
14. Simpson, J.L.; Scott, R.J.; Boyle, M.J.; Gibson, P.G. Inflammatory subtypes in asthma: Assessment and identification using induced sputum. *Respirology* **2006**, *11*, 54–61. [CrossRef] [PubMed]
15. McDonald, V.M.; Gibson, P.G. Exacerbations of severe asthma. *Clin. Exp. Allergy* **2012**, *42*, 670–677. [CrossRef]
16. Ordonez, C.L.; Shaughnessy, T.E.; Matthay, M.A.; Fahy, J.V. Increased neutrophil numbers and IL-8 levels in airway secretions in acute severe asthma: Clinical and biologic significance. *Am. J. Respir. Crit. Care Med.* **2000**, *161*, 1185–1190. [CrossRef] [PubMed]
17. Green, R.H.; Brightling, C.E.; Woltmann, G.; Parker, D.; Wardlaw, A.J.; Pavord, I.D. Analysis of induced sputum in adults with asthma: Identification of subgroup with isolated sputum neutrophilia and poor response to inhaled corticosteroids. *Thorax* **2002**, *57*, 875–879. [CrossRef]
18. Zhang, X.-Y.; Simpson, J.L.; Powell, H.; Yang, I.A.; Upham, J.W.; Reynolds, P.N.; Hodge, S.; James, A.L.; Jenkins, C.; Peters, M.J.; et al. Full blood count parameters for the detection of asthma inflammatory phenotypes. *Clin. Exp. Allergy* **2014**, *44*, 1137–1145. [CrossRef]
19. Takeshita, S.; Kanai, T.; Kawamura, Y.; Yoshida, Y.; Nonoyama, S. A comparison of the predictive validity of the combination of the neutrophil- to-lymphocyte ratio and platelet-to-lymphocyte ratio and other risk scoring systems for intravenous immunoglobulin (ivig)- resistance in Kawasaki disease. *PLoS ONE* **2017**, *12*, e0176957. [CrossRef]
20. Pilaczynska-Cemel, M.; Golda, R.; Dabrowska, A.; Przybylski, G. Analysis of the level of selected parameters of inflammation, circulating immune complexes, and related indicators (neutrophil/lymphocyte, platelet/lymphocyte, CRP/CIC) in patients with obstructive diseases. *Centr. Eur. J. Immunol.* **2019**, *43*, 292–298. [CrossRef]
21. Ha, E.K.; Park, J.H.; Lee, S.J.; Yon, D.K.; Kim, J.H.; Jee, H.M.; Lee, K.S.; Sung, M.; Kim, M.A.; Shin, Y.H.; et al. Shared and unique individual risk factors and clinical biomarkers in children with allergic rhinitis and obstructive sleep apnea syndrome. *Clin. Respir. J.* **2020**, *14*, 250–259. [CrossRef]
22. Moosmann, J.; Krusemark, A.; Dittrich, S.; Ammer, T.; Rauh, M.; Woelfle, J.; Metzler, M.; Zierk, J. Age-and sex-specific pediatric reference intervals for neutrophil-to-lymphocyte ratio, lymphocyte-to-monocyte ratio, and platelet-to-lymphocyte ratio. *Int. J. Lab. Hematol.* **2022**, *44*, 296–301. [CrossRef] [PubMed]
23. Mochimaru, T.; Ueda, S.; Suzuki, Y.; Asano, K.; Fukunaga, K. Neutrophil-to-lymphocyte ratio as a novel independent predictor of severe exacerbation in patients with asthma. *Ann. Allergy Asthma Immunol.* **2019**, *122*, 337–339.e1. [CrossRef] [PubMed]
24. Imtiaz, F.; Shafique, K.; Mirza, S.S.; Ayoob, Z.; Vart, P.; Rao, S. Neutrophil lymphocyte ratio as a measure of systemic inflammation in prevalent chronic diseases in Asian population. *Int. Arch. Med.* **2012**, *5*, 2. [CrossRef] [PubMed]
25. Esmaeilzadeh, H.; Nouri, F.; Nabavizadeh, S.H.; Alyasin, S.; Mortazavi, N. Can eosinophilia and neutrophil–lymphocyte ratio predict hospitalization in asthma exacerbation? *Allergy Asthma Clin. Immunol.* **2021**, *17*, 16. [CrossRef] [PubMed]
26. Dogru, M.; Yesiltepe Mutlu, R.G. The evaluation of neutrophil-lymphocyte ratio in children with asthma. *Allergol. Immunopathol.* **2016**, *44*, 292–296. [CrossRef]
27. Zhu, X.; Zhou, L.; Li, Q.; Pan, R.; Zhang, J.; Cui, Y. Combined score of C-reactive protein level and neutrophil-to-lymphocyte ratio: A novel marker in distinguishing children with exacerbated asthma. *Int. J. Immunopathol. Pharmacol.* **2021**, *35*, 20587384211040641. [CrossRef]
28. Pan, R.; Ren, Y.; Li, Q.; Zhu, X.; Zhang, J.; Cui, Y.; Yin, H. Neutrophil–lymphocyte ratios in blood to distinguish children with asthma exacerbation from healthy subjects. *Int. J. Immunopathol. Pharmacol.* **2023**, *37*, 03946320221149849. [CrossRef]
29. Allon, R.; Feldman, O.; Karminsky, A.; Steinberg, C.; Leiba, R.; Shavit, I. Validity of the Pediatric Canadian Triage Acuity Scale in a tertiary children's hospital in Israel. *Eur. J. Emerg. Med.* **2018**, *25*, 270–273. [CrossRef]
30. Galie, N.; Hoeper, M.M.; Humbert, M.; Torbicki, A.; Vachiery, J.L.; Barbera, J.A.; Beghetti, M.; Corris, P.; Gaine, S.; Gibbs, J.S.; et al. Guidelines for the diagnosis and treatment of pulmonary hypertension: The Task Force for the Diagnosis and Treatment of Pulmonary Hypertension of the European Society of Cardiology (ESC) and the European Respiratory Society (ERS), endorsed by the International Society of Heart and Lung Transplantation (ISHLT). *Eur. Heart J.* **2009**, *30*, 2493–2537.25.
31. Shennan, A.T.; Dunn, M.S.; Ohlsson, A.; Lennox, K.; Hoskins, E.M. Abnormal pulmonary outcomes in premature infants. Prediction from oxygen requirement in the neonatal period. *Pediatrics.* **1988**, *82*, 527–532. [CrossRef]
32. Higgins, R.D.; Jobe, A.H.; Koso-Thomas, M.; Bancalari, E.; Viscardi, R.M.; Hartert, T.V.; Ryan, R.M.; Kallapur, S.G.; Steinhorn, R.H.; Konduri, G.G.; et al. Bronchopulmonary Dysplasia: Executive Summary of a Workshop. *J. Pediatr.* **2018**, *197*, 300–308 [CrossRef] [PubMed]

33. Jensen, E.A.; Dysart, K.; Gantz, M.G.; McDonald, S.; Bamat, N.A.; Keszler, M.; Kirpalani, H.; Laughon, M.M.; Poindexter, B.B.; Duncan, A.F.; et al. The Diagnosis of Bronchopulmonary Dysplasia in Very Preterm Infants. An Evidence-based Approach. *Am. J. Respir. Crit. Care Med.* **2019**, *200*, 751–759. [CrossRef] [PubMed]
34. Du, Y.; Wang, A.; Zhang, J.; Zhang, X.; Li, N.; Liu, X.; Wang, W.; Zhao, X.; Bian, L. Association Between the Neutrophil-to-Lymphocyte Ratio and Adverse Clinical Prognosis in Patients with Spontaneous Intracerebral Hemorrhage. *Neuropsychiatr. Dis. Treat.* **2022**, *18*, 985–993. [CrossRef] [PubMed]
35. Pan, L.; Li, Z.; Li, C.; Dong, X.; Hidru, T.H.; Liu, F.; Xia, Y.; Yang, X.; Zhong, L.; Liu, Y. Stress hyperglycemia ratio and neutrophil to lymphocyte ratio are reliable predictors of new-onset atrial fibrillation in patients with acute myocardial infarction. *Front. Cardiovasc. Med.* **2022**, *9*, 1051078. [CrossRef] [PubMed]
36. Pilcher, J.; Ploen, L.; McKinstry, S.; Bardsley, G.; Chien, J.; Howard, L.; Lee, S.; Beckert, L.; Swanney, M.; Weatherall, M.; et al. A multicentre prospective observational study comparing arterial blood gas values to those obtained by pulse oximeters used in adult patients attending Australian and New Zealand hospitals. *BMC Pulm. Med.* **2020**, *20*, 7. [CrossRef] [PubMed]
37. Gao, J.; Wu, F. Association between fractional exhaled nitric oxide, sputum induction and peripheral blood eosinophil in uncontrolled asthma. *Allergy Asthma Clin. Immunol.* **2018**, *14*, 21. [CrossRef]
38. Shilovskiy, I.P.; Nikolskii, A.A.; Kurbacheva, O.M.; Khaitov, M.R. Modern View of Neutrophilic Asthma Molecular Mechanisms and Therapy. *Biochem. Mosc.* **2020**, *85*, 854–868. [CrossRef]
39. Ben-Shimol, S.; Dagan, R.; Givon-Lavi, N.; Bar-Ziv, Y.; Greenberg, D. Community acquired pneumonia (CAP) in children younger than 5 years of age in southern Israel. *Harefuah* **2010**, *149*, 137–142+196. (In Hebrew)
40. Horwitz, D.; Kestenbom, I.; Goldbart, A.; Chechik, T.; Dizitzer, Y.; Golan-Tripto, I. The effect of a coaching program on asthma control and health care utilization in children with asthma. *J. Asthma* **2021**, *58*, 240–247. [CrossRef]

Disclaimer/Publisher's Note: The statements, opinions and data contained in all publications are solely those of the individual author(s) and contributor(s) and not of MDPI and/or the editor(s). MDPI and/or the editor(s) disclaim responsibility for any injury to people or property resulting from any ideas, methods, instructions or products referred to in the content.

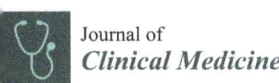 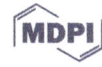

Article

Role of Lung Ultrasonography (LUS) as a Tool for Evaluating Children with Pediatric Inflammatory Multisystem Syndrome Temporally Associated with SARS-CoV-2 (PIMS-TS)

Jolanta Tomczonek-Moruś [1,*], Natalia Krysiak [1], Agnieszka Blomberg [1], Marta Depczyk-Bukała [1], Marcin Tkaczyk [1,2] and Krzysztof Zeman [1,2]

[1] Department of Pediatrics, Immunology and Nephrology, Institute of the Polish Mother's Memorial Hospital in Lodz Poland, 93-338 Lodz, Poland
[2] Department of Pediatrics Nephrology and Immunology, Medical University of Lodz, 90-151 Lodz, Poland
* Correspondence: jolanta.tomczonek-morus@iczmp.edu.pl

Abstract: Background: Pediatric inflammatory multisystem syndrome temporally associated with SARS-CoV-2 (PIMS-TS) is a novel entity. The inflammatory process involves the circulatory, digestive, respiratory, and central nervous systems, as well as the skin. Making a diagnosis requires extensive differential diagnoses, including lung imaging. The aim of our study was to retrospectively assess the pathologies found in lung ultrasound (LUS) in children diagnosed with PIMS-TS and to evaluate the usefulness of the examination in diagnostics and monitoring. Methods: The study group consisted of 43 children diagnosed with PIMS-TS, in whom LUS was performed at least three times, including on admission to hospital, on discharge, and 3 months after disease onset. Results: Pneumonia (mild to severe) was diagnosed in 91% of the patients based on the ultrasound image; the same number had at least one pathology, including consolidations, atelectasis, pleural effusion, and interstitial or interstitial-alveolar syndrome. By the time of discharge, the inflammatory changes had completely regressed in 19% of the children and partially in 81%. After 3 months, no pathologies were detected in the entire study group. Conclusion: LUS is a useful tool for diagnosing and monitoring children with PIMS-TS. Inflammatory lesions of the lungs resolve completely when the generalized inflammatory process subsides.

Keywords: lung ultrasound; PIMS-TS; MIS-C; pneumonia; intensive care; children; adolescents

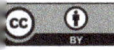

1. Introduction

In 2019 reports of a previously unknown set of clinical symptoms appeared in the pediatric population. An association with SARS-CoV-2 was observed. On 7 April 2020, the first case of a novel entity was registered, called multisystem inflammatory syndrome in children (MIS-C) or adolescents (MIS-A) by the United States Centers for Disease Control (CDC) and the World Health Organization (WHO). At the same time, the Royal College of Pediatrics and Child Health (RCPCH) used the term pediatric inflammatory multisystem syndrome temporally associated with SARS-CoV-2 (PIMS-TS), with slightly different criteria [1–3]. We will use this name in our article, but both terms function in parallel in the literature. It is coded with 'U10' in the International Classification of Diseases [4].

Symptoms of PIMS-TS appear 4–8 weeks after SARS-CoV-2 infection and are the result of the immune system's reaction to the infectious agent. Cytokine-dependent inflammation of small vessels occurs. The leading symptom of PIMS-TS is fever. Children also present manifestations from the digestive system (abdominal pain, vomiting, or diarrhea), the cardiovascular system (tachycardia, low-output syndrome, or coronary artery aneurysm), the central nervous system (headache, photophobia, meningeal syndrome, or hyperaesthesia), the respiratory system (cough, shortness of breath, or respiratory failure) or the skin and mucous membranes (erythema, exanthema, or aphthae). The general condition of patients is moderate or severe, often requiring treatment in the pediatric intensive care unit due to circulatory and/or respiratory failure. The variety of clinical symptoms and their concurrence, as well as the lack of specific laboratory markers, necessitates a thorough and extensive differential diagnosis. According to the current criteria, making a diagnosis of PIMS-TS requires that other infectious and non-infectious causes be excluded, e.g., sepsis, toxic shock syndrome (TSS), meningitis, acute abdominal diseases, pneumonia, myocarditis, or other multi-organ inflammatory diseases, such as hemophagocytic syndrome or Kawasaki disease [5–13]. It requires many laboratory and imaging tests confirming the involvement of at least two systems. There are still few articles focussing on the analysis of lung imaging findings and their evolution in the acute state, and even fewer on lung residues after PIMS-TS.

In the last decade, the role of ultrasound in assessing the lungs and pleura in children has increased [14]. This tool is easily accessible, repeatable, and—compared to X-ray—safer, more sensitive, and specific in the imaging of inflammatory lung changes and pleural effusion [15]. Incomplete skeletal ossification in children and the typically sparse adipose tissue make it possible to use additional acoustic windows [14].

The aim of our study was to evaluate pathologies on LUS in children with PIMS-TS and to assess the usefulness of this examination in the diagnosis pathway and monitoring.

2. Materials and Methods

The study was conducted from November 2019 to March 2022 among patients hospitalized at the Department of Pediatrics, Immunology, and Nephrology of the Polish Mother's Memorial Hospital Research Institute in Łódź, Poland. We retrospectively evaluated the lung ultrasound (LUS) images of all patients hospitalized with fever for more than 3 days and symptoms associated with PIMS-TS from at least two systems. The examinations were performed with a linear or curvilinear probe (Philips Affiniti 70G eL18-4 and C8-2, respectively) by only four pediatric specialists with certified LUS training and extensive experience in ultrasound imaging. After use, all materials were disinfected correctly.

The examination included the assessment of the entire lung fields on the anterior, lateral, and posterior surfaces of the chest and in the sagittal and frontal planes. LUS was carried out at least twice—in all patients on the first day after admission and before discharge—but most had it performed 3–4 times, depending on their clinical condition.

Inflammatory lesions of the lungs were diagnosed on the basis of applicable parenchymal, pleural, and vascular criteria [15–18]. They were classified as B-line artifacts, interstitial syndrome, interstitial-alveolar syndrome, consolidations, and atelectatic lesions. The presence of fluid in the pleural cavity was also assessed, typically in the sitting position, unless the patient's clinical condition did not allow it, in which case it was done in the lateral or supine position (e.g., in ICU patients). In our study, we estimated the pleural effusion layer in millimeters but not in total volume. A normal ultrasound image of the lungs was classified as the presence of all the following criteria: sliding sign visible over the entire surface of the lungs, A-line artifacts visible over the entire surface of the lungs, a continuous, smooth pleural line over the entire surface of the lungs, no consolidation, no pleural effusion, a visible layer of fluid <2 mm, and single (1–2) B-line artifacts at the base of the lungs. No LUS score was used to assess the severity of lung involvement.

LUS was repeated in all patients before hospital discharge and 3 months after discharge. The assessment was made according to the same methodology as given above. All study participants underwent a typical physical examination of the respiratory system on each day of hospitalization. Routine chest radiographs were not performed, as this was not the subject of our analysis.

The study was approved by our institute's ethics committee (No. 45/2021). Parental consent for the study was obtained.

3. Results

In the given period, 47 children met the criteria for a PIMS-TS diagnosis, and 43 met all evaluation criteria (30 boys and 13 girls, aged from 11 months to 17 years 4 months; average: 6 years 7 months; median: 6 years). Abnormalities on physical examination were found in 21 subjects (49%). These included tachypnoea and asymmetry of respiratory murmurs or crackles. 39 of the 43 patients (91%) were diagnosed with pneumonia based on ultrasound criteria. The same number of children (39/43; 91%) had more than one pathology, and 28 of them (65%) had bilateral lesions. The most common pathologies were consolidations with air bronchogram or mixed bronchogram, which were observed in 37 respondents (86%) [Figure 1a]. These were followed, in descending order, by fluid in the pleura (36/43 [84%]) in the amount of 2 to 55 mm (average 11.5 mm: median 24.3 mm) [Figure 1b,c], interstitial syndrome (30/43 [70%]) [Figure 1(d1,d2), atelectasis (28/43 [65%]) [Figure 1(f1,f2)], and interstitial-alveolar syndrome (19/43 [44%]) [Figure 1e]. For other abnormalities, an image of so-called 'white lungs' was observed in five patients (12%). A normal LUS image was found in only three of the children (7%). By the day of discharge, total regression of inflammatory changes was observed in eight (19%) and partial regression in 35 (81%) patients. Three months after discharge from the hospital, a normal ultrasound image of the lungs was found in all respondents (43/43 [100%]) (Tables 1 and 2).

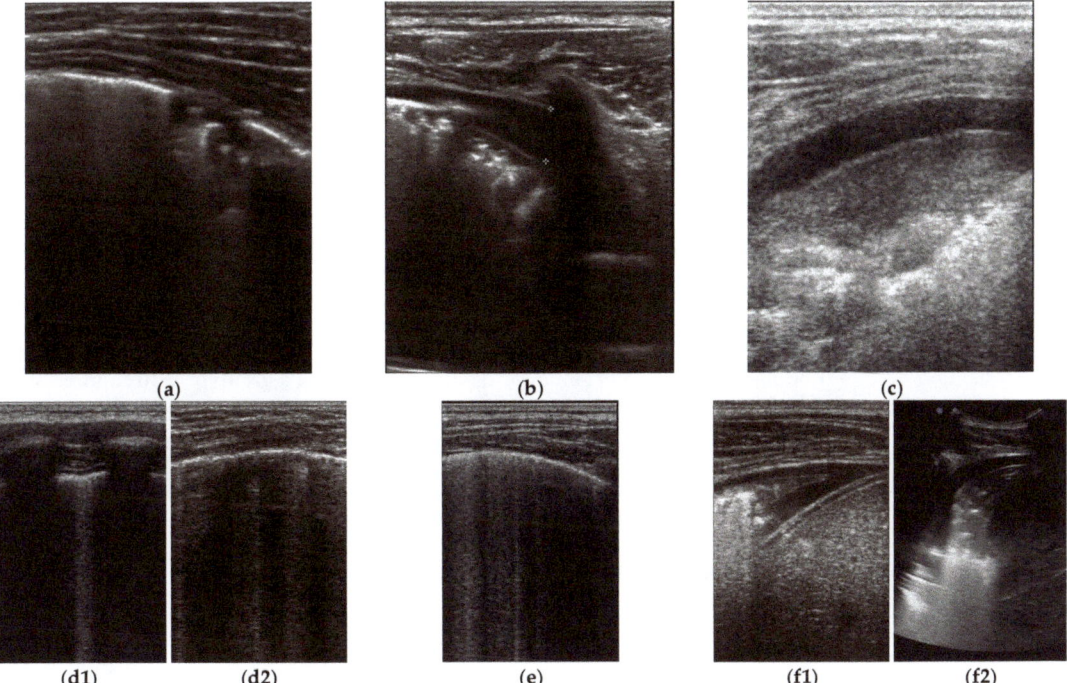

Figure 1. LUS images (**a**)—consolidation; (**b,c**)—consolidation and fluid in pleural cavity; (**d1**)—interstitial syndrome—a longitudinal projection; (**d2**)—interstitial syndrome—a transversal projection; (**e**)—interstitial-alveolar syndromes; (**f1**)—atelectasis with consolidation and pleural effusion/linear probe/; (**f2**)—atelectasis with consolidation and pleural effusion/curvilinear probe/.

Table 1. Study group.

age (years), mean (median)	6 7/12 (6)
sex, n (%)	
FEMALE	13 (30)
MALE	30 (70)
respiratory abnormalities signs n (%)	21 (49)
pneumonia criteria n (%)	
on admission	39 (91)
>1 pathology n (%)	39 (91)
bilateral lesions, n (%)	28 (65)
Normal LUS image, n (%)	3 (7)
by the day of discharge	
Total regression, n (%)	8 (19)
Partial regression, n (%)	35 (81)

Table 2. LUS findings.

	1-SIDED (TOT 43; %)	2-SIDED (TOT 43; %)	TOTAL (TOT 43; %)	AFTER 3 MONTHS
B-Lines Artifacts	0 (0)	40 (93)	40 (93)	0 (0)
Interstitial Syndrome	0 (0)	30 (70)	30 (70)	0 (0)
Interstitial-alveolar syndrome	0 (0)	19 (44)	19 (44)	0 (0)
Consolidations	7 (16)	30 (70)	37 (86)	0 (0)
Atelectasis	9 (21)	19 (44)	28 (65)	0 (0)
Pleural effusion	0 (0)	36 (84)	36 (84)	0 (0)

4. Discussion

Inflammatory lung changes are one of the diagnostic criteria for PIMS-TS. In our study, on the basis of USG criteria, inflammatory changes in the lungs were diagnosed in the majority of patients (91%), while respiratory symptoms were present in less than half of them (49%). Daniel A. Lichtenstein promoted LUS and proved its superiority over lung auscultation and classical X-ray diagnostics in acute respiratory failure (ARDS) in adults almost 20 years ago [19]. In recent years, LUS has also been used in the pediatric population [14]. A meta-analysis of studies involving a group of 1510 children showed that LUS has similar sensitivity and specificity to chest radiographs in the diagnosis of inflammatory changes in the lungs of children [20].

Part of the chest ultrasound examination is also pleural imaging and evaluation of the presence of fluid in the pleural cavities. LUS is characterized by 100% sensitivity and 97.7% specificity, while chest radiography demonstrates 71% and 88%, respectively [15]. So far, CT remains the gold standard in lung imaging. Due to the impact of ionizing radiation, as well as high operating and maintenance costs, it should not be performed routinely. In addition, in younger children, CT usually requires sedation. Moreover, studies comparing LUS and chest CT in the assessment of inflammatory lung lesions in children are not yet known.

As mentioned in the introduction, the clinical picture of MIS-C/PIMS-TS is quite heterogeneous. With the exception of fever, which is the leading symptom, the symptoms occur with different coincidences, and the diagnosis requires a broad differential diagnosis. Due to the heterogeneity of the clinical signs and symptoms, diagnosis of PIMS-TS is difficult. Based on a systematic review from 2021, it was found that in the course of PIMS-TS, cough occurred in almost 24% of patients and dyspnea in 26.7%. Respiratory symptoms were not the leading ones, as cardiac symptoms occurred in almost 80% of patients, and abdominal symptoms presented in more than 70% [21]. In our work, 21 children (49%) had abnormalities on physical examination of the respiratory system (tachypnoea, asymmetry of breath murmur, or crackles). Although almost half of the patients with PIMS-TS did not show any respiratory symptoms, most of them were found to have abnormalities on LUS.

The first reported use of LUS in PIMS-TS patients was an Italian paper published in early 2022. Musolino et al. found pathologies in LUS in 10/10 patients (100%) with PIMS-TS, most often as an abnormal pleural image and disseminated B-line artifacts, in 8/10 (80%) interstitial syndrome was visible, in 7/10 (70%) there were subpulmonary consolidations, and in half of the subjects, interstitial-alveolar changes were found. It is worth mentioning that symptoms such as cough or shortness of breath were found in less than half of the respondents (4/10 [40%]) [22]. The results of this work strongly indicate that even in the absence of clinical signs, the lungs are usually involved in the inflammatory process during PIMS-TS. The limitations of that publication are its small study group and lack of follow-up.

In another publication, only 2/24 children (8%) had a normal ultrasound image of the lungs [23]. Another work using point-of-care lung ultrasound (PoCUS-LUS) found pleural fluid in 6/9 subjects (67%) with PIMS-TS [24]. In our publication, abnormal LUS images were found in 91% of the subjects. Compared to the cited publications, ours included a larger group—43 respondents. These reports show that the majority of children with PIMS-TS had pathologies in LUS, while less than 30% of them presented symptoms from the respiratory system [21].

These data differ from classical radiological examinations. Depending on the methodology and the size of the study group, normal chest X-ray images were found in 16–64% of subjects with PIMS-TS [25–27]. The systematic review by Hoste et al. reported that disseminated radiological changes were found in 35% of respondents [21]. Even larger discrepancies were found while analyzing chest CT scans. Abnormalities were found in 39–83% of patients, predominantly (>80%) the appearance of milky glass and the presence of consolidation. Pleural effusion was detected in 30–58%, while atelectasis was in 26% [25,26,28].

In our study group, we did not routinely perform chest radiograms. X-rays or CTs were only used for clinical indications, for example, in patients in serious condition or to assess the position of the vascular catheter. Based on our own work and the publications cited herein, it seems that there are currently no indications for routine X-rays or CTs for respiratory assessment in children with PIMS-TS (too much discrepancy between clinic and imaging). Examination by LUS provides quick, repeatable diagnostic information at the bedside that complements physical examination. However, as with other lung imaging modalities, some knowledge and skill are required to use lung ultrasound. If the team is inexperienced in performing lung ultrasounds, the choice of classic chest X-ray seems obvious. Furthermore, accurate imaging of the mediastinum, especially in older and obese children, is impossible. Our team suggests consideration for chest CTs in patients with respiratory failure requiring intubation, with extensive inflammatory changes in the lungs, or in patients with an unclear clinical picture.

An advantage of our study is the fairly large, age-diverse, and clinically heterogeneous study group. We found that the inflammatory lesions of the lungs regressed totally or significantly in all children after effective immunosuppressive treatment. Often, an abnormal LUS image—especially involving bilateral inflammatory lesions with pleural effusion in a patient with fever and in moderate or severe overall condition—directed our diagnostics towards PIMS-TS despite the absence of signs and/or symptoms suggesting respiratory involvement. At the same time, with an ambiguous clinical picture, the use of LUS allowed for a faster diagnosis of PIMS-TS. Currently, it is not known whether similar changes in the lungs are observed in other acute multisystem, hyperinflammatory diseases, such as Kawasaki disease or hemophagocytic syndrome [5,6,22]. So far, there are no data on how long LUS changes persist in the course of PIMS-TS. During our observation, 3 months after discharge from the hospital, normal LUS imagery was found in all patients. From these observations, we conclude that inflammatory changes in the lungs in the course of PIMS-TS are acute.

5. Conclusions

LUS, despite its limitations, is a useful tool that can be easily used in the diagnosis, differentiation, and monitoring of inflammatory changes in the lungs. Ultrasound pathologies occur in most patients with PIMS-TS in the acute stage and regress completely with the extinction of the generalized inflammatory process. Ultrasound pathologies and inflammatory changes in the lungs are present in most patients with PIMS-TS, even if respiratory symptoms and signs are absent. In our team, we agree on the need to disseminate LUS as a 'point-of-care' in children. As PIMS-TS is still a new entity, patients should be carefully followed up.

Author Contributions: Conceptualization J.T.-M. and A.B.; methodology N.K.; formal analysis N.K.; investigation, J.T.-M., A.B., M.D.-B. and N.K.; writing—J.T.-M.; writing review and editing—A.B.; supervision M.T. and K.Z. All authors have read and agreed to the published version of the manuscript.

Funding: The study was supported by the Internal Grant PMMH-RI no 10GW/2021 funded by the Ministry of Science and Higher Education in Poland.

Informed Consent Statement: Informed consent was obtained from all subjects involved in the study.

Data Availability Statement: The data that support the findings of this study are available from the corresponding author upon reasonable request.

Conflicts of Interest: The authors declare no conflict of interest.

References

1. World Health Organization. Multisystem Inflammatory Syndrome in Children and Adolescents with COVID-19. 2020. Available online: https://www.who.int/publications/i/item/multisystem-inflammatory-syndrome-in-children-and-adolescents-with-covid-19 (accessed on 15 May 2020).
2. Centers for Disease Control and Prevention. Emergency Preparedness and Response: Health Alert Network. 2020. Available online: https://emergency.cdc.gov/han/index.asp (accessed on 14 May 2020).
3. Royal College of Pediatrics and Child Health. Guidance: Pediatric Multisystem Inflammatory Syndrome Temporally Associated with COVID-19. 2020. Available online: https://www.rcpch.ac.uk/resources/paediatric-multisystem-inflammatory-syndrome-temporally-associated-covid-19-pims-guidance (accessed on 1 May 2020).
4. Available online: https://icd.who.int/browse10/2019/en#/U00-U49 (accessed on 1 September 2020).
5. Gupta, A.; Gill, A.; Sharma, M.; Garg, M. Multi-System Inflammatory Syndrome in a Child Mimicking Kawasaki Disease. *J. Trop. Pediatr.* **2021**, *67*, fmaa060. [CrossRef] [PubMed]
6. Marino, A.; Varisco, T.; Quattrocchi, G.; Amoroso, A.; Beltrami, D.; Venturiello, S.; Ripamonti, A.; Villa, A.; Andreotti, M.; Ciuffreda, M.; et al. Children with Kawasaki disease or Kawasaki-like syndrome (MIS-C/PIMS) at the time of COVID-19: Are they all the same? Case series and literature review. *Reumatismo* **2021**, *73*, 48–53. [CrossRef]
7. Opoka-Winiarska, V.; Grywalska, E.; Roliński, J. PIMS-TS, the New Paediatric Systemic Inflammatory Disease Related to Previous Exposure to SARS-CoV-2 Infection-"Rheumatic Fever" of the 21st Century? *Int. J. Mol. Sci.* **2021**, *22*, 4488. [CrossRef] [PubMed]
8. Lad, S.S.; Kait, S.P.; Suryawanshi, P.B.; Mujawar, J.; Lad, P.; Khetre, R.; Jadhav, L.M.; Bhor, A.; Balte, P.; Kataria, P.; et al. Neurological Manifestations in Pediatric Inflammatory Multisystem Syndrome Temporally Associated with SARS-CoV-2 (PIMS-TS). *Indian J. Pediatr.* **2021**, *88*, 294–295. [CrossRef] [PubMed]
9. Walker, E.T.; Humphrey, H.N.; Daniels, I.R.; McDermott, F.D. COVID-19 and the paediatric acute abdomen—The emerging dilemma of PIMS-TS. *BJS Open* **2022**, *6*, zrac049. [CrossRef] [PubMed]
10. Meshaka, R.; Whittam, F.C.; Guessoum, M.; Eleti, S.; Shelmerdine, S.C.; Arthurs, O.J.; McHugh, K.; Hiorns, M.P.; Humphries, P.D.; Calder, A.D.; et al. Abdominal US in Pediatric Inflammatory Multisystem Syndrome Associated with SARS-CoV-2 (PIMS-TS). *Radiology* **2022**, *303*, 173–181. [CrossRef]
11. Di Nardo, M.; De Piero, M.E.; Hoskote, A.; Belohlavek, J.; Lorusso, R.; Thiruchelvam, T.; Lillie, J.; Stanley, V.; StJohn, L.; Amodeo, A.; et al. EuroECMO neonatal and paediatric COVID-19 Working Group and EuroELSO Steering Committee. Extracorporeal membrane oxygenation in children with COVID-19 and PIMS-TS during the second and third wave. *Lancet Child Adolesc. Health* **2022**, *6*, e14–e15. [CrossRef]
12. Waterhouse, M.A.; Villion, A.; Manougian, T.; Salik, I. The Perfect Cytokine Storm: Utilization of Lung Ultrasound During Urgent Surgery in an Infant with Multisystem Inflammatory Syndrome in Children and Hemophagocytic Lymphohistiocytosis. *Cureus* **2021**, *13*, e15640. [CrossRef]

13. Okarska-Napierała, M.; Ludwikowska, K.; Szenborn, L.; Dudek, N.; Mania, A.; Buda, P.; Książyk, J.; Mazur-Malewska, K.; Figlerowicz, M.; Szczukocki, M.; et al. Pediatric Inflammatory Multisystem Syndrome (PIMS) Did Occur in Poland during Months with Low COVID-19 Prevalence, Preliminary Results of a Nationwide Register. *J. Clin. Med.* **2020**, *9*, 3386. [CrossRef]
14. Musolino, A.M.; Tomà, P.; De Rose, C.; Pitaro, E.; Boccuzzi, E.; De Santis, R.; Morello, R.; Supino, M.C.; Villani, A.; Valentini, P.; et al. Ten Years of Pediatric Lung Ultrasound: A Narrative Review. *Front. Physiol.* **2022**, *12*, 721951. [CrossRef]
15. Jaworska, J.; Buda, N.; Ciuca, I.M.; Dong, Y.; Fang, C.; Feldkamp, A.; Jüngert, J.; Kosiak, W.; Mentzel, H.J.; Pienar, C.; et al. Ultrasound of the pleura in children, WFUMB review paper. *Med. Ultrason.* **2021**, *23*, 339–347. [CrossRef] [PubMed]
16. Dietrich, C.F.; Buda, N.; Ciuca, I.M.; Dong, Y.; Fang, C.; Feldkamp, A.; Jüngert, J.; Kosiak, W.; Mentzel, H.J.; Pienar, C.; et al. Lung ultrasound in children, WFUMB review paper (part 2). *Med. Ultrason.* **2021**, *23*, 443–452. [CrossRef] [PubMed]
17. Dietrich, C.F.; Mathis, G.; Blaivas, M.; Volpicelli, G.; Seibel, A.; Atkinson, N.S.; Cui, X.W.; Mei, F.; Schreiber-Dietrich, D.; Yi, D. Lung artefacts and their use. *Med. Ultrason.* **2016**, *18*, 488–499. [CrossRef] [PubMed]
18. Volpicelli, G.; Elbarbary, M.; Blaivas, M.; Lichtenstein, D.A.; Mathis, G.; Kirkpatrick, A.W.; Melniker, L.; Gargani, L.; Noble, V.E.; Via, G.; et al. International Liaison Committee on Lung Ultrasound (ILC-LUS) for International Consensus Conference on Lung Ultrasound (ICC-LUS). International evidencebased recommendations for point-of-care lung ultrasound. *Intensive Care Med.* **2012**, *38*, 577–591. [CrossRef] [PubMed]
19. Lichtenstein, D.; Goldstein, I.; Mourgeon, E.; Cluzel, P.; Grenier, P.; Rouby, J.-J. Comparative diagnostic performances of auscultation, chest radiography, and lung ultrasonography in acute respiratory distress syndrome. *Anesthesiology* **2004**, *100*, 9–15. [CrossRef]
20. Balk, D.S.; Lee, C.; Schafer, J.; Welwarth, J.; Hardin, J.; Novack, V.; Yarza, S.; Hoffmann, B. Lung ultrasound compared to chest X-ray for diagnosis of pediatric pneumonia: A meta-analysis. *Pediatr. Pulmonol.* **2018**, *53*, 1130–1139. [CrossRef]
21. Hoste, L.; Van Paemel, R.; Haerynck, F. Multisystem inflammatory syndrome in children related to COVID-19: A systematic review. *Eur. J. Pediatr.* **2021**, *180*, 2019–2034. [CrossRef]
22. Musolino, A.M.; Boccuzzi, E.; Buonsenso, D.; Supino, M.C.; Mesturino, M.A.; Pitaro, E.; Ferro, V.; Nacca, R.; Sinibaldi, S.; Palma, P.; et al. The Role of Lung Ultrasound in Diagnosing COVID-19-Related Multisystemic Inflammatory Disease: A Preliminary Experience. *J. Clin. Med.* **2022**, *11*, 234. [CrossRef]
23. Camporesi, A.; Gemma, M.; Buonsenso, D.; Ferrario, S.; Mandelli, A.; Pessina, M.; Diotto, V.; Rota, E.; Raso, I.; Fiori, L.; et al. Lung Ultrasound Patterns in Multisystem Inflammatory Syndrome in Children (MIS-C)-Characteristics and Prognostic Value. *Children* **2022**, *9*, 931. [CrossRef]
24. Kennedy, T.M.; Dessie, A.; Kessler, D.O.; Malia, L.; Rabiner, J.E.; Firnberg, M.T.; Ng, L. Point-of-Care Ultrasound Findings in Multisystem Inflammatory Syndrome in Children: A Cross-Sectional Study. *Pediatr. Emerg. Care* **2021**, *37*, 334–339. [CrossRef]
25. Caro-Domínguez, P.; Navallas, M.; Riaza-Martin, L.; Mahani, M.G.; Charcape, C.F.U.; Valverde, I.; D'Arco, F.; Toso, S.; Shelmerdine, S.C.; van Schuppen, J.; et al. Imaging findings of multisystem inflammatory syndrome in children associated with COVID-19. *Pediatr. Radiol.* **2021**, *51*, 1608–1620. [CrossRef] [PubMed]
26. Hameed, S.; Elbaaly, H.; Reid, C.E.L.; Santos, R.M.F.; Shivamurthy, V.; Wong, J.; Jogeesvaran, K.H. Spectrum of Imaging Findings at Chest Radiography, US, CT, and MRI in Multisystem Inflammatory Syndrome in Children Associated with COVID-19. *Radiology* **2021**, *298*, E1–E10. [CrossRef] [PubMed]
27. Rostad, B.S.; Shah, J.H.; Rostad, C.A.; Jaggi, P.; Richer, E.J.; Linam, L.E.; Alazraki, A.L.; Riedesel, E.L.; Milla, S.S. Chest radiograph features of multisystem inflammatory syndrome in children (MIS-C) compared to pediatric COVID-19. *Pediatr. Radiol.* **2021**, *51*, 231–238. [CrossRef] [PubMed]
28. Rostami-Maskopaee, F.; Ladomenou, F.; Razavi-Amoli, S.-K.; Navaeifar, M.R.; Hajialibeig, A.; Shahbaznejad, L.; Hosseinzadeh, F.; Aski, B.H.; Anari, A.M.; Mohammadi, M.; et al. Clinical characteristics and outcomes of the multisystem inflammatory syndrome in children (MIS-C) following COVID-19 infection in Iran: A multicenter study. *PLoS ONE* **2022**, *17*, e0274104. [CrossRef] [PubMed]

Disclaimer/Publisher's Note: The statements, opinions and data contained in all publications are solely those of the individual author(s) and contributor(s) and not of MDPI and/or the editor(s). MDPI and/or the editor(s) disclaim responsibility for any injury to people or property resulting from any ideas, methods, instructions or products referred to in the content.

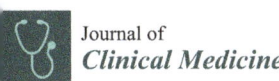

Article

Airway Findings in Patients with Hunter Syndrome Treated with Intravenous Idursulfase

Richard De Vuyst [1,*], Elizabeth Jalazo [1], Tamy Moraes Tsujimoto [2], Feng-Chang Lin [2], Joseph Muenzer [1] and Marianne S. Muhlebach [1,3]

1. Department of Pediatrics, University of North Carolina, Chapel Hill, NC 27599, USA
2. Department of Biostatistics, UNC Gillings School of Global Public Health, Chapel Hill, NC 27599, USA
3. Marsico Lung Institute, University of North Carolina, Chapel Hill, NC 27599, USA
* Correspondence: richard_devuyst@med.unc.edu; Tel.: +1-806-662-1412

Abstract: People with Hunter syndrome are known to be affected by a variety of airway pathologies. Treatment of Hunter syndrome with the enzyme replacement therapy (ERT) idursulfase is now the standard of care. However, it is not known how ERT changes the progression of airway involvement. To evaluate this, we performed a retrospective analysis of bronchoscopies performed on children with Hunter syndrome who were part of intrathecal ERT trials. Findings for airway pathology were extracted from bronchoscopy reports and analyses were performed for cross-sectional and longitudinal changes in airway disease. One-hundred and thirty bronchoscopies from 23 subjects were analyzed. Upper airway disease (adenoid hypertrophy and/or pharyngomalacia) was reported in 93% and 87% of bronchoscopies, respectively. Laryngeal abnormalities were recognized in 46% of cases. There were lower airway (tracheal and or bronchial) findings in 64% of all bronchoscopies and prevalence increased with age. Evaluations over time adjusted for repeat evaluations showed that increasing airway involvement was associated with older age ($p = 0.0007$) despite ongoing ERT. No association was discovered between age of intravenous ERT initiation and progression of airway disease. Individuals with Hunter syndrome who are receiving intravenous enzyme replacement therapy showed the progression of airways disease supporting the need for regular airway monitoring and intervention.

Keywords: tracheopathy; Hunter syndrome; lysosomal storage disease; bronchoscopy; airway severity score; enzyme replacement therapy

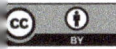

1. Introduction

Mucopolysaccharidosis II (Hunter syndrome, MPS II) is an X-linked recessive lysosomal storage disease with multiple organ involvement and variable progression. It is caused by a deficiency of the enzyme iduronate-2-sulfatase [1]. This results in the accumulation of the glycosaminoglycans (GAG) dermatan sulfate and heparan sulfate within lysosomes which results in gradual physiologic and anatomic dysfunction. GAG accumulation leads to progressive cardiac valvular disease, pulmonary dysfunction, and skeletal deformities. Two thirds of individuals with MPS II have the severe or neuronopathic form of the disease which manifests as early cognitive impairment with progressive neurological decline; without treatment, this leads to death in the first or second decade of life. Breathing impairment is recognized as a major cause of morbidity and mortality, with respiratory failure representing a common cause of death in affected patients [2–4]. Upper airway complications are a common presenting problem and individuals are frequently treated for upper airway problems prior to diagnosis of MPS II [5–7]. The upper airway manifestations include adenoidal and tonsillar hypertrophy, macroglossia, and laryngomalacia [6–9]. Lower airway dysfunction includes tracheomalacia, bronchomalacia, narrowing of airways due to deposition of GAG, and restrictive lung disease due to decreased chest wall compliance [6,8].

The development of the intravenous (IV) enzyme replacement therapy (ERT) idursulfase has provided a treatment option for individuals with MPS II since 2006. Intravenous idursulfase has been shown to be well tolerated and in clinical trials demonstrated decreased liver and spleen sizes and decreased urinary GAG levels, and either stabilized or improved several clinical parameters, including walking ability (6-min walk test), lung volume as measured by forced vital capacity (FVC), left ventricular mass index, and joint range of motion (shoulder) [4,10,11]. However there has been a paucity of research into intravenous idursulfase effects on specific airway findings associated with MPS II.

We had previously shown a high incidence of airway complications in individuals naïve to IV ERT [6]. We hypothesized that ERT in MPS II would prevent progression of airway pathology. The aims of this study were to describe the incidence and longitudinal course of airway pathology in a population of individuals with the severe phenotype of MPS II treated with IV ERT.

2. Materials and Methods

Study Setting and Subjects

This study is a retrospective analysis of individuals with the severe or the neuronopathic form of MPS II, who participated in the phase I/II (NCT00920647 and NCT01506141) or phase II/III (NCT00937794 and NCT00920647) intrathecal enzyme replacement clinical trials at the University of North Carolina at Chapel Hill site since 2011. As part of their annual clinical trial evaluations requiring general anesthesia, the participants underwent airway evaluation by flexible bronchoscopy and if needed, fiberoptic intubation to decrease the risk of airway complications with general anesthesia. Recruitment criteria for the phase I/II MPS II intrathecal enzyme replacement clinical study included individuals' ages 3 to 17 years, cognitive impairment and at least 6 months of IV idursulfase at enrollment into the study. Recruitment criteria for the phase II/III MPS II intrathecal enzyme replacement clinical study included individuals' ages 2 to 17 years, cognitive impairment and at least 4 months of IV idursulfase at enrollment into the study. All subjects were treated with weekly IV and monthly intrathecal ERT throughout the period in which data for the current study were collected.

Clinical information collected from medical records included patient demographics, age at MPS II diagnosis, age at first bronchoscopy, age at IV ERT initiation, number of bronchoscopies and age at each bronchoscopy, history of prior airway surgery, and airway findings on bronchoscopy.

Ethics

The airway findings analyzed in this report were from MPS II patients who were enrolled in intrathecal ERT studies at the University of North Carolina at Chapel. These studies were approved by the University of North Carolina Institutional Review Board (IRB) with consent obtained from the parents or guardians of each subject. For this retrospective airway study, IRB approval at the University of North Carolina was obtained (20-2178) but was deemed exempt from consent due to posing no more than a minimal risk to the subjects.

Assessment of Airway Disease

To analyze the relationship between ERT and the degree of airway involvement, we developed a grading system of airway severity for statistical analysis. The airway severity score system was developed to include the wide variety of airway pathology seen in MPS II individuals while preventing the overrepresentation of any single anatomic area. To determine how each area of the airway contributed to progression of anatomical changes, bronchoscopy findings were analyzed for the three anatomic divisions: upper, laryngeal, and lower airway. Findings were typically expressed as mild, moderate, or severe in bronchoscopy reports and we graded all findings on a scale from 1 to 3. If severity of abnormal findings was not specified in the bronchoscopy report as mild, moderate, or severe, it was given a score of 1. Each anatomic location could only contribute a maximum of

3 points, for a maximum total score of 9. Upper airway diagnoses included in the score were adenoidal hypertrophy, phayngomalacia, and glossoptosis. Tonsillar hypertrophy was not included in the score as a description of incidence and severity showed high interobserver variation; however, it was reported in our description of findings. Laryngeal findings included in the score were epiglottal thickening, arytenoid thickening, and laryngomalacia. Vocal cord thickening was not scored as it was inconsistently recorded. Lower airway pathology scores included tracheomalacia, bronchomalacia, and tracheal or bronchial deposits. Bronchitis was often incidentally observed but not included in the score as it was not considered a static or progressive finding and could occur due to other reasons, e.g., infection. An example of common findings and of the airway severity score is seen in Figure 1.

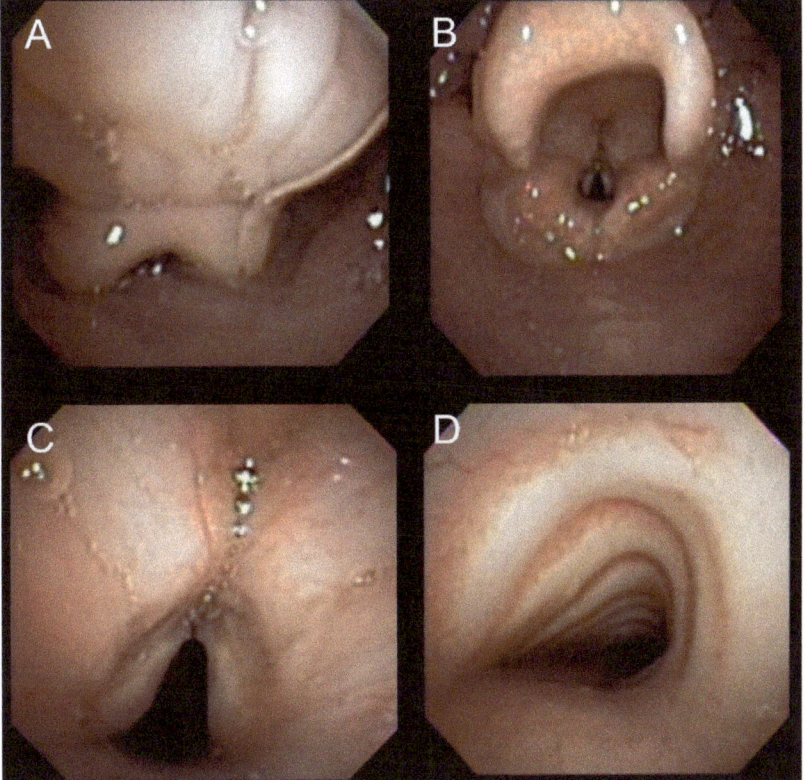

Figure 1. Airway scoring. (**A**) Shows moderate pharyngeal collapse, which would be +2 on the score. (**B**) Shows epiglottal thickening which would be +1 on the score, and mild arytenoid thickening, which would be +1 on the score. (**C**) Shows vocal cord thickening, which is not a finding incorporated into the airway severity score, but is clinically relevant and was inconsistently reported. (**D**) Shows moderate tracheopathy which would be a +2 on the score. Therefore, the total airway severity score for this bronchoscopy would be 6.

Statistical Analysis

Summary statistics were computed for subject level clinical and demographic variables. For the airway findings from the bronchoscopy, the proportion of individuals with a condition in at least one evaluation and the total of positive bronchoscopy for each of abnormal findings were computed. The plot of cumulative incidence of lower airway findings was constructed.

Linear models were fitted via generalized estimation equations (GEE), with an exchangeable working correlation matrix to assess the association between airway severity score and age at bronchoscopy, while accounting for the correlation between repeated measures within patient.

We defined the airway disease progression as the slope of the simple linear regression model using the airway severity score as the response, and age at bronchoscopy as the covariate for each one of the observations. The association between airway disease progression and age at start of ERT was assessed using simple linear regression.

All statistical analyses were performed in Excel Professional Plus 2013, Graph pad prism 9.0.1, and R version 4.0.2 (R Core Team, 2018). Complete case analysis was considered, with $p < 0.05$ determining statistical significance.

3. Results

Subjects

Twenty-three male subjects (MPS II is an X-linked recessive disorder primarily affecting males) were included in the IV and intrathecal ERT group. All individuals had the severe or neuronopathic form of Hunter syndrome. Most individuals, 17/23, had been diagnosed prior to the age of 3 years old, with a median (range) age of 2.0 (0–4.5) years at diagnosis. The youngest two subjects were diagnosed early due to positive family history. The median age at time of initiation of IV ERT was 2.6 (0.13–4.7) years and median age at first bronchoscopy was 4.7 (2.3–9.7) years. Number of bronchoscopies per subject averaged 5.6 (2–10). Seven subjects whose data were collected as part of a previous study prior to the advent of ERT were used as a control. These subjects were 2.4–12.6 years old at the time of bronchoscopy.

Cross-sectional Bronchoscopy findings

A total of 130 bronchoscopies were included that occurred between August 2011 and February 2020; no bronchoscopies were excluded. No child experienced complications during bronchoscopy. The airway evaluations were almost all abnormal (129 out of 130 bronchoscopies), and all subjects developed an additional airway abnormality through the course of the observed period. Bronchoscopy findings are summarized in Table 1.

Table 1. Abnormal airway findings diagnosed via bronchoscopy.

Abnormal Findings	Number of Total Bronchoscopies Positive for Condition (% Positive)	% of Individuals Positive for Condition on at Least One Bronchoscopy
Upper airway	129/130 (99)	100
Adenoidal hypertrophy	122/130 (93)	100
Pharyngomalacia	114/130 (87)	100
Glossoptosis	40/130 (30)	52
Laryngeal	60/130 (46)	65
Laryngomalacia	29/130 (22)	52
Arytenoid thickening	6/130 (5)	22
Epiglottis thickened	35/130 (27)	26
Vocal cord thickening	6/130 (5)	17
Lower airway	84/130 (64)	95
Tracheomalacia/tracheopathy	72/130 (55)	86
Bronchomalacia/nodularity	24/130 (18)	54

Legend Table 1: Data are presented for each bronchoscopy including repeat bronchoscopies in subjects with multiple procedures. The column on the left described the proportion of every bronchoscopy performed which was positive for each listed condition. The column on the right describes the percentage of subjects who had the listed finding on at least one evaluation.

Comparisons to ERT-negative subjects

We previously published data concerning airway findings in individuals with MPS II [6]. A subset of seven individuals in this previous study was ERT naïve, and we applied the airway severity score to the bronchoscopy reports of these seven ERT naïve individuals. Linear regression of severity scores against age tended to show worsening with age for each of the groups (Figure 2).

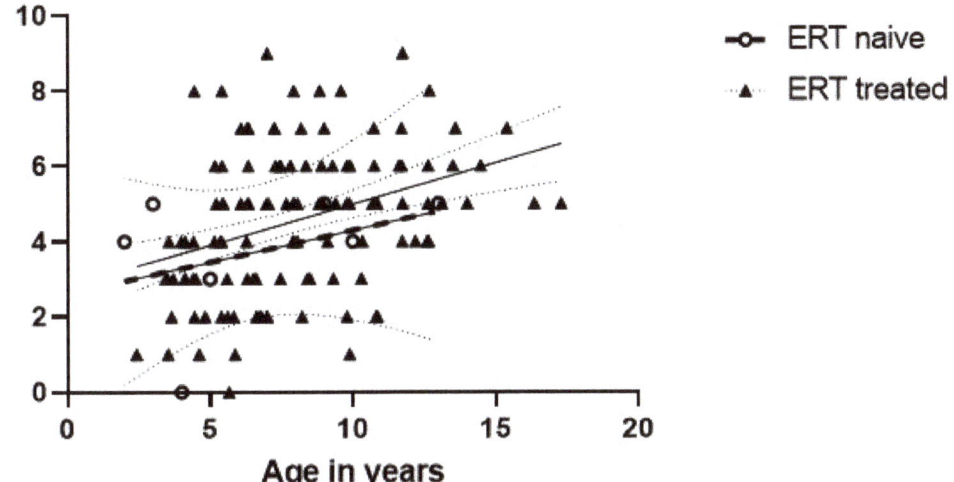

Figure 2. Linear model fitted via generalized estimation equations (GEE) between average airway severity score and age, controlling for ERT group. One year increase in age leads to an expected increase of 0.25 (95% CI: 0.16, 0.33; $p < 0.001$) units in the airway severity score. The dotted lines represent 95% confidence intervals. Open circles are ERT naïve, and closed triangles are ERT treated individuals.

Longitudinal Airway findings

Generalized estimation equations, which account for repeat evaluations for the subjects showed that increasing airway involvement was associated with older age ($p = 0.0007$) (Figure 3). In many individuals, worsening scores were due to increased occurrence of abnormalities in the lower airway over time. Figure 3 shows the increased slope of airway severity score progression in the lower airways compared to upper or laryngeal findings. Specifically, 16 of the 23 subjects had no lower airway pathology described at the time of their first bronchoscopy but 12 of them subsequently developed at least one abnormal lower airway finding. The cumulative occurrence of lower airway findings is shown in Figure 4. To evaluate if age at time of ERT initiation may affect progression of airway disease, we further analyzed for each patient their slope of progression of the airway severity score from first to last bronchoscopy. Individual slopes are shown in Figure 5. Next, a linear model was constructed for slopes of progression against age at time of ERT initiation. There was no correlation between disease progression and age of initiation of ERT, where one year increase in age at the start of ERT led to an expected increase of −0.03 (95% CI: −0.18, 0.12; $p = 0.7$) units in the airway disease progression (Figure 6).

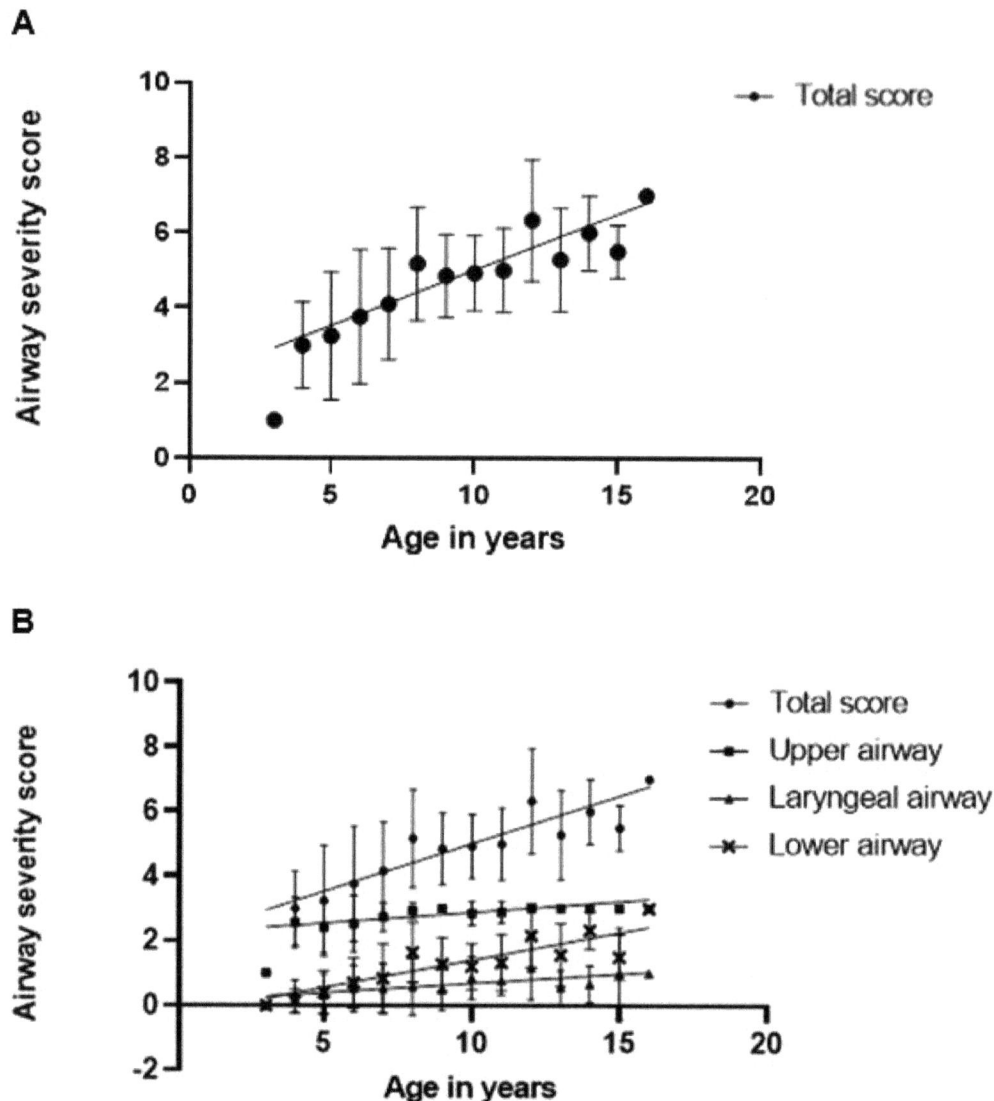

Figure 3. (**A**) Linear model fitted via generalized estimation equations (GEE) between average airway severity score and age. One year increase in age leads to an expected increase of 0.29 (95% CI: 0.2, 0.38; $p < 0.0001$) units in the airway severity score. (**B**) Linear model fitted via GEE between average severity score and age for each anatomic division used in the study. One year increase in age leads to an expected increase of 0.06 for upper airway (95% CI: 0.03, 0.09; $p < 0.0001$) 0.05 for laryngeal airway (95% CI: 0.01, 0.1; $p < 0.0091$) for lower airway 0.16 (0.11, 0.22; $p < 0.0001$) (**A**,**B**) Each point is the combined average airway severity score for bronchoscopies of subjects within this age group in increments of 1 year. Error bars represent standard deviation from the mean.

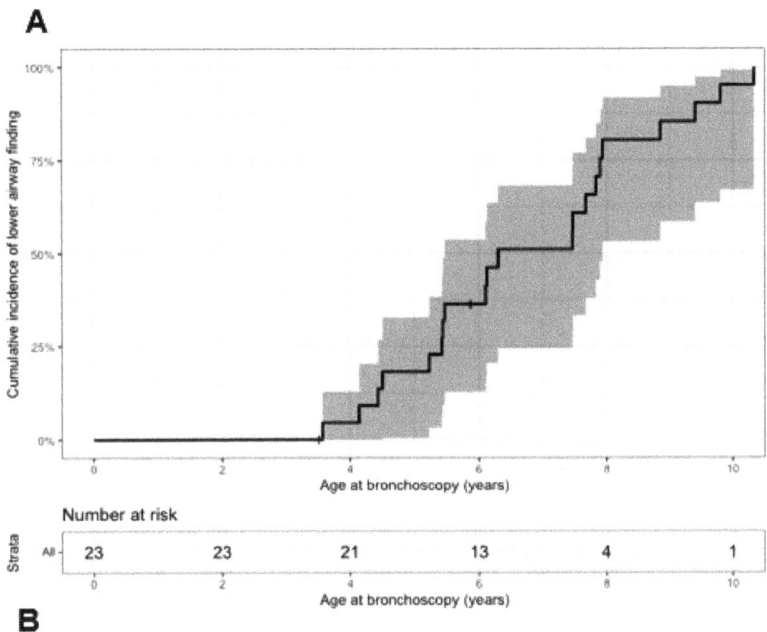

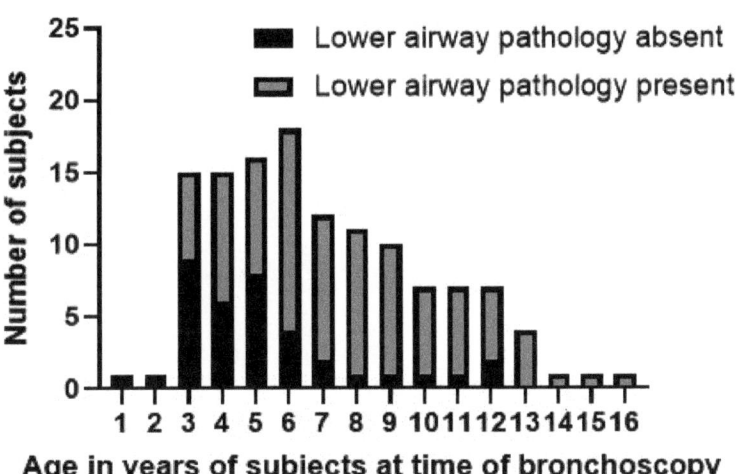

Figure 4. (**A**) Cumulative incidence of lower airway finding with 95% confidence interval. Each deflection point is the entire number of subjects who have bronchoscopies at that age, and the percentage of those subjects which have had bronchoscopies showing lower airway pathology. (**B**) Presence of lower airway findings over time. The dark bars represent bronchoscopies where lower airway pathology is absent, the light bars represent bronchoscopies where lower airway pathology is present. The total number of subjects on the y axis is the number of subjects who underwent bronchoscopy per year of age. Each individual was accounted for only once per year.

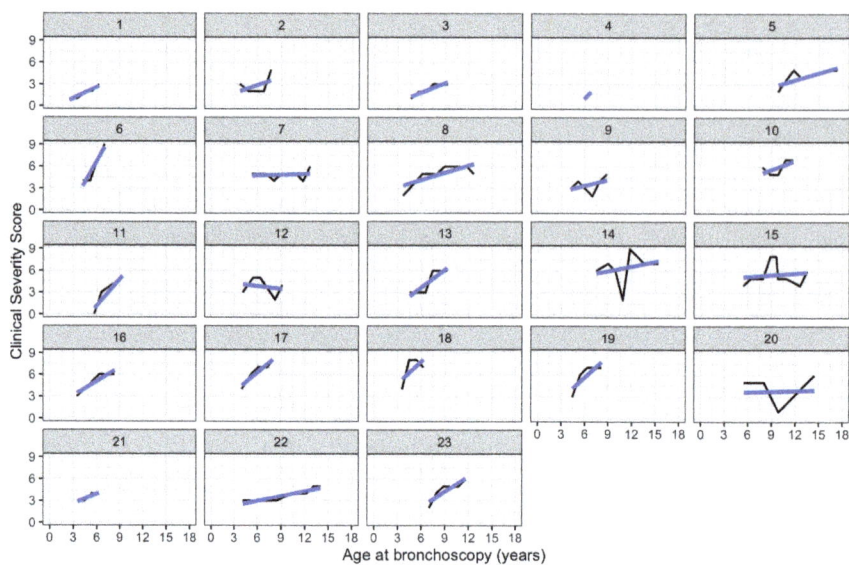

Figure 5. Individual slope of progression of airway disease, expressed as the airway severity score for each subject.

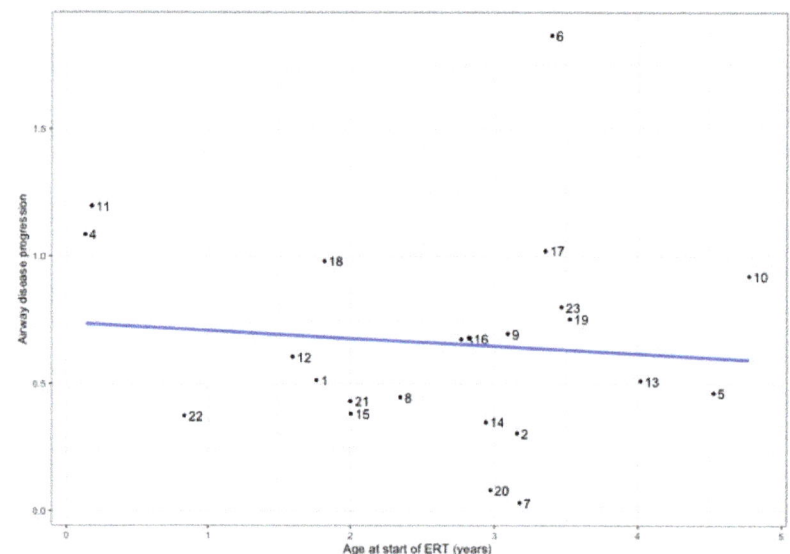

Type	Correlation	p-value
Pearson	−0.09	0.68
Spearman	0	0.99
Kendall	−0.01	0.96

Figure 6. A linear model was fitted with changes in airway severity score as response and age at bronchoscopy as covariate for each one of the $n = 23$ observations. The number indicates subject ID. The association between airway disease progression and age at start of ERT did not reach statistical significance, as one year increase in age at start of ERT leads to an expected increase of −0.03 (95% CI: −0.18, 0.12; $p = 0.7$) units in the airway disease progression.

4. Discussion

All individuals in our study were found to have upper airway abnormalities. Despite all individuals having a history of adenoidectomy prior to the first bronchoscopy, all were found to have adenoidal hypertrophy on at least one bronchoscopy, with 122 of the total 130 bronchoscopies mentioning adenoidal hypertrophy. While adenoidal hypertrophy is a well-known finding in MPS II [12], the mechanism of tissue reaccumulating is not entirely clear. Pharyngomalacia is also common in our study, with all individuals having pharyngomalacia on at least one bronchoscopy. These findings of persistent upper airway abnormalities correlate with the well-known problem associated with MPS II of upper airway obstruction and obstructive sleep apnea.

Laryngeal pathology was common as well (Table 1), with 65% having a laryngeal abnormality on at least one bronchoscopy. A prior study focusing on mucosal alterations of the larynx and hypopharynx had evaluated a detailed score to standardize findings across different types of MPS [9]. Of 55 individuals studied, 15 had MPS II. The MPS II individuals had an age range of 5–45 years, and a mean of 20.8 years. Their score showed a varied response to ERT. In this study, one MPS II subject was noted who was examined before and after ERT initiation and who did not have any improvement. Our study differed in the broadened assessment of the entire airway as opposed to a detailed focus on the laryngeal anatomy.

We found that lower airway pathology became more common with increasing age. Notably, all the subjects who had bronchoscopy at age 14 years or older showed lower airway involvement (Figure 4B). This suggests that close monitoring for lower airway pathology in individuals with MPS II should be recommended, and that lower airway pathology will continue to be a major cause of morbidity and mortality in this patient population.

The most frequent lower airway abnormalities are described as "tracheomalacia." Classic tracheomalacia shows dynamic collapse, generally due to weakening of the tracheal cartilage. However, the trachea in individuals with MPS II is narrowed and tortuous, with evidence of GAG deposition, and is overall different in appearance from classic tracheomalacia. The term tracheopathy is a more accurate descriptor in individuals with MPS II, and we would recommend future use of this term for diagnostic clarity.

We developed a score to compare individuals' airway findings cross-sectionally and longitudinally. The score attempted to be inclusive of all anatomic pathologies while not allowing for one location to be overwhelmingly represented. Upper airway pathology was almost universal (Table 1), often severe, and laryngeal and lower airway pathology would have been less impactful in the overall score had we not limited each anatomic location. Another challenge was that certain findings are more clearly identified earlier in the course of disease than others. For example, pharyngeal collapse is more obvious than subtle nodularity in the trachea. The airway severity score was designed to assess anatomic variation for statistical analysis, not the clinical condition, so the score presently is not designed for clinical implementation. Additionally, upper airway abnormalities are amenable to surgical interventions (e.g., adenoidectomy or tracheostomy) which is very difficult for lower airway pathology. Thus, identification of lower airway lesions prior to an individual's emergency presentation in the setting of an illness is important. For example, the tracheopathy associated with MPS II is likely seen on bronchoscopy before affecting airway function.

In our study, there was a progression of upper and lower airway abnormalities seen on flexible bronchoscopy despite treatment with IV ERT (Figure 3). We also noted heterogeneous progression between individuals as is typical for the overall disease in MPS II. The fact that the age of ERT initiation was not associated with changes in slope of airway disease progression further supports the idea that IV ERT does not eliminate progression of airway involvement but may slow progression. Yet, the lack of systematic studies prior to routine use of ERT does not allow for a direct larger scale comparison of airway progression. Furthermore, even earlier initiation of ERT may prove efficacious in preventing airway pathology [13]. Individuals with MPS II are most often diagnosed due to clinical signs of the disease, with the median age of diagnosis in one study being 3.3 years but newborn screening is needed to improve the age of diagnosis and long-term outcome [14].

A study performed in 2016 involving five adult individuals with MPS II, and which included CTs of the chest to evaluate lower airway involvement, showed thickening of the tracheobronchial tree, and narrowing of the lower airways. The individuals in this study were all adults without CNS disease, and who had been on ERT from 0–6 years at the time the study was performed. This study showed that the degree of narrowing predicted morbidity from airway involvement [15]. The findings in this study of persistent airway thickening and narrowing on the CT chest in individuals with MPS II is similar to our bronchoscopic findings in pediatric subjects. A recent study in adult people with MPS included multiple measures to compile a score of airway severity for clinical use in different types of MPS [16]. This score included exam, upper airway endoscopy, imaging, and if possible, lung function testing. The severity of lower airway involvement with tracheopathy could be well demonstrated on the 3D reconstruction of CT scans. The effect of ERT was not assessed in this retrospective study.

The fact that there were ongoing, progressive airway abnormalities in our study despite consistent use of ERT likely indicates additional mechanisms of injury apart from cellular GAG deposition. This includes uncontrolled inflammation and tissue remodeling due to alterations in signal transduction [17–19], aberrations in immune function [20], activation of inflammatory cascades [21], and abnormal oxidative stress [22,23]. Further studies into the mechanisms of progressive airway deterioration despite ERT are warranted.

MPS II also predisposes to increased mucus sections in upper and lower airways, a finding that has improved with ERT. The cause of increased secretions is likely a combination of factors including aspiration, infection, and increased inflammation due to lysosomal dysfunction [18]. It has been observed by bronchoscopists at our institution that the volume of secretions and of signs of bronchitis has decreased since the initiation of ERT. A previous study reviewing the clinical improvements associated with ERT showed that 22 of the 22 subjects studied had improvement in frequency of respiratory infections [24]. Our expectation is that this decrease in mucus burden represents substantial clinical benefit for people with MPS II, though this was not directly measured in our study given the different possible contributors to increased secretions.

The subjects in our study have been receiving intrathecal ERT throughout. This is a potentially confounding factor. However, based on our understanding of the somatic manifestations of MPS II, and the action of idursulfase, we would not expect the addition of intrathecal ERT to substantially affect the airway pathology. However, it is possible that increased airway tone due to improvement in neurologic function would cause improvements in airway patency.

Our study was limited by variability among reporters, as data were collected from bronchoscopy reports from multiple providers. We addressed this variability by careful review of the bronchoscopy reports and by developing a bronchoscopy scoring system that addressed different terminology. While our institution has performed a number of bronchoscopies in individuals with MPS II prior to initiation of ERT, the number and bronchoscopies was small, and lacked longitudinal data for each ERT-naïve subject [6]. A larger subset of ERT-naïve individuals with similar longitudinal observations would have improved comparisons; however, as ERT is now the standard of care, it would be difficult to find a cohort of individuals who had undergone bronchoscopy prior to ERT initiation. Individuals with MPS II can develop antibodies to idursulfase. These antibodies are associated with increased GAG in treated patients and are associated with attenuation of the improvement seen in pulmonary function [25,26]. The efficacy of ERT in preventing airway pathology may be affected by these antibodies. However, we were not able to evaluate anti-idursulfase antibodies' effects on airway pathology in this study since the antibody data are not available to the authors.

To enhance comparability in reporting MPS II-specific airway anomalies among bronchoscopists, we suggest that providers review the potential airway findings of MPS prior to bronchoscopies. This would enhance identification of subtle manifestations of MPS II such as vocal cord thickening or mucosal nodularity. It is possible that bronchoscopists without experience in MPS II populations may not recognize certain findings as developing pathologies.

The strengths of this study were its unprecedented access to a large number of bronchoscopies which examined the upper and lower airway, and which were consistently performed yearly over extended periods of time. The original study from which these data were collected included visits for intrathecal injection of enzyme (idursulfase-IT), as such compliance with enzyme replacement therapy treatment for the individuals included was excellent, and we could confidently rule out adherence to therapy as a potential source for error.

5. Conclusions

In individuals with mucopolysaccharidosis II, treatment with intravenous ERT did not prevent progression or development of lower airway pathology. Individuals with MPS who are receiving ERT will continue to have progressive airway disease and will need continued monitoring and intervention by their medical providers. Future studies investigating the role of inflammation and other mechanisms of airway disease and the effect of ERTs in the airway are warranted. We are hopeful that widespread adoption of newborn screening for MPS II with early initiation of ERT will more effectively prevent airway pathology in this population.

Author Contributions: Conceptualization, M.S.M., R.D.V., J.M. and E.J.; methodology, R.D.V. and M.S.M.; formal analysis, R.D.V., M.S.M., T.M.T. and F.-C.L.; data curation, R.D.V. and M.S.M.; writing—original draft preparation, R.D.V.; writing—review and editing, M.S.M., J.M., E.J., T.M.T. and F.-C.L.; supervision, M.S.M. All authors have read and agreed to the published version of the manuscript.

Funding: The project described was supported by the National Center for Advancing Translational Sciences (NCATS), National Institutes of Health, through Grant Award Number UL1TR002489. The content is solely the responsibility of the authors and does not necessarily represent the official views of the NIH.

Institutional Review Board Statement: The study was conducted in accordance with the Declaration of Helsinki and approved by the Institutional Review Board of the University of North Carolina Chapel Hill (20-2178).

Informed Consent Statement: Patient consent was waived due to study due to posing no more than minimal risk for subjects.

Data Availability Statement: Data sharing is not available due to the possibility of identifying research subjects.

Conflicts of Interest: The authors declare no conflict of interest.

References

1. Bach, G.; Eisenberg, F.; Cantz, M.; Neufeld, E.F. The defect in the Hunter syndrome: Deficiency of sulfoiduronate sulfatase. *Proc. Natl. Acad. Sci. USA* **1973**, *70*, 2134–2138. [CrossRef]
2. Jones, S.A.; Almássy, Z.; Beck, M.; Burt, K.; Clarke, J.T.; Giugliani, R.; Hendriksz, C.; Kroepfl, T.; Lavery, L.; Lin, S.P.; et al. Mortality and cause of death in mucopolysaccharidosis II-A historical review based on data from the Hunter Outcome Survey (HOS). *J. Inherit. Metab. Dis.* **2009**, *32*, 534–543. [CrossRef] [PubMed]
3. Tulebayeva, A.; Sharipova, M.; Boranbayeva, R. Respiratory dysfunction in children and adolescents with mucopolysaccharidosis types I, II, IVA, and VI. *Diagnostics* **2020**, *10*, 1–8. [CrossRef] [PubMed]
4. Burton, B.K.; Jego, V.; Mikl, J.; Jones, S.A. Survival in idursulfase-treated and untreated patients with mucopolysaccharidosis type II: Data from the Hunter Outcome Survey (HOS). *J. Inherit. Metab. Dis.* **2017**, *40*, 867–874. [CrossRef] [PubMed]
5. Martin, R.; Beck, M.; Eng, C.; Giugliani, R.; Harmatz, P.; Muñoz, V.; Muenzer, J. Recognition and diagnosis of mucopolysaccharidosis II (Hunter syndrome). *Pediatrics* **2008**, *121*, e377–e386. [CrossRef]
6. Muhlebach, M.S.; Shaffer, C.B.; Georges, L.; Abode, K.; Muenzer, J. Bronchoscopy and airway management in patients with mucopolysaccharidoses (MPS). *Pediatr. Pulmonol.* **2013**, *48*, 601–607. [CrossRef]

7. Lenka, M.; Michal, J.; Pavel, J.; Malinova, V.; Bloomfield, M.; Zeman, J.; Magner, M. Otorhinolaryngological manifestations in 61 patients with mucopolysaccharidosis. *Int. J. Pediatr. Otorhinolaryngol.* **2020**, *135*, 110137. [CrossRef]
8. Muhlebach, M.S.; Wooten, W.; Muenzer, J. Respiratory Manifestations in Mucopolysaccharidoses. *Paediatr. Respir. Rev.* **2011**, *12*, 133–138. [CrossRef]
9. Keilmann, A.; Bendel, F.; Nospes, S.; Lampe, C.; Läßig, A.K. Alterations of mucosa of the larynx and hypopharynx in patients with mucopolysaccharidoses. *J. Laryngol. Otol.* **2016**, *130*, 194–200. [CrossRef]
10. Parini, R.; Deodato, F. Intravenous enzyme replacement therapy in mucopolysaccharidoses: Clinical effectiveness and limitations. *Int. J. Mol. Sci.* **2020**, *21*, 1–30. [CrossRef]
11. Muenzer, J.; Giugliani, R.; Scarpa, M.; Tylki-Szymańska, A.; Jego, V.; Beck, M. Clinical outcomes in idursulfase-treated patients with mucopolysaccharidosis type II: 3-year data from the hunter outcome survey (HOS). *Orphanet J. Rare Dis.* **2017**, *12*, 1–11. [CrossRef] [PubMed]
12. Mendelsohn, N.J.; Harmatz, P.; Bodamer, O.; Burton, B.K.; Giugliani, R.; Jones, S.A.; Lampe, C.; Malm, G.; Steiner, R.D.; Parini, R. Importance of surgical history in diagnosing mucopolysaccharidosis type II (Hunter syndrome): Data from the Hunter Outcome Survey. *Genet. Med.* **2010**, *12*, 816–822. [CrossRef]
13. Grant, N.; Sohn, Y.B.; Ellinwood, N.M.; Okenfuss, E.; Mendelsohn, B.A.; Lynch, L.E.; Braunlin, E.A.; Harmatz, P.R.; Eisengart, J.B. Timing is everything: Clinical courses of Hunter syndrome associated with age at initiation of therapy in a sibling pair. *Mol. Genet. Metab. Rep.* **2022**, *30*, 100845. [CrossRef]
14. Parini, R.; Jones, S.A.; Harmatz, P.R.; Giugliani, R.; Mendelsohn, N.J. The natural history of growth in patients with Hunter syndrome: Data from the Hunter Outcome Survey (HOS). *Mol. Genet. Metab.* **2016**, *117*, 438–446. [CrossRef] [PubMed]
15. Rutten, M.; Ciet, P.; van den Biggelaar, R.; Oussoren, E.; Langendonk, J.G.; van der Ploeg, A.T.; Langeveld, M. Severe tracheal and bronchial collapse in adults with type II mucopolysaccharidosis. *Orphanet J. Rare Dis.* **2016**, *11*, 1–6. [CrossRef] [PubMed]
16. Gadepalli, C.; Stepien, K.M.; Sharma, R.; Jovanovic, A.; Tol, G.; Bentley, A. Airway abnormalities in adult mucopolysaccharidosis and development of salford mucopolysaccharidosis airway score. *J. Clin. Med.* **2021**, *10*, 3275. [CrossRef]
17. Costa, R.; Urbani, A.; Salvalaio, M.; Bellesso, S.; Cieri, D.; Zancan, I.; Filocamo, M.; Bonaldo, P.; Szabò, I.; Tomanin, R.; et al. Perturbations in cell signaling elicit early cardiac defects in mucopolysaccharidosis type II. *Hum. Mol. Genet.* **2017**, *26*, 1643–1655. [CrossRef]
18. Bellesso, S.; Salvalaio, M.; Lualdi, S.; Tognon, E.; Costa, R.; Braghetta, P.; Giraudo, C.; Stramare, R.; Rigon, L.; Filocamo, M.; et al. FGF signaling deregulation is associated with early developmental skeletal defects in animal models for mucopolysaccharidosis type II (MPSII). *Hum. Mol. Genet.* **2018**, *27*, 2262–2275. [CrossRef]
19. Settembre, C.; Fraldi, A.; Medina, D.L.; Ballabio, A.; Children, T. Signals from the lysosome. *Nat. Rev. Mol. Cell Biol.* **2013**, *14*, 283–296. [CrossRef]
20. Parker, H.; Bigger, B.W. The role of innate immunity in mucopolysaccharide diseases. *J. Neurochem.* **2019**, *148*, 639–651. [CrossRef]
21. Azambuja, A.S.; Pimentel-Vera, L.N.; Gonzalez, E.; Poletto, E.; Pinheiro, C.V.; Matte, U.; Giugliani, R.; Baldo, G. Evidence for inflammasome activation in the brain of mucopolysaccharidosis type II mice. *Metab. Brain Dis.* **2020**, *35*, 1231–1236. [CrossRef] [PubMed]
22. Jacques, C.E.D.; Donida, B.; Mescka, C.P.; Rodrigues, D.G.; Marchetti, D.P.; Bitencourt, F.H.; Burin, M.G.; de Souza, C.F.; Giugliani, R.; Vargas, C.R. Oxidative and nitrative stress and pro-inflammatory cytokines in Mucopolysaccharidosis type II patients: Effect of long-term enzyme replacement therapy and relation with glycosaminoglycan accumulation. *Biochim. Biophys. Acta-Mol. Basis Dis.* **2016**, *1862*, 1608–1616. [CrossRef] [PubMed]
23. Filippon, L.; Vanzin, C.S.; Biancini, G.B.; Pereira, I.N.; Manfredini, V.; Sitta, A.; Peralba, M.d.C.R.; Schwartz, I.V.D.; Giugliani, R.; Vargas, C.R. Oxidative stress in patients with mucopolysaccharidosis type II before and during enzyme replacement therapy. *Mol. Genet. Metab.* **2011**, *103*, 121–127. [CrossRef] [PubMed]
24. Lampe, C.; Bosserhoff, A.-K.; Burton, B.K.; Giugliani, R.; De Souza, C.F.; Bittar, C.; Muschol, N.; Olson, R.; Mendelsohn, N.J. Long-term experience with enzyme replacement therapy (ERT) in MPS II patients with a severe phenotype: An international case series. *J. Inherit. Metab. Dis.* **2014**, *37*, 823–829. [CrossRef]
25. Vollebregt, A.A.M.; Hoogeveen-Westerveld, M.; Ruijter, G.J.; Hout, H.V.D.; Oussoren, E.; van der Ploeg, A.T.; Pijnappel, W.P. Effect of Anti-Iduronate 2-Sulfatase Antibodies in Patients with Mucopolysaccharidosis Type II Treated with Enzyme Replacement Therapy. *J. Pediatr.* **2022**, *248*, 100–107. [CrossRef]
26. Muenzer, J.; Beck, M.; Eng, C.M.; Giugliani, R.; Harmatz, P.; Martin, R.; Ramaswami, U.; Vellodi, A.; Wraith, J.E.; Cleary, M.; et al. Long-term, open-labeled extension study of idursulfase in the treatment of Hunter syndrome. *Genet. Med.* **2011**, *13*, 95–101. [CrossRef]

Disclaimer/Publisher's Note: The statements, opinions and data contained in all publications are solely those of the individual author(s) and contributor(s) and not of MDPI and/or the editor(s). MDPI and/or the editor(s) disclaim responsibility for any injury to people or property resulting from any ideas, methods, instructions or products referred to in the content.

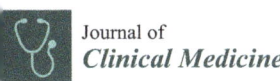

Article

Lactose-Containing Dry-Powder Inhalers for Patients with Cow's Milk Protein Allergy—The Conundrum; A National Survey of Pediatric Pulmonologists and Allergologists

Ophir Bar-On [1,*], Hagit Levine [1,2], Patrick Stafler [1,2], Einat Shmueli [1,2], Eyal Jacobi [1], Ori Goldberg [1,2], Guy Steuer [1], Dario Prais [1,2] and Meir Mei-Zahav [1,2]

1 Pulmonology Institute, Schneider Children's Medical Center of Israel, Petach Tikva 4920235, Israel
2 Sackler Faculty of Medicine, Tel-Aviv University, Tel-Aviv 6997801, Israel
* Correspondence: ophirbo@clalit.org.il

Abstract: Introduction: Several dry-powder inhalers (DPIs) contain lactose which may be contaminated with milk proteins. Confusion exists pertaining to DPI use in patients with cow's milk protein allergy (CMPA). **Methods:** A computerized survey sent via e-mail to pediatric pulmonologists and allergologists. **Results:** A total of 77 out of 232 (33.2%) doctors replied, of whom 80.5% were pediatric pulmonologists. A total of 69 of 77 (89.6%) were specialists, 37.6% with more than 15 years of experience. The most commonly used DPIs were formoterol + budesonide and vilanterol + fluticasone. A total of 62 out of 77 (80.5%) responders knew these DPIs contained lactose. A total of 35 out of 77 (45.5%) doctors who replied did not know that DPI leaflets list CMPA as a contra-indication to DPI administration. Of these, 4 (11.4%) stated that they would instruct patients with CMPA to stop DPIs, and 7 (20%) would avoid recommending DPIs. A total of 42 out of 77 (54.5%) responders were aware of this warning, yet 13 of these 42 (30.9%) continued to recommend lactose-containing DPIs without hesitation and 18 of these 42 (42.8%) responders prescribed DPIs but considered allergy severity. **Conclusions:** Almost half of certified, experienced pediatric pulmonologists and allergologists were unaware of the warning to administer DPIs to patients with CMPA. Most doctors who do know of this warning still continue to prescribe these DPIs.

Keywords: dry-powder inhalers; lactose; cow's milk protein allergy

1. Introduction

Asthma affects millions of people worldwide, both children and adults [1]. Many of these patients additionally suffer from aeroallergen sensitivities and food allergies, including cow's milk protein allergy (CMPA) [2].

Asthmatic patients use many different types of inhalers. For example, dry-powder inhalers (DPIs) containing bronchodilators and inhaled corticosteroids (ICSs) are frequently used as controllers and reliever therapies in asthma [3].

Many DPIs contain the excipient lactose, an inactive ingredient frequently found in various medications. Lactose is a carbohydrate, milk sugar, and should not be confused with milk proteins. Nevertheless, many web-based medication databases [4] and some DPI leaflets [5–7] list CMPA as a contraindication, probably because, during manufacturing, the purification process of lactose could theoretically result in contamination with milk proteins and thus may hypothetically induce an allergic reaction in patients with CMPA.

Approximately 2–3% of infants and young children suffer from CMPA [8]. Approximately 80% of them outgrow it by age five, yet some continue to suffer from CMPA into adult life [9], with a reported prevalence of approximately 0.5%. Some reports stated that CMPA is more prevalent in asthmatic children [10].

Adverse reactions to lactose-containing DPIs in patients with CMPA are seemingly rare, and so some authors have stated that patients with CMPA "need not avoid" DPIs

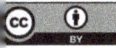

containing lactose [11]. However, a meagre few case reports [12–16] over the last two decades described patients with CMPA who developed an allergic reaction due to lactose-containing DPIs and thus advised against their use in asthmatic subjects with CMPA.

Due to this wide variability, we decided to evaluate the knowledge, experience, and approach of pediatric pulmonologists and allergologists to treating patients with CMPA with lactose-containing DPIs.

2. Methods

A computerized Google Forms questionnaire link was sent via e-mail to all participants. The message included a short explanation about the survey and a request to comply. The mail was sent to all pediatric pulmonologists in the country via their society mailing list, which includes 82 doctors. A similar e-mail was sent to all allergologists in the country via their society mailing list, which included 150 doctors (part of which are immunologists). In Israel, allergologists occasionally treat patients with asthma, both adult and pediatric. The e-mails were sent to specialists and fellows indiscriminately.

The questionnaire was written in Hebrew by the principal investigator, with the aid of clinical pharmacists and the co-authors. Almost all questions were multiple choice questions, some permitting only one answer, while other questions accepted multiple answers, as appropriate. The final two questions were open for free text answers.

The first section of the questionnaire included three basic questions regarding the speciality type, years of experience, and the number of asthma patients seen per week (to assess the overall patient number). The doctors were also asked whether they usually inquire about aeroallergen and food allergen sensitization.

Next, the doctors were asked which dry-powder inhalers they routinely recommended. The following question evaluated doctors' awareness of the excipients found in dry-powder inhalers. The subsequent section started with a question about the familiarity of doctors with the warning of administering DPIs to patients with CMPA. This question was a split point, i.e., if the reply was "yes", the participant was forwarded to a specific question, while if the reply was "no", the participant was forwarded to a different question. Both paths continued to ask about the doctors' strategy to use or avoid DPIs while treating asthmatic patients with CMPA. The last two questions were "free text"; the first question appeared to participants who chose that they knew about allergic reactions to DPIs, and requested them to describe the event. The final question was an open request for comments.

All the participants answered all the questions. The participant details were anonymized. The results are presented as absolute numbers and percentages. The data are also presented as bar graphs where appropriate. Only descriptive statistics were used.

3. Results

The poll was sent via e-mail to 232 doctors, 82 pediatric pulmonologists, and 150 allergologists, of whom only 77 responded. That is, the overall response rate was 33.2%. Most responders, 62 of 77 (80.5%), were pediatric pulmonologists.

Most responders (n = 69, 89.6%) were specialists, i.e., licensed and board certified. Only eight responders (10.4%) were residents in their fields, either pediatric pulmonology or allergy.

Of all the doctors who answered, 29 (37.6%) were specialists with over 15 years of experience, 24 (31.1%) were specialists with 5–15 years of experience, and 16 (20.7%) were young specialists with up to 5 years of experience. Eight residents (10.4%), who were in their pulmonology or allergology subspeciality training at the time of the survey, also responded.

Overall, forty-two doctors (54.5%) reported seeing approximately 1–20 patients per week with a diagnosis of asthma or an asthma-like illness (33 of 62 pediatric pulmonologists, 53.2%, and 9 of 15 allergologists, 60%). Overall, 29 doctors (37.6%) reported seeing approximately 20 to 50 patients per week with a diagnosis of asthma or an asthma-like illness (25 of 62 pediatric pulmonologists, 40.3%, and 4 of 15 allergologists, 26.7%). Overall, three doctors (3.9%) reported seeing more than 50 patients with asthma or an asthma-like illness per week (2 of 62 pediatric pulmonologists, 3.2%, and 1 of 15 allergologists, 6.7%). Three additional doctors (3.9%) reported they do not see patients with a diagnosis of asthma at all (2 of 62 pediatric pulmonologists, 3.2%, and 1 of 15 allergologists, 6.7%). Two of these three doctors were residents, which probably meant they did not see patients by themselves; the last doctor of the three was an experienced pediatric pulmonologist, and thus we regarded his response as a selection/technical error.

We asked all participants about their routine medical patient interviews in regards to allergies, specifically aeroallergens, and food allergens, including cow's milk protein allergy (CMPA) specifically, and lactose intolerance. A total of 11 (14.2%) out of all the doctors reported they inquired about aeroallergen sensitization. In total, 53 (68.8%) out of all the doctors reported they inquired about aeroallergen sensitization and food allergies, including CMPA specifically. Nine (11.7%) doctors stated that they asked about aeroallergen sensitizations, food allergies, including CMPA, and lactose intolerance. Two (2.6%) doctors reported they asked only about lactose intolerance, and only one (1.3%) doctor reported that they asked only about CMPA during a routine interview. Finally, one doctor (1.3%) out of all doctors who responded stated that they did not routinely inquire about allergies during history taking. To summarize, overall, 73 of 77 doctors (94.8%) who replied reported they asked about aeroallergen sensitization and 63 (81.8%) of all doctors who replied also asked about food allergies, including CMPA specifically.

When asked about Dry-Powder Inhalers (DPIs) in all dose ranges, that doctors routinely and frequently recommend for patients with a diagnosis of asthma or an asthma-like illness, 68 doctors (88.3%) stated that they routinely recommend a combined long-acting beta-agonist (LABA) plus an inhaled corticosteroid (ICS) inhaler, such as formoterol + budesonide (branded as Symbicort[R] Turbuhaler[R]); 60 (77.9%) stated that they normally recommend an ultra-LABA/ICS combination of vilanterol + fluticasone furoate (branded as Breo[TM] or Relvar[R] Ellipta), and 17 doctors (22%) recommend DuoResp Spiromax, also a combined LABA and ICS inhaler, containing formoterol and budesonide. A total of 29 doctors (37.6%) recommend salbutamol, a short-acting beta-agonist (SABA), in a dry-powder inhaler formulation (branded as Ventolin[R] Diskus), 29 doctors (37.6%) recommend fluticasone (Flixotide) in a discus dry-powder inhaler formulation, 29 doctors (37.6%) recommend a combined LABA and ICS discus (salmeterol + fluticasone), branded as Seretide[R] or Advair[R]. The cumulative percentages mentioned are larger than 100% since multiple answers were allowed, and most doctors indicated they recommend more than one type of inhaler on a regular basis. The results are displayed in Figure 1. Several metered dose inhalers (MDIs) also appeared in the responses, such as salbutamol (Ventolin), fluticasone (Flixotide), formoterol + fluticasone (Flutiform), and formoterol + beclomethasone (Foster), but for the purpose of this study, these MDIs were disregarded.

The doctors were then asked if they knew what excipients, that is, the non-active ingredients, are routinely found in dry-powder inhalers. Sixty-two doctors (80.5%) indicated they knew that DPIs contain milk sugar (lactose). Nineteen doctors (24.6%) indicated they knew that DPIs contain milk protein. Some responders indicated that DPIs contained certain excipients which they do not, as follows: eleven doctors (14.3%) indicated they knew that DPIs contain CFC (Chloro-Fluoro-Carbons); eight (10.4%) indicated magnesium, and seven (9%) indicated ethanol. The results are displayed in Figure 2. The cumulative percentage is larger than 100% since multiple answers were allowed, and most doctors marked more than one excipient.

The next question was a major one and inquired whether doctors are familiar with the warning written in DPI leaflets and web-based drug databases regarding DPI administration to patients with cow's milk protein allergy. It was phrased as follows: "in the medication leaflet of some dry-powder inhalers, a warning exists about administration to patients who have cow's milk protein allergy; did you ever hear about this warning?". In total, 35 doctors (45.5%) answered that they had never heard about this warning and 42 (54.5%) answered that they knew and heard about this contraindication.

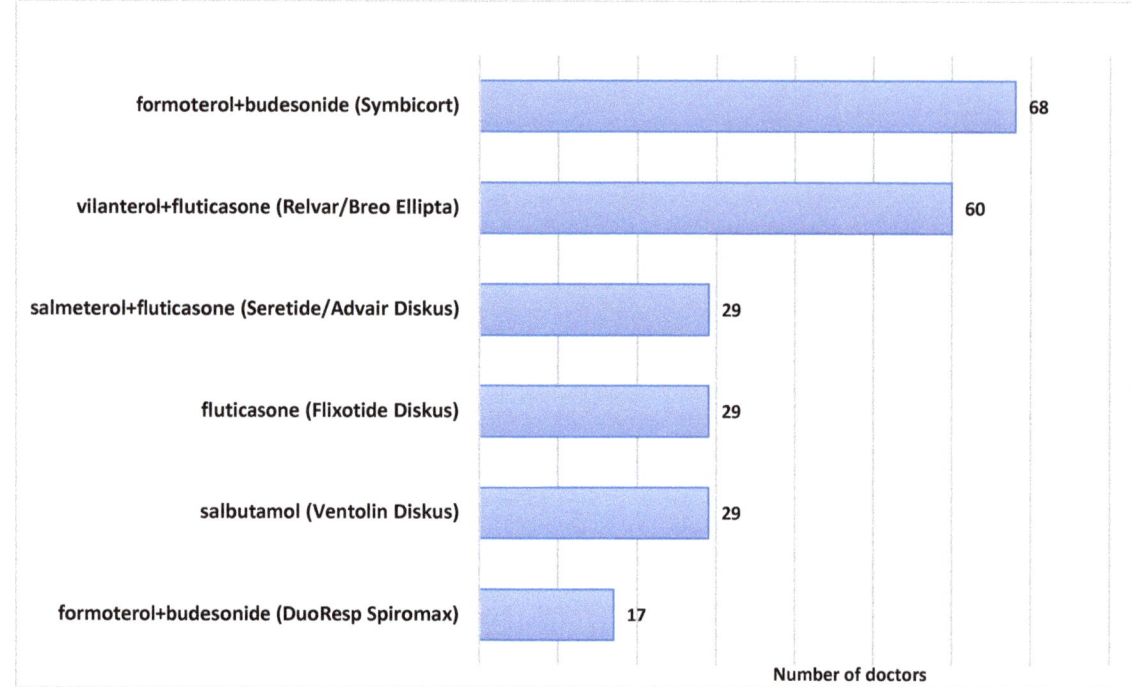

Figure 1. Frequently prescribed Dry-Powder Inhalers for asthma.

The sub-divisions of these responses, according to the speciality, are displayed in Figure 3. The pediatric pulmonologists (62 total) were fairly equally divided between those who have heard (32 doctors, 51.6%) to those who have not heard (30 doctors, 48.4%) of this warning; A total of 10 of the 15 (66.6%) of the allergologists who responded were aware of this warning.

Of the 42 doctors who confirmed they were familiar with the warning of milk proteins within DPIs, 13 doctors (30.9%) stated that they still continued to recommend and prescribe DPIs to patients known to be allergic to the cow-milk protein, despite this clear contraindication to administering dry-powder inhalers to patients allergic to milk protein. Eighteen doctors (42.8%) stated that they continued to recommend and prescribe DPIs to these patients, but they took the allergy severity into consideration. Eleven doctors (26.2%) stated that they stopped prescribing DPIs to patients with cow's milk protein allergy once they learned of this warning.

Of the 35 doctors who replied that they had not heard of the warning, 4 doctors (11.4%) stated that they would now stop prescribing DPIs for patients with cow's milk protein allergy and think of an alternative treatment. Seven doctors (20%) stated that they would not start DPIs for these patients but rather would find an alternative. Nine (25.7%) doctors reported they would continue prescribing DPIs for patients with cow's milk protein allergy, despite this warning. Fifteen doctors (42.8%) stated that they would consider stopping DPIs in cow's milk protein allergic patients, depending on their personal allergy levels.

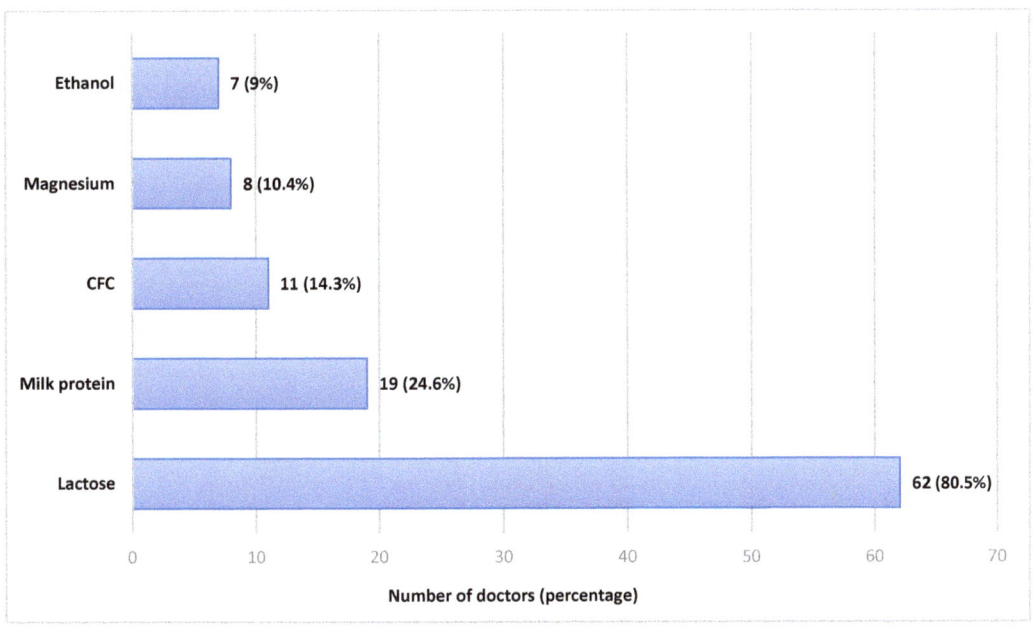

Figure 2. Responses regarding the excipients in Dry-Powder Inhalers. CFC—Chlorofluorocarbons.

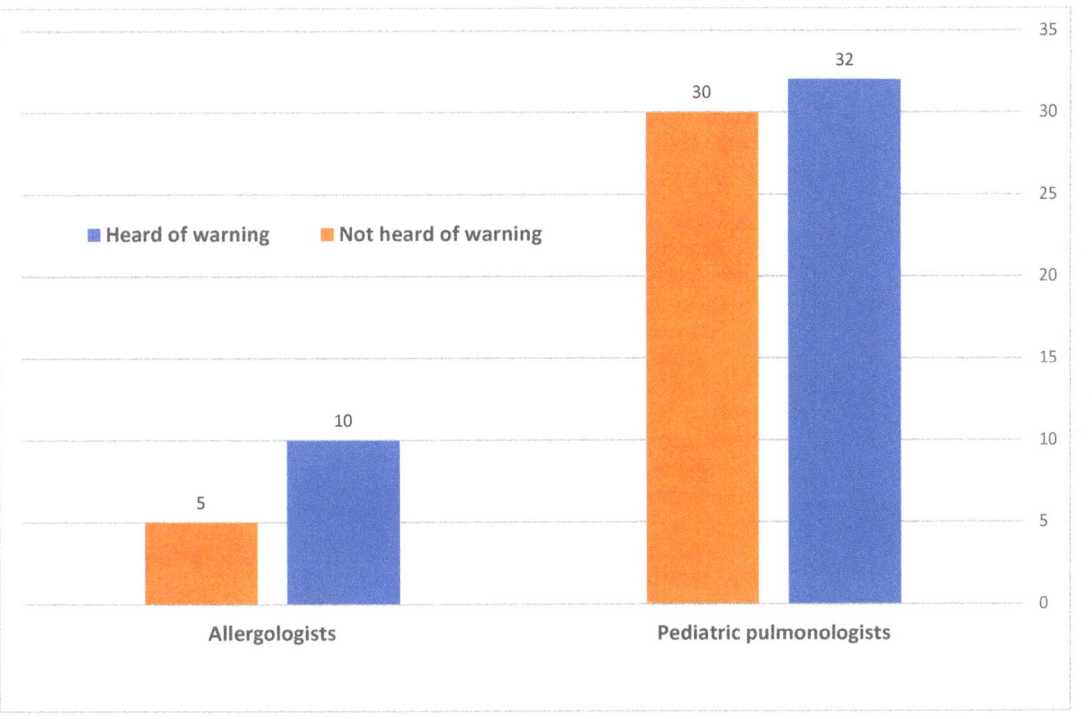

Figure 3. Division of the awareness to the warning of Dry-Powder Inhaler administration in CMPA, according to speciality.

Finally, we asked all doctors to recall, to the best of their knowledge and memory, if any of their patients who suffer from cow's milk protein allergy and have received lactose-containing DPIs, developed an allergic reaction. One doctor (1.3%) did not respond to this question. However, the majority of responders, 54 doctors (70.1%), answered that they were not aware of any allergic reactions that occurred to any of their patients who received DPIs. Fifteen doctors (19.5%) answered that they did not prescribe DPIs to these patients. Seven doctors (9%) answered that they did prescribe DPIs in the past, and there were suspicious allergic reactions. Five of these doctors elaborated with free text and described the allergic reactions as a "mild worsening of asthma symptoms"; no comment mentioned a severe systemic allergic reaction that required systemic steroids or epinephrine administration.

4. Discussion

The most striking result of our survey is the fact that approximately half of the certified, experienced pulmonologists and allergologists surveyed, who regularly treat asthmatic patients, declared that they had never heard of the warning to administer lactose-containing DPIs to patients with known CMPA. This contraindication is clearly stated in the medical leaflet of these inhalers and also appears on internet-based medication databases, although occasionally in confusing phrasing. Interestingly, most doctors, including those who declared they were aware of this warning, stated that they continue to recommend lactose-containing DPIs without hesitation to patients with CMPA. On the other hand, some doctors, after participating in this survey, announced they would change their practice and, from now on, would avoid lactose-containing DPIs in patients with CMPA.

None of our survey participants, with a collective experience of hundreds of years, and tens of thousands of patients, reported they were aware of any systemic adverse effects, especially not anaphylactic reactions, in patients with CMPA who received lactose-containing DPIs. Similarly, in the literature, there are just a few reports about such events.

Nowak-Wegrzyn [12] et al. in 2004 wrote a letter to the JACI editor, reporting about an 8-year-old boy with proven severe CMPA who used Advair Diskus, a lactose-containing DPI, without any adverse events for several months. However, upon switching to a new batch, he developed chest tightness which required anti-allergic medication; this was further proven by a supervised challenge that eventually also required intramuscular epinephrine. They obtained the powder from that specific inhaler and powder from other lactose-containing DPIs and tested them for the presence of milk proteins using silver staining and via the immuno-labeling of monoclonal anti-β-lactoglobulin, anti-α-casein, and anti-β-casein antibodies. They indeed demonstrated the presence of milk proteins in all DPIs, with wide lot-to-lot variability. They concluded that the purification process of lactose might have unpredictable protein contamination and therefore advised to avoid, or at least "use with caution" lactose-containing DPIs in patients with CMPA.

Morisset et al. [13] described an adult female with CMPA who presented with asthma exacerbation after exposure to a lactose-containing DPI (formoterol). They concluded that there was a risk of anaphylaxis in patients with CMPA who use lactose-containing DPIs.

Sa et al. [14] reported a 10-year-old boy with known CMPA, who also had asthma symptoms, and thus was started on a fluticasone lactose-containing DPI. Firstly, this administration caused peri-oral urticaria. After a second administration, he developed bronchospasms requiring systemic steroids. They concluded that the contamination of lactose by milk proteins should not be neglected due to the potential risk of allergic reactions.

Robles et al. [15] also reported a case of a 9-year-old child with CMPA who had asthma exacerbation following an administration of a lactose-containing DPI and also concluded that lactose-containing inhaled medications should not be administered to patients with CMPA.

Morikawa et al. [16] described a 6-year-old female with CMPA who developed an anaphylactic reaction after inhalation with Inavir^R (laninamivir) to treat the flu. An analysis with a skin-prick test and silver staining of the powder, plus Western blotting, proved the presence of trace amounts of β-lactoglobulin in the lactose excipient. They concluded that lactose-containing DPIs may trigger an allergic reaction in patients with CMPA.

Besides these five reports, despite a meticulous search of PubMed, Google Scholar, and other databases (using keywords such as dry-powder inhalers, lactose, milk allergy, allergic/anaphylactic reaction, and others), we did not find any other case reports describing a possible adverse reaction to milk proteins contaminating lactose in DPIs. Therefore, considering the large number of patients worldwide with CMPA who have most probably received DPIs, this is indeed an extremely uncommon phenomenon, or perhaps an under-reported one.

Spiegel et al. [17] performed a chart review of 8418 asthmatics, of whom 278 had CMPA. Of these, 21 took lactose-containing DPIs and were exposed to a total of 616 inhalers during a total of 715 months. According to the charts, they did not identify any reaction attributable to inadvertent milk protein exposure through these DPIs. Their data suggested that allergic reactions in patients with CMPA taking these DPIs are rare. They concluded that the "watchful vigilance for reactions, not avoidance of these medications, is appropriate".

In our opinion, this strategy of watchfulness is unacceptable in potential life-threatening allergic reactions. Coinciding with this, current inhaler leaflets clearly state that a severe hypersensitivity to milk proteins is a contraindication to administering lactose-containing DPIs, yet our survey of professional physicians who regularly treat asthmatic patients indicated there was insufficient awareness of this possible hazardous effect. More so, many physicians know of this warning yet choose to ignore it. With all this considered, true life-threatening anaphylactic reactions to these inhalers are apparently very rare, possibly because pharmaceutical companies have improved the lactose purification process over the years or due to exposure route variability, i.e., the inhalation of milk proteins is different from the ingestion of milk proteins and theoretically less immunogenic and allergenic.

Our study has limitations, firstly being a questionnaire study, which relies on the memory of past events. Additionally, only a minority of allergologists answered the study, predisposing the study to a response bias, as the answers might not represent this group. However, overall, the majority of participants in our study were pediatric pulmonologists, with a high rate of response.

To conclude: lactose-containing DPIs may theoretically occasionally contain milk proteins and are therefore officially contraindicated for patients with severe CMPA. In common practice, as evident from our single-nation survey of certified pulmonologists and allergologists, approximately half were unaware of this warning and continued to prescribe these DPIs to patients with CMPA. More so, many doctors who knew of the warning chose to ignore it. Consequently, innumerable patients with CMPA have received these inhalers in recent years. Remarkably, the medical literature of the past 20 years, and the collaborative experiences of our surveyed doctors, contained just a few single reports describing adverse reactions, suggesting that the true contamination of lactose with milk proteins causing anaphylactic reactions is either indeed very rare, under-reported, or confounded by varied allergic phenotypes. Clear, updated regulatory statements should be re-published, and larger studies are required to further assess the safety of DPIs in patients with CMPA.

Author Contributions: Conceptualization, O.B.-O., M.M.-Z. and D.P.; methodology, O.B.-O., M.M.-Z. and D.P.; formal analysis, O.B.-O.; writing—original draft preparation, O.B.-O.; writing—review and editing, M.M.-Z., D.P., H.L., P.S., G.S., E.S., E.J. and O.G.; supervision, D.P. and M.M.-Z.; project administration, O.B.-O. All authors have read and agreed to the published version of the manuscript.

Funding: This research received no external funding.

Institutional Review Board Statement: According to local guidelines, Institutional Review Board (IRB) approval is not required for doctor surveys, but still, approval was requested and provided (RMC-1055-20).

Conflicts of Interest: The authors declare no conflict of interest.

References

1. GINA Main Report 2022. Available online: https://ginasthma.org/wp-content/uploads/2022/07/GINA-Main-Report-2022-FINAL-22-07-01-WMS (accessed on 15 July 2022).
2. Mousan, G.; Kamat, D. Cow's Milk Protein Allergy. *Clin. Pediatr.* **2016**, *55*, 1054–1063. [CrossRef] [PubMed]
3. Cloutier, M.M.; Dixon, A.E.; Krishnan, J.A.; Lemanske, R.F.; Pace, W.; Schatz, M. Managing Asthma in Adolescents and Adults: 2020 Asthma Guideline Update From the National Asthma Education and Prevention Program. *JAMA Netw.* **2020**, *324*, 2301–2317. [CrossRef] [PubMed]
4. UpToDate. Seretide Contraindications. 2022. Available online: https://www-uptodate-com.beilinson.idm.oclc.org/contents/fluticasone-propionate-and-salmeterol-drug-information?search=seretide&source=search_result&selectedTitle=1~{}4&usage_type=default&display_rank=1#F173420 (accessed on 8 November 2022).
5. AstraZeneca. Formoterol-Budesonide (Symbicort) Product Information. 2021. Available online: https://www.astrazeneca.ca/content/dam/az-ca/downloads/productinformation/symbicort-turbuhaler-product-monograph-en (accessed on 23 April 2022).
6. GlaxoSmithKline. Vilanterol-Fluticasoe (Breo/Relvar) Prescribing Information. 2019. Available online: https://www.accessdata.fda.gov/drugsatfda_docs/label/2019/204275s017lbl (accessed on 23 April 2022).
7. US Food and Drug Administration. Salmeterol+Fluticasoe (Advair/Seretide) Prescribing Information. 2008. Available online: https://www.accessdata.fda.gov/drugsatfda_docs/label/2008/021077s029lbl (accessed on 23 April 2022).
8. Harvey, L.; Ludwig, T.; Hou, A.Q.; Hock, Q.S.; Tan, M.L.; Osatakul, S.; Bindels, J.; Muhardi, L. Prevalence, cause and diagnosis of lactose intolerance in children aged 1-5 years: A systematic review of 1995–2015 literature. *Asia. Pac. J. Clin. Nutr.* **2018**, *27*, 29–46. [CrossRef] [PubMed]
9. Caffarelli, C.; Baldi, F.; Bendandi, B.; Calzone, L.; Marani, M.; Pasquinelli, P. Cow's milk protein allergy in children: A practical guide. *Ital. J. Pediatr.* **2010**, *36*, 5. [CrossRef] [PubMed]
10. Høst, A.; Halken, S.; Jacobsen, H.P.; Christensen, A.E.; Herskind, A.M.; Plesner, K. Clinical Course of Cow's Milk Protein Allergy/Intolerance and Atopic Diseases in Childhood. *Blackwell Munksgaard. Pediatr. Allergy Immunol.* **2002**, *13*, 23–28. [CrossRef] [PubMed]
11. Kelso, J.M. Potential food allergens in medications. *J. Allergy Clin. Immunol.* **2014**, *133*, 1509–1518. [CrossRef] [PubMed]
12. Nowak-Wegrzyn, A.; Shapiro, G.; Beyer, K.; Bardina, L.; Sampson, H. Contamination of dry powder inhalers for asthma with milk proteins containing lactose. *J. Allergy Clin. Immunol.* **2004**, *113*, 558–560. [CrossRef] [PubMed]
13. Morisset, M.; Moneret-Vautrin, D.; Commun, N.; Schuller, A.; Kanny, G. Allergy to Cow Milk Proteins Contaminating Lactose, Common Excipient of Dry Powder Inhalers for Asthma. *J. Allergy Clin. Immunol.* **2006**, *117*, S95. [CrossRef]
14. Sa, A.B.; Oliveira, L.C.L.; Miyagi, K.V.M.; Mello, Y.A.M.F.; Cabral, E.C.; Carvalho, A.P.E.; Komaroff, F.F.; Gonçalves, R.F.F. Reaction Due to Milk Proteins Contaminating Lactose Added to Inhaled Corticosteroid. *J. Allergy Clin. Immunol.* **2011**, *127*, 241. [CrossRef]
15. Robles, J.; Motheral, L. Hypersensitivity Reaction After Inhalation of a Lactose-Containing Dry Powder Inhaler. *J. Pediatr. Pharmacol. Ther.* **2014**, *19*, 206–211. [CrossRef] [PubMed]
16. Morikawa, M.; Kanemitsu, Y.; Tsukamoto, H.; Morikawa, A.; Tomioka, Y. A Case of Anaphylaxis in the Pediatric Patient with Milk Allergy Due to Traces of Milk Protein in the Lactose Used as an Excipient of Inavir Inhalation. *Jpn. J. Allergol.* **2016**, *65*, 200–205. [CrossRef]
17. Spiegel, W.A.; Anolik, R. Lack of Milk Protein Allergic Reactions in Patients Using Lactose Containing Dry Powder Inhalers (DPIs). *J. Allergy Clin. Immunol.* **2010**, *125*, AB69. [CrossRef]

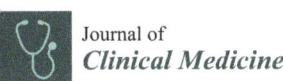

Article

Reversible Bronchial Obstruction in Primary Ciliary Dyskinesia

Hagit Levine [1,2,*,†], Ophir Bar-On [1,2,†], Vered Nir [3], Nicole West [2], Yotam Dizitzer [4], Huda Mussaffi [1,2] and Dario Prais [1,2]

1. Pulmonary Institute, Schneider Children's Medical Center, Petah-Tikva 49100, Israel
2. Sackler Faculty of Medicine, Tel Aviv University, Tel Aviv 6997801, Israel
3. Department of Pediatrics, Hillel-Yaffe Medical Center, Hadera 3810101, Israel
4. Department of Pediatrics, Schneider Children's Medical Center, Petah-Tikva 4920235, Israel
* Correspondence: hagitlevine@gmail.com; Tel.: +97-23-925-3654; Fax: +97-23-925-3308
† These authors contributed equally to this work.

Abstract: Background: Inhaled bronchodilators are frequently used among patients with primary ciliary dyskinesia (PCD), although neither the effectiveness nor the prevalence of their use is known, due to the paucity of relevant studies. Methods: This is a retrospective analysis of pre- and post-bronchodilator spirometry results, of patients with PCD from two centers. Correlations were examined of bronchodilator response, with asthma and atopy markers. Results: Of 115 patients, 46 (40%) completed spirometry pre- and post-bronchodilation. Of these, 26 (56.5%) demonstrated reversible airway obstruction (increase in %FEV_1 predicted $\geq$ 10%). Obstruction reversibility was not found to be associated with a family history of asthma, blood eosinophil level, elevated IgE, or atopy symptoms. Of the 46 patients who completed bronchodilator spirometry, 29 (63%) were regularly using bronchodilators and inhaled corticosteroids. Conclusions: More than half of patients with PCD presented with reversible airway obstruction, without any correlation to markers of personal or familial atopy. Inhaled bronchodilators and corticosteroid therapies are commonly used for treating PCD. Evaluating bronchodilator response should be considered, and its effectiveness should be further studied.

Keywords: primary ciliary dyskinesia; airway hyperreactivity; airway obstruction; asthma; bronchodilators; inhaled corticosteroids; spirometry

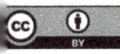

1. Introduction

Primary ciliary dyskinesia (PCD) is an uncommon, genetically heterogeneous disorder, with a prevalence of approximately 1 in 15,000 births. The inheritance is usually autosomal-recessive and results in dysfunction of motile cilia, leading to mucus stasis. Mutations in more than 40 genes have been reported to cause PCD; the involvement of many other genes is likely to be discovered. As PCD is more common in populations with closed genetic pools, genetic heterogeneity is seen in socially isolated consanguineous populations. Estimates of prevalence are scarce in populations outside of Europe, but the disease is expected to be more common in certain populations, such as in Arab countries [1].

In the lungs, PCD manifests as a chronic progressive airway disease starting in the neonatal period or during infancy, which then gradually advances to suppurative lung disease with bronchiectasis in adult life [1,2]. About 50% of patients have situs inversus (Kartagener's syndrome). Situs ambiguus, including heterotaxy, is reported in up to 12% of patients. Chronic rhinosinusitis, recurrent otitis media until conductive hearing impairment and infertility are also common [1]. Airway pathology stems from a dysregulated cycle of infection (with pathogenic bacteria including *Pseudomonas aeruginosa*) and inflammation [3]. Indeed, airway inflammation is common in PCD, as in cystic fibrosis (CF) and asthma; however, the pathomechanisms are different. In PCD, the inflammation is mostly neutrophilic; whereas in asthma, eosinophilic Th2 inflammation is more common [4].

Individuals with PCD frequently use inhaled beta2-agonists, with or without saline inhalations, to soothe shortness of breath and to enhance bronchodilation before chest physiotherapy. However, the effectiveness of bronchodilators in PCD has not been documented, due to the paucity of relevant studies [5].

Our study aimed to identify the frequency of airway reversibility following inhaled bronchodilators in individuals with PCD. Furthermore, we aimed to correlate bronchodilator response with markers of personal or family atopy.

2. Methods

This study reviewed medical charts of patients diagnosed with PCD who were followed at Schneider Children's Medical Center and Hillel Yaffe Medical Center. Inclusion criteria: a diagnosis of PCD, based on electron microscopic examination or genetic diagnosis of a defect in the dynein arm, according to accepted criteria; [2] and spirometry performed before and after inhaled bronchodilators, according to ATS/ERS guidelines [6,7].

Standardization of pulmonary function tests:

Spirometry, performed both before and after inhaled bronchodilators, was evaluated during routine follow-up visits. Spirometry was also conducted during exacerbations that were marked by symptoms such as wheezing or dyspnea. For the purpose of this study, the test that demonstrated the largest increase in %FEV$_1$ following bronchodilator administration was used.

Prediction equations that were used by both centers were the Knudson or ECCS/ERS for patients aged 18 years and above, and Polgar for children younger than age 18 years. All the patients followed standard instructions before performing spirometry, namely avoiding the use of bronchodilators (short-acting beta2 agonists (SABA) at least 6 h prior the test, and long-acting beta-agonists (LABA)/combined LABA and inhaled corticosteroids (ICS) at least 12 h prior the test).

Definition:

Reversible airway obstruction was defined as an increase in the percentile predicted FEV$_1$, (%FEV$_1$) by 10% or more [7].

Patient data:

The data collected included demographic details and measurements of weight and height at the best-recorded increase in %FEV$_1$ on spirometry. The atopy markers considered were: known allergies, the highest value of serum IgE, and eosinophil count. First-degree relative history of asthma was also documented. Other medical information collected from the patient files included: respiratory symptoms after birth, the presence of situs-inversus, recurrent wheezing, and the presence of consanguinity. Lastly, we documented whether patients were receiving inhaled bronchodilators: SABA, LABA or ICS.

Statistics:

Demographic and clinical data were described using medians and ranges, or means and standard deviations, as appropriate, according to group characteristics. To identify differences between groups, Pearson's chi-square test or Fisher exact test (two-tailed) were used for categorical variables, and t-tests for normally distributed continuous variables. The Mann–Whitney test was used for the distribution of continuous variables (such as age across categories). Significant differences were defined as a p-value (a two-sided alpha level) ≤ 0.05. The statistical analysis was performed with SPSS 22.0 (IBM, Armonk, NY, USA) for Windows.

The Rabin Medical Center and Hillel-Yaffe Medical Center Research Ethics Committees approved this retrospective study (*Rabin IRB number:* 0392-17-RMC; *Hillel-Yaffe IRB number:* 0087-22-HYMC).

3. Results

Of 115 patients with PCD who were followed during the study period, 46 (40%) fulfilled the inclusion criterion of at least one recorded spirometry test pre- and post-bronchodilator use. Demographic and anthropometric characteristics are presented in Table 1. The patients who were excluded were too young to perform satisfactory spirometry or had not performed spirometry following bronchodilation. The median age at the best-recorded spirometry was 12 years; the range was 5–48 years.

Table 1. Demographic and anthropometric characteristics of patients with primary ciliary dyskinesia, according to airway reversibility.

	Total $n = 46$ (100%)	Without Airway Reversibility $n = 20$ (43.5%)	With Airway Reversibility $n = 26$ (56.5%)	p-Value
Sex (female)	20 (43.5%)	7 (35.0%)	13 (50.0%)	0.309
Ethnicity ($n = 29/46$, 63%)				
Jewish	13 (44.8%)	7 (58.3%)	6 (35.3%)	0.379
Arabic	15 (51.7%)	5 (41.7%)	10 (58.8%)	
Other	1 (3.4%)	0	1 (5.9%)	
Consanguineous ($n = 28/46$, 61%)	14 (50.0%)	6 (50.0%)	8 (50.0%)	1.000
Height (cm) (mean (SD))	149 (19.6)	146.7 (22.0)	151.5 (16.3)	0.24
Weight (kg) (mean (SD))	44.6 (18.3)	42.9 (20.2)	46.6 (16.0)	0.345
BMI (kg/m^2) (mean (SD))	19.1 (3.9)	18.6 (3.9)	19.7 (3.8)	0.899

Airway obstruction reversibility:

Airway obstruction reversibility following inhaled bronchodilators, expressed as an increase larger than 10% in %FEV$_1$ of that predicted, was documented in 26 (56.5%) patients. The median %FEV$_1$ at baseline, predicted for age, was 72% (range 32–109%) among all the patients, and 60% among those with bronchodilator reversibility (range 32–92%) during the best-recorded spirometry. The median change pre- and post-bronchodilator use was 16% (range 10–27%). Significant differences were not observed in the proportions of patients with airway reversibility, between males and females, between ethnic groups (Jewish vs. non-Jewish), nor between patients with and without documented familial consanguinity (Table 1).

The median age was 13.5 (5–41) years among the patients with %FEV$_1$ predicted $\geq 10\%$, and age 11 (5–48) years among those with %FEV$_1$ predicted < 10%; this difference was not statistically significant. In an analysis that matched patients according to age, airway reversibility correlated with worse %FEV$_1$ predicted ($p = 0.039$) (Figure 1).

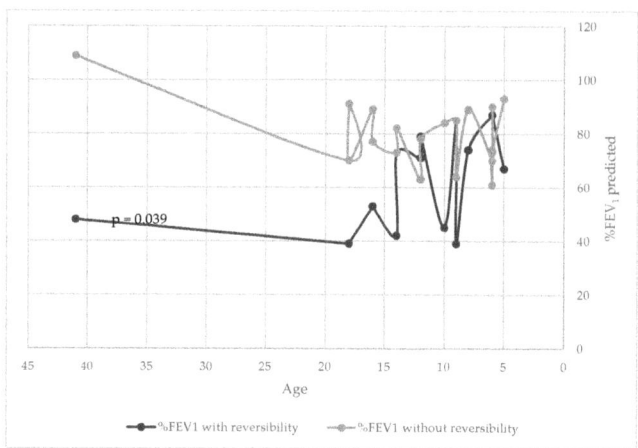

Figure 1. %FEV$_1$ predicted for age comparing patient with primary ciliary dyskinesia with or without airway reversibility.

Asthma and atopy correlation:

Prevalences of self-recorded asthma and of asthma among first-degree family members did not differ between patients with and without reversible airway obstruction (Table 2). Family asthma data were missing for some patients, yet laboratory parameters of atopy were available for most. Nonetheless, differences were not detected in maximal IgE levels, or in eosinophil counts, between patients with and without reversible bronchial obstruction.

Table 2. Respiratory and asthma/allergy characteristics of patients with primary ciliary dyskinesia, according to airway reversibility.

	Total $n = 46$ (100%)	Without Airway Reversibility $n = 20$ (43.5%)	With Airway Reversibility $n = 26$ (56.5%)	p-Value
Spirometry:				
%FEV$_1$ predicted (median, range)	72 (32–109)	77 (61–109)	60 (32–92)	0.07
Reversibility in %FEV$_1$ (median, range)	11.5 (0–27)	5 (0–8)	16 (10–27)	<0.001
Age (years) (median, range)	12 (5–48)	At best-recorded spirometry 11 (5–48)	At best reversibility 13.5 (5–41)	0.301
Asthma/Atopy:				
Familial asthma	6 (13.0%)	2 (10.0%)	4 (15.4%)	0.591
Atopy/allergy	4 (8.7%)	2 (10.0%)	2 (7.7%)	0.783
Eosinophils $\geq$ 5%	28 (62.2%)	14 (70.0%)	14 (56.0%)	0.336
IgE $\geq$ 100 IU	9 (20.0%)	5 (25.0%)	4 (16.0%)	0.453
Neonatal/Childhood characteristics:				
Neonatal tachypnea or pneumonia ($n = 25/46, 54\%$)	19 (76.0%)	11 (91.7%)	8 (61.5%)	0.078
Recurrent wheezing ($n = 22/46, 48\%$)	15 (68.2%)	4 (40.0%)	11 (91.7%)	0.010

ICS–inhaled corticosteroids.

Significant associations were not found of prior transient respiratory symptoms in the newborn or of neonatal pneumonia, with airway reversibility. Notably, however, 91.7% of the patients with documented airway reversibility also had previous documentation of recurrent wheezing ($p = 0.010$).

The association of reversible airway obstruction with medication use

Of the 46 patients evaluated, 29 (63%) were using bronchodilators (Figure 2). Of them, 21 (72%) demonstrated reversible airway obstruction. Of the 26 patients with reversible airway obstruction, 21 (80%) were using inhaled bronchodilators ($p = 0.005$) (Figure 2).

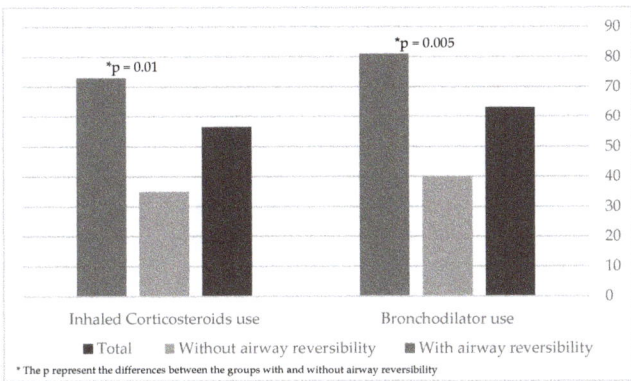

Figure 2. Inhaled bronchodilator and corticosteroid usage among patients with primary ciliary dyskinesia.

ICS usage was also common among the patients. Of the 46 with available data, 26 (56.5%) were using ICS therapy regularly. Of them, 19 (73%) demonstrated reversible airway obstruction. Of the 26 patients with reversible airway obstruction, only 7 (27%) were not using ICS therapy ($p = 0.01$) (Figure 2).

4. Discussion

In this study of individuals with PCD, post-bronchodilator reversible airway obstruction was a common finding. Reversibility of airflow was found to be significantly associated with prior documented recurrent wheezing. However, correlations were not found of reversible bronchial obstruction with atopy, elevated IgE, increased eosinophils, or a family history of atopy. This study highlights the relations of the consistent use of bronchodilators and ICS therapy, with the presence of reversible airway obstruction.

Of note, Phillips et al. [8] did not find a significant difference in the airway response to exercise after bronchodilators (Salbutamol), between healthy people and people with PCD. However, only 12 people were included in each group.

Airway reversibility was previously reported in about half of individuals with CF who were receiving bronchodilator therapy [9]. Galodé et al., reported higher prevalence of airway reversibility among younger patients: 73.5%, 48.5%, and 52.9%, in the 6–8 year, 10–12 year, and 15–17 year age groups, respectively. [10] Mitchell et al., reported a positive response to methacholine in 51% of patients with CF, compared to 98% of patients with a single diagnosis of asthma. [11] In that study, different dose–response curves highlighted differences between the pathophysiologic mechanisms of the two diseases. Van Haren et al. suggested a possible mechanism of increased vagal bronchomotor tone in CF, after demonstrating a bronchodilator response to ipratropium bromide following exercise. [12]

In contrast to the documentations in individuals with CF, [9] this study revealed no correlation between gender and airway reversibility among patients with PCD. However, similar to the study on CF, [9] this study found no correlations of airway reversibility with a family or personal history of asthma, or with atopy. The mechanisms suggested in both CF and PCD are not related to asthma.

Bronchial airway reversibility has also been described in non-CF bronchiectasis. Singh et al. showed bronchodilator reversibility in 30.4% of patients with non-CF bronchiectasis, even after excluding those with asthma, allergic bronchopulmonary aspergillosis, and chronic obstructive pulmonary disease, to avoid false-positive cases [13]. Furthermore,

Guan et al. observed that patients with other reasons for bronchiectasis, who exhibited significant bronchodilator reversibility, commonly shared a few important characteristics: a higher bronchiectasis severity index, a higher prevalence of *Pseudomonas aeruginosa* isolation and infection, and poorer lung function at baseline [14]. Therefore, chronic infection has been suggested as responsible for bronchial hyperreactivity in bronchiectasis [15]. Given its clinical significance, Bulcun et al., proposed that bronchial hyperreactivity should be considered part of routine clinical evaluation in all patients with bronchiectasis [16].

The reason and mechanism for airway reversibility after bronchodilator use in bronchiectasis, and in PCD specifically, is still unclear. The mechanism responsible for this reversibility is probably different from that in patients with asthma or CF. One hypothesis relates to chronic airway inflammation, and effects of toxins, through infected or inflamed bronchial mucosa, on bronchial muscle cells. Bronchial hyperreactivity possibly affects the clearance mechanism, and perpetuation of the cycle of colonization of microbes and subsequent inflammation [17].

Another hypothesis suggests that bronchodilators are responsible for slightly improving the residual function of cilia in patients with mild cilia mutations and symptoms. Bronchodilators are known for their ability to enhance mucociliary clearance, [18] and could be beneficial for patients with PCD who have some residual ciliary movement. One might ask whether the mucus removal effect that clears the airways between spirometries, before and after inhaled bronchodilators, may be the cause for such difference. These hypotheses should be re-evaluated in vitro.

As no curative option for PCD is currently available, treatment is directed at preventing and managing disease complications. No recommendations have been issued for the administration of bronchodilators, ICS, or combination therapy in the guidelines of PCD treatment. [18] Some studies presented substantial heterogeneity in the management of PCD, within and between countries [19].

We report that over half our patients used bronchodilators, and a similar proportion used ICS therapy. Likewise, another study found that ICS are commonly prescribed in PCD, often without evidence of type 2 airway inflammation [20]. The benefits of long-term bronchodilators or ICS treatment in patients with PCD have not been demonstrated.

Notably, the BESTCILIA multicenter trial showed dramatically reduced pulmonary exacerbations in patients with PCD treated with azithromycin than in a placebo group [21]. Macrolides are known to have bacteriostatic properties, as well as anti-inflammatory and immunomodulatory effects. Several studies have researched the use of azithromycin for treating other chronic respiratory suppurative diseases that are dominated by neutrophilic inflammation [22]. As the effectiveness of other treatments has recently been investigated, the long-term effects of bronchodilators and ICS should be further studied.

A strength of this study is its focus on objective measurements of maximal airway reversibility over the entire course of a patient's documented history. Additionally, the patient data were accessed from two large PCD centers.

Limitations of our study include those of any retrospective study design, the lack of a challenge test, variations in data availability among the numerous parameters investigated, and the limited utilization of pre- and post-bronchodilator spirometry. In addition, this study did not discern whether the maximal bronchodilator response occurred during a stable disease period, during an acute pulmonary exacerbation, or during a viral infection when a patient may be more prone to a positive response.

In addition to its presentation of the prevalence of bronchial reactivity among rare diseases such as PCD, this study raises the question as to whether spirometry tests before and after bronchodilators may lead to misdiagnosis of asthma instead of PCD. This issue is important due to the high frequency of spirometry performed worldwide, before and after bronchodilator use, to establish a diagnosis of asthma.

To conclude, reversible airway obstruction appears to be a central feature of PCD lung disease. At present, the associated pathophysiology is poorly understood. However, further research into this topic may inform future decision-making regarding inhaled bronchodilators and ICS therapy. Testing for bronchodilator response in bronchiectasis is important, as it can assess prognosis and guide treatment [14]. The presence of bronchodilator reversibility should be considered an indication for prescribing bronchodilators and ICS to all patients with PCD.

Author Contributions: Conceptualization, H.L. and O.B.-O.; Methodology, H.L.; Software, Y.D.; Formal analysis, Y.D.; Investigation, H.L., O.B.-O., V.N. and N.W.; Resources, O.B.-O., V.N., H.M. and D.P.; Data curation, H.L., V.N. and N.W.; Writing—original draft, H.L.; Writing—review & editing, O.B.-O., V.N., N.W., H.M. and D.P.; Supervision, D.P. All authors have read and agreed to the published version of the manuscript.

Funding: This research received no external funding.

Institutional Review Board Statement: The Rabin Medical Center and Hillel-Yaffe Medical Center Research Ethics Committees approved this retrospective study: *Rabin IRB number:* 0392-17-RMC; *Hillel-Yaffe IRB number:* 0087-22-HYMC.

Informed Consent Statement: Not applicable.

Data Availability Statement: Not applicable.

Conflicts of Interest: The authors declare no conflict of interest.

References

1. Lucas, J.S.; Davis, S.D.; Omran, H.; Shoemark, A. Primary ciliary dyskinesia in the genomics age. *Lancet Respir. Med.* **2020**, *8*, 202–216. [CrossRef]
2. Lucas, J.S.; Barbato, A.; Collins, S.A.; Goutaki, M.; Behan, L.; Caudri, D.; Dell, S.; Eber, E.; Escudier, E.; Hirst, R.A.; et al. European Respiratory Society guidelines for the diagnosis of primary ciliary dyskinesia. *Eur. Respir. J.* **2017**, *49*, 1601090. [CrossRef] [PubMed]
3. Piatti, G.; De Santi, M.M.; Farolfi, A.; Zuccotti, G.V.; D'Auria, E.; Patria, M.F.; Torretta, S.; Consonni, D.; Ambrosetti, U. Exacerbations and Pseudomonas aeruginosa colonization are associated with altered lung structure and function in primary ciliary dyskinesia. *BMC Pediatr.* **2020**, *20*, 158. [CrossRef] [PubMed]
4. Bousquet, J.; Jeffery, P.K.; Busse, W.W.; Johnson, M.; Vignola, A.M. Asthma from Bronchoconstriction to Airways Inflammation and Remodeling. *Am. J. Respir. Crit. Care Med.* **2000**, *161*, 1720–1745. [CrossRef]
5. Koh, Y.Y.; Park, Y.; Jeong, J.H.; Kim, C.K.; Min, Y.G.; Chi, J.G. The effect of regular salbutamol on lung function and bronchial responsiveness in patients with primary ciliary dyskinesia. *Chest* **2000**, *117*, 427–433. [CrossRef]
6. Miller, M.R.; Hankinson, J.A.; Brusasco, V.; Burgos, F.; Casaburi, R.; Coates, A.; Crapo, R.; Enright, P.; Van Der Grinten, C.P.; Gustafsson, P.; et al. Standardisation of spirometry. *Eur. Respir. J.* **2005**, *26*, 319–338. [CrossRef]
7. Pellegrino, R.; Viegi, G.; Brusasco, V.; Crapo, R.O.; Burgos, F.; Casaburi, R.E.; Coates, A.; Van Der Grinten, C.P.; Gustafsson, P.; Hankinson, J.; et al. Interpretative strategies for lung function tests. *Eur. Respir. J.* **2005**, *26*, 948–968. [CrossRef]
8. Phillips, G.E.; Thomas, S.; Heather, S.; Bush, A. Airway response of children with primary ciliary dyskinesia to exercise and β2-agonist challenge. *Eur. Respir. J.* **1998**, *11*, 1389–1391. [CrossRef]
9. Levine, H.; Cohen-Cymberknoh, M.; Klein, N.; Hoshen, M.; Mussaffi, H.; Stafler, P.; Breuer, O.; Kerem, E.; Blau, H. Reversible airway obstruction in cystic fibrosis: Common, but not associated with characteristics of asthma. *J. Cyst. Fibros.* **2016**, *15*, 652–659. [CrossRef]
10. Galodé, F.; Ladipo, O.; Andrieux, A.; Feghali, H.; Bui, S.; Fayon, M. Prevalence and Determinants of Wheezing and Bronchodilatation in Children with Cystic Fibrosis: A Retrospective Cohort Study. *Front. Pediatr.* **2022**, *10*, 856840. [CrossRef]
11. Eggleston, P.A.; Rosenstein, B.J.; Stackhouse, C.M.; Alexander, M.F. Airway Hyperreactivity in Cystic Fibrosis. *Chest* **1988**, *94*, 360–365. [CrossRef] [PubMed]
12. Van Haren, E.H.; Lammers, J.W.; Festen, J.; Van Herwaarden, C.L. Bronchial vagal tone and responsiveness to histamine, exercise and bronchodilators in adult patients with cystic fibrosis. *Eur. Respir. J.* **1992**, *5*, 1083–1088. [CrossRef] [PubMed]
13. Singh, P.; Katoch, C.S.; Vardhan, V.; Chopra, M.; Singh, S.; Ahuja, N. Functional impairment in bronchiectasis: Spirometry parameters versus St. George's Respiratory Questionnaire scores: Any co-relation? *Lung India* **2021**, *38*, 545–551. [CrossRef] [PubMed]
14. Guan, W.J.; Gao, Y.H.; Xu, G.; Li, H.M.; Yuan, J.J.; Zheng, J.P.; Chen, R.C.; Zhong, N.S. Bronchodilator response in adults with bronchiectasis: Correlation with clinical parameters and prognostic implications. *J. Thorac. Dis.* **2016**, *8*, 14–23. [CrossRef] [PubMed]
15. King, P.T.; Daviskas, E. Pathogenesis and diagnosis of bronchiectasis. *Breathe* **2010**, *6*, 342–351. [CrossRef]
16. Bulcun, E.; Arslan, M.; Ekici, A.; Ekici, M. Quality of life and bronchial hyper-responsiveness in subjects with bronchiectasis: Validation of the seattle obstructive lung disease questionnaire in bronchiectasis. *Respir. Care* **2015**, *60*, 1616–1623. [CrossRef]

17. Sevgili, S.; Hasanoğlu, H.C.; Karalezli, A.; Er, M. Bronchial reversibility in the patients with bronchiectasis. *Tuberk. Toraks* **2009**, *57*, 38–47.
18. Frohock, J.I.; Wijkstrom-Frei, C.; Salathe, M. Effects of albuterol enantiomers on ciliary beat frequency in ovine tracheal epithelial cells. *J. Appl. Physiol.* **2002**, *92*, 2396–2402. [CrossRef]
19. Strippoli, M.P.; Frischer, T.; Barbato, A.; Snijders, D.; Maurer, E.; Lucas, J.S.; Eber, E.; Karadag, B.; Pohunek, P.; Zivkovic, Z.; et al. Management of primary ciliary dyskinesia in European children: Recommendations and clinical practice. *Eur. Respir. J.* **2012**, *39*, 1482–1491. [CrossRef]
20. Dehlink, E.; Richardson, C.; Marsh, G.; Lee, K.; Jamalzadeh, A.; Bush, A.; Hogg, C.; Carr, S.B. Are inhaled corticosteroids prescribed rationally in primary ciliary dyskinesia? *Eur. Respir. J.* **2018**, *51*, 1702221. [CrossRef]
21. Kobbernagel, H.E.; Buchvald, F.F.; Haarman, E.G.; Casaulta, C.; Collins, S.A.; Hogg, C.; Kuehni, C.E.; Lucas, J.S.; Moser, C.E.; Quittner, A.L.; et al. Efficacy and safety of azithromycin maintenance therapy in primary ciliary dyskinesia (BESTCILIA): A multicentre, double-blind, randomised, placebo-controlled phase 3 trial. *Lancet Respir. Med.* **2020**, *8*, 493–505. [CrossRef]
22. Kanoh, S.; Rubin, B.K. Mechanisms of action and clinical application of macrolides as immunomodulatory medications. *Clin. Microbiol. Rev.* **2010**, *23*, 590–615. [CrossRef] [PubMed]

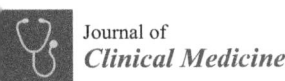

Article

Risk Factors Affecting Development and Persistence of Preschool Wheezing: Consensus Document of the Emilia-Romagna Asthma (ERA) Study Group

Roberto Grandinetti [1], Valentina Fainardi [1], Carlo Caffarelli [1], Gaia Capoferri [1], Angela Lazzara [1], Marco Tornesello [1], Aniello Meoli [1], Barbara Maria Bergamini [2], Luca Bertelli [3], Loretta Biserna [4], Paolo Bottau [5], Elena Corinaldesi [6], Nicoletta De Paulis [7], Arianna Dondi [3], Battista Guidi [8], Francesca Lombardi [9], Maria Sole Magistrali [7], Elisabetta Marastoni [10], Silvia Pastorelli [11], Alessandra Piccorossi [12], Maurizio Poloni [13], Sylvie Tagliati [14], Francesca Vaienti [15], Giuseppe Gregori [16], Roberto Sacchetti [16], Sandra Mari [17], Manuela Musetti [17], Francesco Antodaro [18], Andrea Bergomi [18], Lamberto Reggiani [19], Fabio Caramelli [20], Alessandro De Fanti [10], Federico Marchetti [4], Giampaolo Ricci [3], Susanna Esposito [1,*] and on behalf of the Emilia-Romagna Asthma (ERA) Study Group [†]

1. Pediatric Clinic, Department of Medicine and Surgery, University of Parma, 43126 Parma, Italy
2. Paediatric Unit, Department of Medical and Surgical Sciences of Mothers, Children and Adults, University of Modena and Reggio Emilia, 41125 Modena, Italy
3. Pediatric Clinic, Scientific Institute for Research and Healthcare (IRCCS) Azienda Ospedaliero-Universitaria di Bologna, 40138 Bologna, Italy
4. Paediatrics and Neonatology Unit, Ravenna Hospital, AUSL Romagna, 48121 Ravenna, Italy
5. Paediatrics Unit, Imola Hospital, 40026 Imola, Italy
6. Paediatric Unit, Carpi Hospital, 41012 Carpi, Italy
7. Paediatrics and Neonatology Unit, Guglielmo da Saliceto Hospital, 29121 Piacenza, Italy
8. Hospital and Territorial Paediatrics Unit, Pavullo, 41026 Pavullo Nel Frignano, Italy
9. Paediatrics Unit, Maggiore Hospital, 40133 Bologna, Italy
10. Paediatrics Unit, Santa Maria Nuova Hospital, AUSL-IRCCS of Reggio Emilia, 42123 Reggio Emilia, Italy
11. Paediatrics Unit, Sassuolo Hospital, 41049 Sassuolo, Italy
12. Paediatrics and Paediatric Intensive Care Unit, Cesena Hospital, AUSL Romagna, 47521 Cesena, Italy
13. Paediatrics Unit, Rimini Hospital, AUSL Romagna, 47921 Rimini, Italy
14. Paediatric Clinic, Ferrara Hospital, 44124 Ferrara, Italy
15. Paediatrics Unit, G.B. Morgagni—L. Pierantoni Hospital, AUSL Romagna, 47121 Forlì, Italy
16. Primary Care Pediatricians, AUSL Piacenza, 29121 Piacenza, Italy
17. Primary Care Pediatricians, AUSL Parma, 43126 Parma, Italy
18. Primary Care Pediatricians, AUSL Modena, 41125 Modena, Italy
19. Primary Care Pediatricians, AUSL Imola, 40026 Imola, Italy
20. Pediatric Intensive Care Unit, IRCCS Azienda Ospedaliero-Universitaria di Bologna, 40138 Bologna, Italy
* Correspondence: susannamariaroberta.esposito@unipr.it
† Membership of the ERA Study Group is provided in the Acknowledgments.

Abstract: Wheezing at preschool age (i.e., before the age of six) is common, occurring in about 30% of children before the age of three. In terms of health care burden, preschool children with wheeze show double the rate of access to the emergency department and five times the rate of hospital admissions compared with school-age asthmatics. The consensus document aims to analyse the underlying mechanisms involved in the pathogenesis of preschool wheezing and define the risk factors (i.e., allergy, atopy, infection, bronchiolitis, genetics, indoor and outdoor pollution, tobacco smoke exposure, obesity, prematurity) and the protective factors (i.e., probiotics, breastfeeding, vitamin D, influenza vaccination, non-specific immunomodulators) associated with the development of the disease in the young child. A multidisciplinary panel of experts from the Emilia-Romagna Region, Italy, addressed twelve key questions regarding managing preschool wheezing. Clinical questions have been formulated by the expert panel using the PICO format (Patients, Intervention, Comparison, Outcomes). Systematic reviews have been conducted on PubMed to answer these specific questions and formulate recommendations. The GRADE approach has been used for each selected paper to assess the quality of the evidence and the degree of recommendations. Based on a panel of experts and extensive updated literature, this consensus document provides insight into the pathogenesis, risk and protective factors associated with the development and persistence of preschool wheezing. Undoubtedly, more research is needed to improve our understanding of the disease and confirm the associations between certain factors and the risk of wheezing in early life. In addition, preventive strategies must be promoted to avoid children's exposure to risk factors that may permanently affect respiratory health.

Keywords: allergen sensitization; episodic viral wheezing; multiple trigger wheezing; paediatric pulmonology; wheezing

1. Introduction

Wheezing at preschool age (i.e., before age six) is common, occurring in about 30% of children before age three [1]. In terms of health care burden, preschool children with wheeze show a doubled rate of emergency department access and five times the rate of hospital admissions compared with school-age asthmatics [2]. An audit performed in the UK among children with acute wheezing/asthma admitted to the hospital showed that wheezing only with colds was common in younger children peaking at around three years, whereas children between 12 and 24 months of age accounted for a quarter of admissions [3].

Preschool wheezing can be described as a multifactorial disease influenced by various genetic and environmental factors. At present, the understanding of the pathophysiology and risk factors that contribute to the onset and persistence of wheezing in preschool children is limited. Increasing evidence shows that it is a combination of different factors that contribute to the development of wheezing. Early viral infections [4], bacterial colonisation [5] and allergen sensitisation [6] are among the most important in causing wheeze and the subsequent development of asthma. These early life exposures, coupled with genetically determined susceptibility, can affect the immune system in the early stages of life and have a major impact on the natural history of the disease. In particular, early and multiple sensitisation predicts a severe asthma trajectory [7]. Identifying risk factors may allow the identification of measures and interventions to prevent the development of preschool wheezing and, eventually, its evolution into childhood asthma.

This consensus document aims to analyse the underlying mechanisms involved in the pathogenesis of preschool wheezing and define the risk factors (i.e., allergy, atopy, infection, bronchiolitis, genetics, indoor and outdoor pollution, tobacco smoke exposure, obesity, prematurity) and the protective factors (i.e., breastfeeding, vitamin D, probiotics) associated with the development of the disease in the young child.

2. Materials and Methods

We set up a multidisciplinary panel of experts that included all the Heads of the Paediatric Units of Emilia-Romagna Region, Italy, the Heads of the outpatient clinics for pulmonology and allergology, a sample of primary care paediatricians (identified in each province based on the number of the paediatric population according to ISTAT 2018 data) and a patients' association (Respiro Libero, Parma, Italy). This study group (named Emilia-Romagna Asthma Study Group and described in detail in a previous publication on the management of children with acute asthma attacks [8] included members with previous experience in the development of documents and recommendations with the Grading of Recommendations Assessment, Development, and Evaluation [9,10].

In order to assess risk factors and protective factors influencing the development of preschool wheezing, clinical questions have been formulated by the expert panel using the PICO format (Patients, Intervention, Comparison, Outcomes). Systematic reviews have been conducted on PubMed from January 2008 to December 2021 using different search strategies focused on wheezing pathogenesis (in particular atopy and respiratory infections), risk factors associated with preschool wheeze onset or persistence and protective factors that may reduce the risk of developing the disease. Prospective or retrospective cohort and case-control studies were included. Included studies investigated patients <6 years of age (preschool age). Letters, comments, editorials and case reports were excluded. Only full manuscripts published in the English language were included. Search strategies and extended evidence tables are available in Supplementary Material S1.

Clinical questions were divided into 3 sections:

(1) Pathogenesis of preschool wheezing

Question 1. What is the role of infection in the pathogenesis of preschool wheezing?
Question 2. What is the role of atopy in the pathogenesis of preschool wheezing?

(2) Risk factors for wheeze development

Question 3. Does the presence of risk factors such as allergy/atopy influence the onset and the evolution of preschool wheezing?
Question 4. Does the presence of risk factors such as previous respiratory tract infection/bronchiolitis influence the onset and evolution of preschool wheezing?
Question 5. Does pollution influence the onset and evolution of preschool wheezing?
Question 6. Does genetics influence the onset and the evolution of preschool wheezing?
Question 7. Does obesity influence the onset and the evolution of preschool wheezing?
Question 8. Do prematurity and other perinatal factors influence the onset and the evolution of preschool wheezing?
Question 9. Does smoke exposure influence the onset and the evolution of preschool wheezing?
Question 10. Is immunodeficiency a risk factor for the onset and the evolution of preschool wheezing?

(3) Protective factors for wheeze development:

Question 11. Are probiotics protective for preschool wheezing development?
Question 12. Is vitamin D supplementation protective for preschool wheezing development?
Question 13. Is breastfeeding protective for preschool wheezing development?
Question 14. Is influenza vaccination protective for preschool wheezing development?
Question 15. Are non-specific immunomodulators protective for preschool wheezing development?

The GRADE approach has been used for each selected paper to assess the confidence in the evidence (quality) and the degree of recommendations [11]. Recommendations are graded as strong or weak after considering the quality of the evidence, the balance of desirable and undesirable consequences of compared management options, the assumptions about the relative importance of outcomes, the implications for resource use, and the acceptability and feasibility of implementation [12]. The panel then decided on the strength of the recommendations. A dedicated voting process (collection of voting forms through individual email messages) was developed for the present guidelines, and an online meeting with the participation of the full voting panel was organized. More specifically, voting panel members were provided with the results of the various literature searches, the evidence summaries, the proposed recommendations, and the related GRADE tables. Each voting member was then allowed to individually vote in favour or against each recommendation, propose possible modifications, and judge each recommendation as strong or weak according to GRADE rules. For recommendations with an agreement of <75%, further voting rounds were conducted after implementing dedicated amendments based on the provided comments. After reaching an agreement of ≥75% for all recommendations, all the authors reviewed and approved the final manuscript and Supplementary Material S1.

3. Results

3.1. Pathogenesis of Preschool Wheezing

3.1.1. PICO Question 1. What Is the Role of Infection in the Pathogenesis of Preschool Wheezing?

Executive Summary

In young children, viral infections are the most important triggers of wheezing, particularly for the phenotype called episodic viral wheezing (EVW). These viral infections are mostly due to human rhinovirus (HRV), respiratory syncytial virus (RSV), human metapneumovirus (HMPV) and influenza virus (IV) [13–16]. If respiratory tract infections (RTIs) are the main reason for wheeze development is unclear. Some studies suggested that certain children are more prone to be severely infected because of dysregulation of the innate immune response, such as low antiviral interferon-gamma (IFN-γ) production in response to viral infection or structural airway pathologies [17]. Interestingly, Chawes et al. showed that bronchial hyperresponsiveness in at-risk neonates precedes severe acute bronchiolitis in response to respiratory viral infections [18].

HRV is the most commonly identified virus involved in wheezing exacerbations in preschool and school-aged children [19]. HRV is usually predominant in patients with no history of wheezing [14]. HRV infection at one year of age has been proven to be the strongest predictor for wheezing episodes at three years of age [14,20–22] and recurrent wheezing development [13,15,16,23–25]. HRV infections may increase airway sensitisation and inflammation by different mechanisms: altering the epithelial barrier [26], inducing the release of epithelial cytokines (i.e., interleukin [IL]-25 and IL-33) with T-helper (Th2) inflammation and production of IL-4, IL-5 and IL-13 [27], stimulating the production of granulocyte-macrophage colony-stimulating factor (GM-CSF), IL-6, IL-8, IL-1α, IL-1β and eventually contributing to airway remodelling by stimulating angiogenesis and differentiation of myofibroblasts with the release of extracellular matrix proteins [28,29].

On the other hand, RSV is the most frequent cause of lower RTI, mainly bronchiolitis, in infants [19]. Several epidemiological studies demonstrated that a history of severe RSV bronchiolitis is associated with subsequent persistent wheezing, childhood asthma or both [10,26]. RSV infection causes necrosis of the bronchiolar epithelium with subsequent submucosal oedema, recruitment of polymorphonuclear leukocytes and massive release of pro-inflammatory mediators, increased mucus secretion and bronchoconstriction. The disproportionate release of pro-inflammatory mediators induces a massive infiltration of monocytes and polymorphonuclear cells that may impair the immune response with a switch towards a Th1 response and a reduced IFN-γ-dependent viral clearance [30].

Respiratory viral infections may precede bacterial colonisation, as shown by positive nasopharyngeal culture for at least one bacterium among *Moraxella catarrhalis*, *Haemophilus influenzae* or *Streptococcus pneumoniae* in 60% of patients with respiratory symptoms lasting more than ten days [31]. The evidence on the role of airway bacterial colonisation and airway microbiome in wheeze and asthma pathogenesis is constantly increasing, with several studies showing that children with preschool wheeze have lower airway infection or colonisation with pathogens like *M. catarrhalis*, *H. influenzae* or *S. pneumoniae* [5,32–36].

In the prospective cohort Childhood Asthma Study (CAS), viral RTIs in the first two years of life have been associated with the prevalence of *M. catarrhalis*, *S. pneumoniae* and *H. influenzae* and persistent wheeze at five years old in those with early allergic sensitisation [36]. Schwerk and colleagues demonstrated with a retrospective analysis that patients with recurrent or persistent wheeze presented chronic bacterial colonisation with bronchoalveolar lavage (BAL) cultured positive for *H. influenzae*, *S. pneumoniae* and *M. catarrhalis* and airway neutrophilia [33]. This finding suggested that children with severe wheezing may be early colonised and may be particularly susceptible to these pathogens, leading to neutrophilia and chronic infection unresponsive to inhaled corticosteroids (ICS) [37]. However, randomised controlled trials showed no difference in the number of wheeze episodes and the need for oral corticosteroids in children treated with antibiotics [38,39].

Moreover, a significant relationship between *Mycoplasma pneumoniae* and *Chlamydophila pneumoniae* with wheezing in preschool children, particularly in subjects with a history of recurrent episodes, has been reported [40]. Children with wheezing and acute *M. pneumoniae* infection seem to have a specific cytokine profile characterised by a significant increase in serum levels of IL-5 [41].

Aberrant respiratory microbiota was evident since birth in children experiencing more than two episodes of respiratory tract infections suggesting a trajectory starting from the first month of life. These patients showed a decreased microbial community stability, a prolonged reduction of *Corynebacterium* and *Dolosigranulum*, and enrichment of *Moraxella* spp. [42]. A complex interplay between environmental factors and genetic predisposition is considered to shape the lung and gut microbiome in early life [43,44].

Recommendation 1. There is evidence that mainly viruses can trigger wheezing in young children. RSV and HRV are the main viruses involved in wheezing pathogenesis. Quality of evidence: Moderate.

3.1.2. PICO Question 2. What Is the Role of Atopy in the Pathogenesis of Preschool Wheezing?

Executive Summary

Compared to school-age asthma, which is typically allergic and characterised by type 2 inflammation, little is known about the immunopathology of preschool wheeze. Many children with EVW are not atopic, show bacterial or viral infection in the airways and do not benefit significantly from corticosteroids that are usually effective in allergic asthma, suggesting allergy is not the main driver of disease [44]. On the other hand, children with severe recurrent multi-trigger wheezing may be atopic and have evidence of increased numbers of eosinophils in BAL and endobronchial biopsies [44–47]. These children might be at higher risk of developing asthma at a later age [46]. Asthma and atopy share many genetic risk variants that dysregulate the expression of immune-related genes [48,49].

Lower airway eosinophilia suggests corticosteroid responsiveness, and in support of this, persistent wheezers show some benefit while taking ICS [7]. A prospective cross-sectional study performed by Guiddir et al. analysed airway inflammation with BAL and characterized a phenotype of severe recurrent wheezers with sensitisation to aeroallergen and response to ICS [50], suggesting that preschool wheezers with aeroallergen sensitization may also have lower airway eosinophilia. Three-year-old children with multi-trigger wheezing showed the classic pathological features of asthma, like submucosal eosinophilia and reticular basement membrane (RBM) thickening [37,47,50,51].

In a prospective study, Just et al. investigated the critical thresholds of common biological markers of atopy in persistent wheezy infants [52]. A cohort of infants (n = 219, <30 months old) with recurrent wheezing were enrolled and followed up until the age of 6. Blood eosinophilia (blood count $\geq 470/mm^3$) and elevated IgE (total serum IgE level ≥ 45 IU/mL) during infancy were associated with persistent wheezing at six years of age. The main discriminative parameter of wheezing persistence was eosinophilia: lack of eosinophilia in infancy could account for 91% of subjects in remission when combined with the absence of allergic sensitisation remission correctly predicted in 96.9% of the study population [52]. Children with aeroallergen sensitisation and/or blood eosinophils >300 cells/mm^3 showed the greatest response to daily ICS in the Individualized Therapy for Asthma in Toddlers (INFANT) [53].

The role of IgE was also assessed during wheezing exacerbation in an observational study by Jartti et al. [54]. In 247 children hospitalised for wheezing (median age 1.6 years), atopy and number of exacerbations were closely related to HRV etiology (OR 4.59; 95% CI 1.78–11.8), followed by aeroallergen sensitisation (OR 4.18; 95% CI 2.00, 8.72), total IgE level (OR 2.06; 95% CI 1.32–3.21), food allergen sensitisation (OR 2.02; 95% CI 1.08, 3.78) and nasal eosinophil count (OR 1.52; 95% CI 1.08–2.13) [54]. Nasal eosinophils were found to increase during RTI in a cohort of 35 young children (age range, 6–33 months) and, after adjustment for age, sex, family history, and allergies were predictive of further episodes of wheezing over the subsequent two months (adjusted OR: 27.618, p = 0.016) [55]. Eosinophils were found to also increase in the sputum of preschoolers with severe wheeze and were associated with high blood eosinophil count, high serum total IgE and high allergen detection rate [56].

On the other hand, Ater et al. did not show any difference in sputum eosinophilia between preschoolers with wheezing and healthy peers but demonstrated that wheezers had higher asthma predictive index (S-API) and greater bronchial hyperresponsiveness [57].

Similarly, a positive API was associated with a higher risk of recurrent wheezing in infants (OR: 5.57; 95%; CI 2.23–7.96) [58].

The role of atopy may start early in utero, as suggested by an interesting case-control study where the cord blood of newborns at risk of atopy (family history of asthma) was stimulated for T cell cytokine production. At two years of age, children with wheezing presented increased production of T-cell cytokines IL-2 and IL-5, with IL-5 being the strongest risk factor associated with the development of wheeze (OR: 35; 95% CI, 5.0–246.7) [59].

Recommendation 2. Recurrent multi-trigger wheezing often presents a severe clinical spectrum, can be associated with atopy more frequently than EVW and might expose the child to a higher risk of developing asthma at a later age. Aeroallergen sensitisation and blood eosinophils can be used as biomarkers to identify responses to ICS in a recurrent preschool wheeze.
Quality of evidence: Moderate.

3.2. Risk Factors for Wheeze Development

3.2.1. PICO Question 3. Does the Presence of Risk Factors Such as Allergy/Atopy Influence the Onset and the Evolution of Preschool Wheezing?
Executive Summary

Multiple aeroallergen sensitisations are associated with persistent wheezing and progression to asthma [60,61]. Atopy and allergy have a pivotal role as risk factors in preschool wheezing, as shown by many studies conducted all over the past years.

In the Urban Environment and Childhood Asthma (URECA) longitudinal birth cohort study, cumulative exposure over the first three years of life to cockroach, mouse and house dust mite allergens in the home environment was associated with sensitisation to those allergens at age three and sensitisation was associated with recurrent wheeze at three years [62]. Particularly, a strong association has been found between atopy and the intermediate onset of wheezing (onset after 18 months of life) [63]. Furthermore, high blood eosinophil count ($\geq 470/\text{mm}^3$), allergic sensitisation and a family member (father) with asthma have been implicated in the persistence of wheezing [64]. A sex-dependent association between parental allergic conditions (asthma) and the prevalence of wheezing in offspring has been found: maternal asthma seems to be associated with asthma in girls but not in boys, while the opposite is seen for paternal asthma [65].

Wheeze, allergic rhinitis and atopic eczema were more frequent in children with high total and specific IgE [66]. In particular, anti-cockroach and anti-mouse IgE were specifically linked with the risk of developing both wheezing and atopy [67]. Interestingly, good control of allergic rhinitis reduced the risk of acute exacerbation of wheezing in the first six years of age [68].

A further correlation has been suggested between eczema and wheezing: eczema, and especially early eczema, has been associated with an increased risk of childhood asthma [69,70] but also with an increased risk of developing allergic airway diseases later in life [71]. Furthermore, the risk of developing asthma increases when eczema is combined with wheezing episodes in infancy [72]. Another study has combined eczema and sensitisation to inhaled allergens with hospital admissions for wheezing in the first three years of life, thus resulting in eczema as a strong predictor of asthma [73]. The combination of eczema and food allergy was associated with an increased risk of asthma at age four years, and this risk was higher if the allergy was proven for two or more foods [74].

Interestingly, Illi et al. investigated the pattern of atopic sensitisation typically associated with the development of asthma in childhood, showing that sensitisation to any allergen early in life and sensitised to inhalant allergens by the age of seven years was associated with a significantly increased risk of being asthmatic and maternal transmission may determine both a certain pattern of sensitisation and the expression of asthma [75]. Moreover, they showed that the chronic course of asthma characterised by airway hyper-responsiveness and impairment of lung function at school age is determined by continuing allergic airway inflammation beginning in the first three years of life [76]. However, children with a non-atopic wheezing phenotype lose their symptoms over school age and retain normal lung function at puberty.

Recommendation 3. Young children with recurrent wheezing and atopic eczema, sensitised to allergens or blood eosinophilia, are at higher risk of asthma at a later age. Quality of evidence: High.

3.2.2. PICO Question 4. Does the Presence of Risk Factors Such as Previous Respiratory Tract Infection or Bronchiolitis Influence the Onset and the Evolution of Preschool Wheezing?

Executive Summary

By applying metatranscriptomic, transcriptomic, and metabolomic approaches to infants with bronchiolitis, recent studies found an interplay between major pathogens, their function, and host response in the airway, and their longitudinal relationship with asthma development [42,43].

Viral RTIs occurring early in life have been accounted for as important triggers of wheezing episodes in infancy, and many studies have shown an association with the subsequent development of persistent wheezing in preschool age. A meta-analysis including 22 cohort studies assessed the association between wheezing and lower RTIs (LRTIs) in childhood, demonstrating that LRTIs before three years of age increased the risk of wheezing development not only in childhood but also in adolescence and adulthood [77]. Other observational studies showed that LRTIs occurring during the first three years of life were associated with increased wheezing episodes and overall respiratory morbidity (i.e., bronchitis, pneumonia) in the following two years [18,78–80]. This was particularly evident in children with a family history of atopy or allergy. The risk of developing wheezing following an LRTI like bronchiolitis increases for children with congenital heart disease [81] or children exposed to tobacco smoke [82].

Bronchiolitis is one of the commonest LRTIs in infancy. Epidemiological data show that 3–5% of infants develop severe bronchiolitis requiring hospitalization during their first year of life and that more than 30% will develop recurrent wheezing and asthma [83]. Being hospitalized for bronchiolitis in the first year of life can be a risk factor for preschool wheezing [84,85], particularly in children with respiratory comorbidities and atopy [86]. The need for intensive care for RSV-induced bronchiolitis or severe infections RSV-related were associated with an increased risk of recurrent wheezing episodes by age three years and asthma by age four years [87,88]. Two systematic reviews and other observational studies confirmed the association between RSV infection requiring hospitalization in infancy and wheezing or asthma development [89–92]. Similar results were obtained when studying children born preterm [93–95]. Recently, a large retrospective study on 68,130 infants reported that those (30.7%) hospitalized for RSV-bronchiolitis had more than a 2-fold risk of developing recurrent in the first year of age [96]. A recent meta-analysis of 35 studies estimated the effect of RSV infections on later wheezing as OR 4.17 (95% CI 2.36–7.37), but after adjustment for genetic and environmental influences, the effect size reduced by about 50% (aOR 2.45 (95% CI 1.23–4.88), suggesting that the association was non-causal [97].

Despite the results of one study where no association was found between other viruses different from RSV and recurrent wheezing at five years [94], increasing evidence shows that HRV is deeply implicated in the development of wheezing and asthma later in life. HRV infection is the most common cause of LRTI and wheezing after six months of age [98] and the most common trigger of acute preschool wheeze episodes [99]. A prospective cohort study comparing the clinical differences between HRV and RSV-induced wheezing showed that children infected by HRV experienced wheezing more often and earlier than children infected by RSV [100]. HRV infection increases the risk of wheezing requiring hospital admission [101], and the risk of wheezing episodes in the following year [25]. If HRV results in bronchiolitis in atopic subjects, there is a major risk of developing recurrent wheezing and subsequent asthma, compared to RSV-infected atopic subjects [102,103]. A recent meta-analysis summarized this evidence and showed that children with HRV-bronchiolitis were more likely to develop recurrent wheeze than subjects affected by RSV-bronchiolitis (OR 4.11; 95% CI 2.24–7.56) [101].

A single prospective cohort study by Reimerink et al. investigated the relationship between early intestinal viral infections and the development of eczema, wheeze and atopic sensitization during the first and the second year of life [104]. Seropositivity for immunoglobulin (Ig)G for Rota- and Norovirus (GGI.1 and GGII.4) at one year of age was related to early allergic sensitization (specific IgE), parental reported eczema and wheeze in the first two years of life. Furthermore, Rotavirus seropositivity was associated with an unexpectedly higher risk of recurrent wheeze in the first and second year of life and persistent and new recurrent wheeze (adjusted OR 2.7 and 95% CI 1.1–6.2) [104].

Recommendation 4. Infants with bronchiolitis represent a high-risk group for recurrent wheezing. Quality of evidence: High.

3.2.3. PICO Question 5. Does Pollution Influence the Onset and the Evolution of Preschool Wheezing?
Executive Summary

Environmental pollution has been consistently associated with negative effects on the respiratory health of children [105]. Children are particularly sensitive to the damages of inhaled pollution since they undergo rapid lung growth, have higher respiratory rates and have the greatest exposure since they spend most time outdoor [105]. However, most of the studies on the association between pollution and wheeze development consist of observational studies.

Increasing attention has been paid to traffic-related air pollution (TRAP) as a risk factor for respiratory diseases. Some studies suggested that exposure to moderate levels of TRAP can favour the development of persistent wheezing [106,107], but the duration of the exposition seems crucial. Exposition to pollutants in the first four years of life leads to an increased risk of wheezing exacerbations, although only a continuous exposition in the first seven years may lead to the development of asthma [108]. Other studies confirmed that a certain degree of correlation exists between TRAP and the incidence of preschool wheezing but not with the incidence of asthma [109]. TRAP exposure may be implicated in more frequent and severe exacerbations in children already suffering from recurrent wheezing, whereas living in green areas may be protective [110].

Some studies on ex vivo bronchial epithelial cells confirm a direct correlation between air pollution, viral infections and wheezing exacerbations. Short-term exposure to high levels of nitrogen dioxide (NO_2) and particulate matter (PM)10 may favour wheezing since this exposure seems associated with reduced interferon-β response to viral infections [111]. The same group demonstrated that in children with wheezing, prolonged exposure to PM10 correlated with RBM thickness and airway eosinophilia, likely contributing to the development of asthma by airway remodelling and inflammation [112].

Other studies have focused particularly on the type and levels of TRAP, trying to deduce differences between different pollutants. Some studies have not found specificity considering PM2.5, PM10 or NO_2 levels involved in wheezing exacerbations [113], while others have found certain differences. Particles with lower diameters (especially PM1 and PM2.5) are associated with higher risk than particles with bigger diameters [114,115]. The role of pollutants deriving from industrial emissions (oil refineries, metals smelters or others types of industry) has been assessed in an interesting study where the exposure has been linked to hospital admission for wheezing diseases [116].

Since defining the burden of a single pollutant on wheeze development is very difficult, studies often take into account the role of co-variables. In a wide case-control study [114], the combination of parental asthma, parental education, maternal smoking during pregnancy, and TRAP has been linked to an increased risk of developing persistent wheezing and asthma. Moreover, RNA-based epigenetic mechanisms—mainly microRNA post-transcriptional regulation—could serve as key epigenetic mediators of the link between air pollution and asthma [117–119]. Heterogeneity in the definitions of TRAP exposure and asthma outcomes has led to confusion in the field [118,119]. However, novel information regarding the molecular characterization of asthma phenotypes, TRAP exposure assessment methods, and epigenetics are revolutionizing the field.

The so-called indoor pollution also has a role in affecting respiratory health. Some studies have investigated household indicators of dampness (visible mould spots, window pane condensation or damp stains) and found they were associated with preschool wheezing [113,120], in particular with early onset wheezing and delayed remission. In a comprehensive prospective cohort Japanese study, mould growth and wood stove/fireplace were related with significantly higher ORs for wheezing (mould growth: 1.13; 95% CI, 1.06–1.22; wood stove/fireplace: 1.23; 95% CI, 1.03–1.46) [121]. The use of household chemicals and other cleaning products may also have a role in respiratory outcomes, but the evidence is still scant [122,123].

Particular attention should be paid to the prenatal and perinatal periods. Urbanization levels (according to various indicators), alongside sex, age and geographic region, have been significantly associated with prematurity and wheezing exacerbations [124]. Furthermore, prenatal exposure to certain molecules (high-molecular-weight phthalates, bisphenol-A) might give rise to wheezing symptoms and respiratory tract infections throughout childhood and asthma later in life [125].

Recommendation 5. Traffic-related air pollution may favour wheezing via a reduced response to viral infections. Both outdoor and indoor pollution can influence the respiratory health of young children from conception and birth.
Quality of evidence: Moderate.

3.2.4. PICO Question 6. Does Genetics Influence the Onset and the Evolution of Preschool Wheezing?
Executive Summary

Genome-wide association studies (GWAS) on preschool wheezing have been gradually published over the years, and evidence has begun to emerge regarding specific loci of susceptibility involved in this disease. Single nucleotide polymorphisms (SNPs) have been identified, and a specific locus of chromosome 17 (17q12-q21) has been the object of many studies [126–133].

One study has linked an SNP, rs7216389, with an increased risk of recurrent wheezing but also with asthma and asthma exacerbations [126]. This correlation is present from preschool to school age, but its role has been ascertained only for early-onset disease and not late-onset. A case-control study goes in the same direction, linking rs7216389 SNP with early-onset wheezing (until five years of age) but not with adult-onset asthma [127].

Many studies have focused on the association of SNPs of inflammatory cytokines with preschool wheezing. IL-10 rs1800896 SNP (in heterozygosity state) is significantly associated with the development of preschool wheezing after a severe LRTI in early infancy [128]. On the other hand, homozygosity for rs1800896 allele G (genotype G/G) represents a protective factor from asthma development [128]. Another SNP regarding IL-4, rs2070874 and specifically the genotype T/T, has been associated with a severe phenotype of viral-induced wheeze [129].

Studies on IL receptors have also been conducted. The homozygous variant of IRAK4 (IL-1 receptor-associated kinase-4), rs4251513, has been constantly associated with post-bronchiolitis wheezing episodes and asthma medication use at school-age [130]. IL-10, IL-4, IRAK-4 and many others are implicated in the inflammation pathways leading to viral respiratory infections.

Some genetic studies have also investigated the role of Toll-like receptors (TLR) after bronchiolitis. In particular, TLR-1 SNP rs5743618 has been associated with increased asthma prevalence during the first six years of life if bronchiolitis had been contracted within the first six years of life [131]. However, TLR-2 SNP rs5743708 did not show any correlation with wheezing [131]. In addition, an SNP in TLR-10, rs4129009, has been associated with preschool wheezing after an episode of bronchiolitis in infancy [132].

Other molecules have been investigated to better explain wheezing development in certain subjects. A case-control study conducted in preschool wheezers prospectively followed until six years of age found that intercellular adhesion molecule 1 (ICAM-1) SNP rs5498 was positively associated with asthma development [133]. A study on filaggrin (FLG) loss-of-function mutations highlighted its role in the pathogenesis of asthma and food sensitization [134].

However, although numerous studies investigated genetic susceptibility, the evidence of important genes being responsible for preschool asthma is low.

Recommendation 6. Some individuals have a genetic susceptibility and are predisposed to develop preschool wheezing at first and eventually asthma later in life. At present, little can be done to modify genetic susceptibility, but environmental exposures can be adjusted to reduce this risk and potentially work on primary asthma prevention. Quality of evidence: Low.

3.2.5. PICO Question 7. Does Obesity Influence the Onset and the Evolution of Preschool Wheezing?

Executive Summary

Obesity is an important risk factor and a disease modifier for many respiratory diseases, including childhood asthma. This condition increases susceptibility to respiratory infections and hospitalization [135].

Excessive weight gain in early life is considered a risk factor for wheezing in preterm and term babies. Preterm babies are at particular risk for this condition since they often experience the so-called catch-up growth, an increased growth rate following low birth weight and intrauterine growth retardation. In a cohort of children born preterm, accelerated foetal growth between the first trimester of pregnancy and birth was associated with increased wheeze-ever [136]. Compared to term-born children without weight gain in the first nine months of life, children born preterm (≤32 weeks of gestational age) with rapid weight gain had a fivefold higher risk of wheeze-ever (OR 5.04; 95% CI 3.36–7.54) [136].

Kotecha et al. specifically studied the effect of catch-up growth on wheezing phenotype, which was associated with early wheezing but not with persistent or late wheezing, suggesting that different mechanisms, such as atopy, may be more important in later age [137]. Rapid weight gain in early life may lead to impaired growth of the lungs, a condition known as dysanapsis, whereby somatic growth exceeds that of lung growth [137]. In addition, the adipose tissue may release pro-inflammatory mediators like leptin, which have been associated with airway remodelling [138].

A similar risk and lower lung function were also found in children born at term with rapid weight gain in early life [139,140]. Some longitudinal studies have investigated the relationship between overweight and respiratory diseases in toddlers and older children [141–144]. A prospective cohort study of 731 children aged three to eight found that increased body mass index (BMI) at three and five years of age was associated with a higher risk of recurrent wheezing with no differences between girls and boys [142]. This was not true in the eight-year-old group, where an increased BMI was associated with an increased risk of recurrent wheezing in girls but not boys [142]. Data analysis from the combination of eight different prospective birth cohort studies, including 12,050 children, demonstrated that children with rapid BMI gain in the first two years of life were at higher risk for incident asthma up to age 6 compared with children with less pronounced weight gain slope in early childhood [143]. In the CHILD Cohort Study including 3154 children followed up from three months to five years of age, higher BMI at one year of age remained an independent risk factor for all the wheeze trajectories (transient wheeze, intermediate-onset wheeze and infantile-onset persistent wheeze) after adjustment for other factors [144].

Recommendation 7. Rapid weight gain in infancy and high BMI is associated with an increased risk of wheezing in preschool age.
Quality of evidence: Low.

3.2.6. PICO Question 8. Do Prematurity and Other Perinatal Factors Influence the Onset and the Evolution of Preschool Wheezing?

Executive Summary

In addressing birth-related risk factors for wheezing and asthma, the impact of premature birth must be considered. The prevalence of premature birth (<37 weeks gestation) is about 10% worldwide [145]. Over the years, many studies investigated the association between gestational age and childhood wheezing disorders [146–149], showing that preterm birth was associated with an increased risk of wheezing [147,148,150]. The population is usually stratified in very preterm (<32 weeks of gestation), late preterm (32–36 weeks of gestation), early term (36–38 weeks of gestation) and term (38–41 weeks of gestation) infants and findings show that the risk of wheezing is proportional to prematurity with the highest risk in children born very preterm, particularly if they develop bronchopulmonary dysplasia [147,148,150,151].

When preterm birth is combined with a personal history of atopy and living with two or more children, the risk of recurrent wheezing increases [152]. However, when interpreting these findings as suggested by a systematic review and meta-analysis on this topic, several factors (i.e., sex, maternal smoking, restricted growth and parental atopy or asthma) may confound the association between preterm birth and wheezing disorders since for example, maternal smoking may be a trigger both for preterm birth and for wheezing as well as intrauterine growth restriction [148].

A growing body of literature has highlighted the importance of prenatal and perinatal factors on the subsequent development of recurrent wheezing and asthma. Considering prenatal factors, many studies sustained that an increased risk of childhood wheezing disorders may begin as early as an in utero exposure to maternal ascending infection [153], chorioamnionitis [154], mother's quality of life (QoL) [155], stress [156–158] or depression [155]. Furthermore, a correlation between caesarean delivery (CD) and the risk of developing wheezing in the first three years and asthma in the first four years has been hypothesized [159,160]. Moreover, asthma exacerbations during pregnancy in women with asthma showed an increased risk of early childhood respiratory disorders in their children [161]. All these factors can result in smaller airways, altered foetal immune responses and low birth weight. Birth weight is one of the main predictors of lung function in infants [162], children [163] and also in later age as demonstrated by the linear relationship with lung function at age 45–50 years found in the Aberdeen Birth cohort [164]. Furthermore, low birth weight, particularly if associated with intrauterine growth restriction, is a well-known risk factor for wheezing and asthma [165]. Perinatal factors, including infections, hyperoxia, and mechanical ventilation, are all associated with premature birth and negatively impact lung development and airway reactivity [148].

Overall, children born preterm experience disruptions in lung development and may experience significant shifts from the physiologic lung function trajectory and are at higher risk for respiratory morbidity throughout life [166]. Especially children born very preterm (<28 weeks of gestational age) are at the highest risk for bronchopulmonary dysplasia and can show obstructive patterns in lung function, eventually developing chronic obstructive pulmonary disease in adult age [166].

Recommendation 8. Preterm birth and low birth weight are important early life risk factors for wheezing disorders in childhood. Extremely preterm infants are at the highest risk for respiratory problems and may have lower lung function trajectories across all ages. Quality of evidence: Moderate.

3.2.7. PICO Question 9. Does Smoke Exposure Influence the Onset and the Evolution of Preschool Wheezing?

Executive Summary

The largest body of evidence on environmental risk factors affecting wheeze development relates to cigarette smoking. Tobacco smoke exposure antenatally in utero was associated with reduced lung function at birth [158] and later in life [167], with wheezing and asthma in childhood [168] and more globally with negative interference in lung function and life trajectories [169,170].

Two large independent meta-analyses documented maternal smoking and passive smoke exposure confer the risk of wheezing and asthma in preschool children, particularly children with a family history of allergy [171]. The risk was highest in children exposed to both passive smoking and mothers smoking actively during pregnancy [171,172]. In a recent French study, 129 infants under two years admitted to the hospital for acute wheezing were assessed for prenatal smoke exposure [173]. Children exposed (36.4%) had a longer length of hospital stay, and the authors estimated that smoking one cigarette/day during pregnancy was associated with an increase in hospitalization duration of 0.055 days/month ($r = 0.238$, $p = 0.006$) [173]. Consequences of prenatal and postnatal smoke exposure on wheezing in childhood have also been confirmed in two recent case-control studies [174,175]. A prospective birth cohort study found that the combination of prematurity and maternal smoking during pregnancy synergistically increases recurrent wheezing and the number of episodes in early childhood [176]. However, future studies are needed to define better and quantify the exposure level since heavy parental smoking may be associated with different phenotypes of wheezing [177]. In a study conducted on 150 children with recurrent wheezing, 91 had been exposed to lower-level second-hand tobacco smoke, 24 were exposed to higher-level second-hand tobacco smoke, and 35 were not exposed to cigarette smoke. Wheezing symptom scores were higher in highly exposed children ($p = 0.03$) [178]. An interesting study has investigated one possible mechanism underlying the relationship between cigarette smoke exposure and preschool wheezing, suggesting an interaction between the genome and this environmental factor. Children with a specific polymorphism of IL-13 and in utero exposure to smoke were at higher risk of wheezing at age four and persisting asthma at age ten years [179].

Passive smoke also includes third-hand smoke, which is the smoke that stays on every surface in the area where someone has been smoking, including on skin, hair, clothing, furniture and flooring [180]. Due to particular habits of children like hand-to-mouth eating, crawling and sucking, these subjects may be particularly vulnerable to the effects of third-hand smoke. At present, there are no studies on the effect of third-hand smoke on wheezing preschool development, but we can speculate that this exposure can contribute to increasing airway reactivity in young children.

Recommendation 9. Maternal smoking during uterine foetal life and subsequent second and third-hand smoke exposure increase the risk of wheezing in preschool children, particularly those with a family history of allergy.
Quality of evidence: Moderate.

3.2.8. PICO Question 10. Is Immunodeficiency a Risk Factor for the Onset and the Evolution of Preschool Wheezing?
Executive Summary

Primary immunodeficiency disorder (PID) is a heterogeneous group of disorders resulting from innate or adaptive immunity defects. The clinical spectrum presented by patients with PID is variable but increased susceptibility to infections is a common feature [181]. PID must be suspected in case of persistent wheeze refractory to therapies and a history of pulmonary or systemic infections with unusual organisms [182], although some data did not show an association between PIDs and recurrent wheezing [183].

Selective IgA deficiency is one of the most common PIDs, occurring in approximately 1 in 300 people [181]. An undetectable level of IgA defines IgA deficiency in the blood and secretions but no other immunoglobulin deficiencies. The IgA antibodies present in the secretions play a major role in protecting from respiratory airways and gastrointestinal tract infections. In children, the main infections associated with IgA deficiency are pharyngotonsillitis, otitis, bronchitis, sinusitis and, less frequently, pneumonia [182].

In a cohort of Swedish children with positive skin prick test to at least one allergen and with circulating IgE antibodies to egg or cat, development of late-onset wheezing (at four years of age) was reduced by high levels of secretory salivary IgA levels ($p = 0.04$) [184]. On the other hand, low levels of IgA in the respiratory mucosa might predispose to develop bronchial hyperresponsiveness and asthma [185]. In addition, IgA deficiency may predispose subjects to allergy, but underlying mechanisms need to be clarified [186].

Transient dysfunctions of the humoral immune system include reduced IgG subclasses (IgG1, IgG2, IgG3, IgG4). The most common IgG1 deficiency results from a generalized deficiency of antibodies, IgG2 deficiency is associated with recurrent viral and bacterial infections, both IgG2 and IgG3 deficiency predisposes to recurrent respiratory tract infections, and IgG4 deficiency has been found in chronic bronchial and lung diseases [187]. Two studies showed that low levels of the IgG4 subclass were associated with recurrent wheezing, requiring hospitalization in infants and young children [188,189].

Recommendation 10. PID must be suspected in case of persistent wheeze refractory to therapies and a history of pulmonary or systemic infections with unusual organisms. IgA deficiency can predispose the child to recurrent respiratory infections, including wheezing in predisposed subjects.
Quality of evidence: Moderate.

3.3. Protective Factors for Wheeze Development

3.3.1. PICO Question 11. Are Probiotics Protective for Preschool Wheezing Development?
Executive Summary

Diversity and maturity of gut and lung microbiota can influence the onset and progression of allergic diseases, including asthma, since early life [190–193]. Bacterial colonisation starts in utero [194]. Then, at birth, skin, gut and lung microbiome start establishing. In the gut with dysbiosis, bacteria of the *Bacteroidetes* phyla are more present than *Firmicutes* phyla, resulting in a reduction of short-chain fatty acids (SCFA) production that may result in the secretion of pro-inflammatory cytokines such as IL-6, IL-8 and TNF-α and reduction of Treg lymphocytes favouring the development of inflammatory disease such as asthma [191].

In the Copenhagen Prospective Studies on Asthma in Childhood 2010 (COPSAC2010), particular bacterial colonisation of the infant's gut in the first month of life was related to the risk of wheezing and asthma at six years of age [195]. In another study, the increase of opportunistic pathogens like *Enterococcus* and the decrease of *Eubacterium*, *Faecalibacterium* and *Bifidobacterium* in early life may increase the risk of respiratory infection [196]. Similarly, in the Asthma Detection and Monitoring (ADEM) study, 202 wheezing children and 50 healthy children aged 2–4 years were studied until the age of six years, showing that bacterial composition and maturation of intestinal microbiota in the first months of life may influence the risk of asthma at school age, especially in children born to asthmatic mothers [197]. In the CHILD (Canadian Healthy Infant Longitudinal Development) birth cohort study, wheezing and atopy at one year of age were associated with decreased abundance of *Faecalibacterium*, *Lachnospira*, *Rothia*, and *Veillonella* in faecal microbiota at three months [198]. On the other hand, in a Swedish study, higher microbial diversity during the first month of life was associated with protection against the development of asthma at seven years of age [199].

Over the last decade, several studies reported on the use of probiotics in order to modulate the gut microbiome composition and development of respiratory disease. The potential beneficial effects of probiotic immunomodulation include increased synthesis of IgA and IL-10, suppression of tumour necrosis factor (TNF)-alfa and the inhibition of casein-induced T-cell activation [200].

Jensen et al., in a randomised controlled trial of 123 five-year-old children, demonstrated that early-life supplementation with probiotics did not change allergic disease prevalence [201]. On the contrary, there was instead a subtle trend in the probiotic group towards developing more recurrent wheezing episodes [201]. Similar results were reported in high-risk infants with oral supplementation of *Lactobacillus rhamnosus* GG during the first six months of life [202]. Further research on the relationship between probiotic supplementation and wheezing risk in three-year-old children was the trial by Berni Canani et al. [203].

In this randomised controlled trial, authors demonstrated that probiotics associated with extensively hydrolysed casein formula (EHCF) could reduce allergic manifestation, including asthma, in children with cow's milk allergy (CMA) and, therefore at high risk of atopy [203]. These studies were included in a recent meta-analysis including 13 trials for a total of 4021 children [204], showing that, despite some effectiveness in eczema prevention, probiotic supplementation during pregnancy or in early life did not reduce the incidence of asthma or wheezing in infants, except for the subgroup of atopic infants [201–203]. Further systematic reviews and meta-analyses did not confirm the protective effect of probiotic administration in the first years of life on the risk of childhood wheezing and asthma [204–206]. The meta-analysis by Wei et al., including 2521 children, showed that compared to placebo, probiotic supplementation reduced wheeze episodes only in a small subgroup of atopic infants [204]. The prophylactic effect was not influenced by other factors (i.e., asthma risk factors such as personal medical history or positive family history, type of probiotic used, timing and duration of intervention and follow-up) [204]. Similar results were obtained when administered antenatally to the mother and postnatally to the child [207].

Studies show controversial results when probiotics are administered in children with wheezing or asthma. A recent meta-analysis found an association with fewer exacerbations but no difference in asthma control test (ACT), respiratory symptoms or lung function [208]. Rose et al. conducted a double-blind, randomised controlled trial, which included 131 infants (aged 6–24 months) with at least two wheezing episodes and a family history of atopy [209]. The supplementation of *Lactobacillus rhamnosus* GG (LGG) did not prevent asthma or wheezing over a six-month follow-up. On the other hand, the study showed that in the subgroup sensitised to aeroallergens, the asthma symptoms score was higher in the LGG-supplemented subgroup than in the placebo group (22.9 vs. 42.5) [209]. The same authors in another trial studied the effects of probiotic supplementation on asthma exacerbations in a longer follow-up (44 months) and demonstrated no difference in terms of exacerbations between the probiotic and placebo group [210]. A meta-analysis of 25 studies demonstrated that probiotics do not influence asthma or wheeze development but may reduce IgE blood levels and the risk of atopic sensitisation when administered early in life [211].

Recommendation 11. Probiotic administration to reduce wheezing development is not recommended.
Quality of evidence: High.

3.3.2. PICO Question 12. Is Vitamin D Supplementation Protective for Preschool Wheezing Development?
Executive Summary

Vitamin D is mainly formed in the skin from 7-dehydrocholesterol after UVB exposure. Many foods are rich in vitamin D, such as plants, fish, eggs and liver [211,212]. The vitamin is then activated, firstly in the liver and then in the kidneys. Vitamin D seems to play a role in asthma control, given its effects on immune cell function, oxidative stress, airway remodelling and corticosteroid responsiveness through various pathways, including those involving IL-10 and IL-17 [213–218].

The potential preventive role of vitamin D starts in utero. Mothers with asthma and vitamin D sufficiency had a lower risk of offspring with asthma or recurrent wheezing by age three years [219–221]. On the contrary, low levels of vitamin D in mothers during gestation are important risk factors for decreased lung function at ages four, five, and six years [222]. In a recent meta-analysis including 6068 subjects, there was an inverse relationship between the intake of vitamin D during pregnancy, and the occurrence of wheezing in offspring (pooled OR: 0.68; 95% CI: 0.55–0.83) found [223]. However, it has been argued that supplementation may not work not for all the mothers since only the presence of maternal 17q21 functional SNP rs12936231 genotype confers a protective effect of high-dose prenatal vitamin D3 supplementation against offspring asthma/recurrent wheeze at age 0–3 years [224].

Considering vitamin D levels in children, higher levels are associated with lower frequency, duration and severity of wheezing attacks [225–232]. In 131 young children with recurrent wheezing, a suboptimal vitamin D status increased the risk of asthma exacerbation in the previous month, and a recent exacerbation was associated with low levels despite oral supplementation [233].

However, conflicting results have been reported for vitamin D supplementation and the prevention of RTIs and wheezing. Ducharme and colleagues investigated the effects of vitamin D supplementation on upper RTIs, asthma exacerbations, OCS use and emergency care evaluation in children between one and five years of age [234]. No difference was found between subjects supplemented with vitamin D and the placebo group. Similarly, oral supplementation for the first six months of life did result in the prevention of asthma, wheezing, and other atopic diseases (food allergy, rhinitis, eczema and allergen sensitization) at 2.5 years [235]. A systematic review and meta-analysis on nutrients included six studies performed in children and found no significant decreased incidence of RTIs with vitamin D supplementation (RR 0.88; 95% CI: 0.66–1.11, $p < 0.0001$) [236].

On the contrary, in a large meta-analysis including both children and adults, vitamin D's overall effect is positive in reducing RTIs, particularly in deficient subjects [237,238]. Interestingly, patients with moderate to severe asthma treated with ICS and with vitamin D supplementation had a reduced risk of asthma exacerbation (pooled RR 0.70; 95% CI, 0.59–0.83; $p < 0.05$) [239].

Recommendation 12. Vitamin D supplementation during the winter season may decrease the risk of RTIs and wheezing exacerbations.
Quality of evidence: Moderate.

3.3.3. PICO Question 13. Is Breastfeeding Protective for Preschool Wheezing Development?
Executive Summary

In a prospective cohort study conducted on 8499 children, breastfeeding for at least three months was associated with a lower risk of asthma between the ages of two and five [240]. Compared to exclusive breastfeeding, any other method of infant feeding was associated with an increased risk of asthma [241]. However, when considering hospitalization of asthma exacerbations in school-aged children, the data failed to demonstrate a protective effect of breastfeeding [242].

In addition to maternal antibodies, breast milk contains other immunomodulatory mediators, including activated T cells and memory T cells, secretory IgA, oligosaccharides, antibacterial proteins such as lactoferrin, lysozyme, beta-lactoglobulin, casein and pro- and anti-inflammatory factors that confer passive protection against incidence and severity of respiratory infections [241].

The protective effect of breastfeeding is particularly evident in the first years of life, as demonstrated by a recent meta-analysis where a lower risk of asthma is seen in children younger than seven years [243]. In the large birth cohort study, ALSPAC (Avon Longitudinal Study of Parents and Children), breastfeeding for at least six months reduced the risk of asthma in the first three years of life but not between the ages of 7 and 8 [244]. These findings were also confirmed by the metanalysis from Dogaru et al., which demonstrated that breastfeeding for more than six months reduced the risk of asthma and wheezing only for children younger than two years of age and not for older children [245].

Recommendation 13. Maternal breastfeeding protects from preschool wheezing.
Quality of evidence: High.

3.3.4. Question 14. Is Influenza Vaccination Protective for Preschool Wheezing Development?

Executive Summary

Influenza virus was detected in 8% of young children with wheeze hospitalized for an LRTI [15]. The risk of influenza infection and wheezing in children with EVW can be reduced through influenza vaccination [246]. All health authorities recommend annual influenza vaccination for subjects ≥6 months of age with asthma [247,248].

In children, the most commonly administered influenza vaccines are inactivated influenza vaccines (IIV), the efficacy of which has also been proven in children with recurrent wheezing on steroids [249]. The quadrivalent live-attenuated influenza vaccine (LAIV4) can be a suitable alternative for children ≥2 years of age [250]. LAIV4 is an intranasally administered vaccine that is very popular among parents and healthcare professionals due to the non-invasive route of administration. However, a diagnosis of asthma or a wheezing episode in the previous 12 months represents a contraindication for LAIV4 in children aged two to four years because of a reported higher incidence of wheezing in LAIV recipients compared with IIV recipients [250,251]. This contraindication has been questioned and many studies also demonstrated the vaccine's safety in the population of preschool wheezers and severe asthmatic patients [252–254]. In a recent UK multicentre, open-label, phase IV intervention study in preschool children with recurrent wheezing, a follow-up of asthma symptoms 72 hours and four weeks later showed no significant change after administration of LAIV in the presence of efficacy against influenza [255,256]. LAIV4 has also been investigated concerning long-term effects, and in a prospective cohort of vaccinated children who were 12 through 35 months of age, there was no evidence of increased risk of subsequent asthma diagnosis at 14 years of age [252].

Recommendation 14. Influenza vaccination is recommended for its efficacy and safety in young children ≥6 months of age with wheezing.
Quality of evidence: High.

3.3.5. Question 15. Are Immunomodulators Protective for Preschool Wheezing Development?

Executive Summary

Recurrent RTIs are one of the most common diseases in children [257–259]. Despite being generally mild, recurrent RTIs may disrupt children's growth, contribute to antibiotic misuse, generate a significant burden of care and be a significant risk factor for asthma in later life [257]. The underlying pathogenesis of recurrent RTIs is complex. Immunological immaturity, genetic characteristics and environmental factors, such as exposure to air pollutants, attendance of daycare and lack of breastfeeding, are considered the most important factors promoting RTIs [258]. Boosting the immune system activity with non-specific immunomodulators can be an option to improve protection against infections [259].

Over the years, clinical evidence for the role of non-specific immunomodulators in reducing recurrent RTIs in the paediatric population has consistently increased [259]. Once administered orally, non-specific immunomodulators stimulate innate and adaptive immunity through different mechanisms. OM-85 is a non-specific lyophilised bacterial lysate of common pathogenic bacteria of the respiratory tract. In the mechanism of action of OM-85, the gut–lung immune axis plays a crucial role. OM-85 induces the maturation of human dendritic cells in gastrointestinal Peyer's patches, stimulates macrophages in the production of proinflammatory cytokines and anti-viral chemokines, up-regulates the Th1 specific cytokine IFN-γ and down-regulate the Th2 specific cytokine IL-4 and increases the activity of B cells with the secretion of salivary IgA, bronchoalveolar IgA, and serum IgA and IgG [259]. A double-blind, randomised, controlled study involving 288 children aged between one and six years with a history of recurrent RTIs (at least six episodes in the previous year) showed that OM-85 reduced the number of new RTI episodes when administered for the first ten days of each month for three months (33% vs. 65.1% in children with placebo, $p < 0.0001$). This was associated with fewer days of absence from daycare for children and working days lost by parents [260]. So far, several meta-analyses have been published on the effect of OM-85, demonstrating that it reduces the frequency and length of RTIs and eventually limits the use of antibiotics. Overall, data suggest that the effect is greater in patients at increased risk of recurrent RTIs. Some authors recently speculated that this non-specific immuno-modulator might also be useful against COVID-19 infection [261–263].

Interestingly, since non-specific immunomodulators correct Th1/Th2 imbalance through activation of T regulatory (Treg) cells and promote the immune system's maturation in children, their use can be associated with the reduction of Th2 atopic responses associated with wheezing and asthma [264]. Razi et al.'s study showed that prophylaxis with OM-85 reduced the duration and incidence of exacerbations in children with a history of recurrent wheezing [265].

Recommendation 15. Prophylaxis with non-specific immunomodulators can be considered in children with recurrent EVW to reduce the number of episodes during the winter season.
Quality of evidence: Moderate.

4. Discussion

This study shows that atopy and respiratory infections are pivotal in preschool wheezing pathogenesis. Multi-trigger wheezing is often associated with atopy and recurrent severe clinical phenotype. The evidence of blood eosinophilia and allergen sensitisation may guide the treatment in favour of ICS. HRV and RSV are the most common viruses associated with a higher risk of developing asthma at later ages. Bacterial colonisation and airway neutrophilia may characterise a unique phenotype of preschool wheezing not responsive to steroids.

Genetics and modifiable risk factors such as obesity, pollution or smoke exposure can affect the onset and evolution of wheezing phenotypes. The first 1000 days of life, including the intrauterine period, are crucial in the organism's physiological growth and the development of respiratory diseases. Prematurity can significantly affect lung development, risk of wheezing and obstructive respiratory disease across all ages. Breastfeeding and vitamin D supplementation may contribute to protecting the child from the development of wheezing.

Table 1 summarises the 15 statements. An extended evidence summary is available in the Supplementary Material.

Table 1. Statements on risk factors affecting development and persistence of preschool wheezing.

Question	Answer
Section 1. Pathogenesis of preschool wheezing	
Q1. What is the role of infection in the pathogenesis of preschool wheezing?	There is evidence that mainly viruses can trigger wheezing in young children. RSV and HRV are the main viruses involved in wheezing pathogenesis.
Q2. What is the role of atopy in the pathogenesis of preschool wheezing?	Recurrent multi-trigger wheezing often presents a severe clinical spectrum, can be associated with atopy more frequently than EVW and might expose the child to a higher risk of developing asthma at a later age. Aeroallergen sensitization and blood eosinophils can be used as biomarkers to identify responses to ICS in a recurrent preschool wheeze.
Section 2. Risk factors for wheeze development	
Q3. Does the presence of risk factors such as allergy/atopy influence the onset and the evolution of preschool wheezing?	Young children with recurrent wheezing with atopic eczema, sensitized to allergens or blood eosinophilia, are at higher risk of asthma at a later age.
Q4. Does the presence of risk factors such as previous respiratory tract infection/bronchiolitis influence the onset and evolution of preschool wheezing?	Infants with bronchiolitis represent a high-risk group for recurrent wheezing.

Table 1. Cont.

Question	Answer
Q5. Does pollution influence the onset and evolution of preschool wheezing?	Traffic-related air pollution may favour wheezing, likely via a reduced response to viral infections. Both outdoor and indoor pollution can influence the respiratory health of young children from conception and birth.
Q6. Does genetics influence the onset and the evolution of preschool wheezing?	Some individuals have a genetic susceptibility and are predisposed to develop preschool wheezing at first and eventually asthma later in life. At present, little can be done to modify genetic susceptibility, but environmental exposures can be adjusted to reduce this risk and potentially work on primary asthma prevention.
Q7. Does obesity influence the onset and the evolution of preschool wheezing?	Rapid weight gain in infancy and high BMI is associated with an increased risk of wheezing in preschool age.
Q8. Do prematurity and other perinatal factors influence the onset and the evolution of preschool wheezing?	Preterm birth and low birth weight are important early life risk factors for wheezing disorders in childhood. Extremely preterm infants are at the highest risk for respiratory problems and may have lower lung function trajectories across all ages.
Q9. Does smoke exposure influence the onset and the evolution of preschool wheezing?	Maternal smoking during uterine fetal life and subsequent second and third-hand smoke exposure increase the risk of wheezing in preschool children, particularly those with a family history of allergy.
Q10. Is immunodeficiency a risk factor for the onset and the evolution of preschool wheezing?	PID must be suspected in case of persistent wheeze refractory to therapies and a history of pulmonary or systemic infections with unusual organisms. IgA deficiency can predispose the child to recurrent infections, including wheezing.
Section 3. Protective factors for wheeze development	
Q11. Are probiotics protective for preschool wheezing development?	Probiotic administration to reduce wheezing development is not recommended.
Q12. Is vitamin D supplementation protective for preschool wheezing development?	Vitamin D supplementation during the winter season may decrease the risk of RTIs and wheezing exacerbations.
Q13. Is breastfeeding protective for preschool wheezing development?	Maternal breastfeeding protects from preschool wheezing.
Q14. Is influenza vaccination protective for preschool wheezing development?	Influenza vaccination is recommended for its efficacy and safety in young children ≥ 6 months of age with wheezing.
Q15. Are non-specific immunomodulators protective for preschool wheezing development?	Prophylaxis with non-specific immunomodulators can be considered in children with recurrent EVW to reduce the number of episodes during the winter season.

5. Conclusions

Based on a panel of experts and extensive updated literature, this consensus document provides insights on the pathogenesis, the risk and protective factors associated with the development and persistence of preschool wheezing. Undoubtedly, more research is needed to improve our understanding of the disease and confirm the associations between certain factors and the risk of wheezing in early life. In addition, preventive strategies must be promoted to avoid children's exposure to risk factors that may permanently affect respiratory health.

Supplementary Materials: The following supporting information can be downloaded at: https://www.mdpi.com/article/10.3390/jcm11216558/s1, Supplementary Material S1: PICO questions and review of the literature.

Author Contributions: R.G., V.F. and C.C. wrote the first draft of the manuscript; G.C., A.L., M.T. and A.M. coordinated the literature analysis; B.M.B., L.B. (Luca Bertelli), L.B. (Loretta Biserna), P.B., E.C., N.D.P., A.D., B.G., F.L., M.S.M., E.M., S.P., A.P., M.P., S.T., F.V., G.G., R.S., S.M., M.M., F.A., A.B., L.R., F.C., A.D.F. and F.M. gave a substantial scientific contribution; G.R. supervised the project and gave a substantial scientific contribution; S.E. designed the study, supervised the project and revised the first draft of the manuscript. All members of Emilia-Romagna Asthma (ERA) Study Group gave a scientific contribution. All authors have read and agreed to the published version of the manuscript.

Funding: This research received no external funding.

Institutional Review Board Statement: Not applicable.

Informed Consent Statement: Not applicable.

Data Availability Statement: Not applicable.

Acknowledgments: In addition to the main authors, the Emilia-Romagna Asthma (ERA) Study Group includes Sara Scavone, Michela Deolmi, Kaltra Skenderaj, Riccardo Morini, Adriana Fracchiolla, Giuliana Gianni, Giulia Antoniol, Giovanna Pisi, Onelia Facini, Aurelia Pantaleo, Claudia Cutrera, Alberto Argentiero, Cosimo Neglia: UOC Clinica Pediatrica, Azienda Ospedaliera-Universitaria, Parma, Italy; Andrea Pession, Marcello Lanari, Emanuela Di Palmo: IRCCS Azienda-Ospedaliera Universitaria di Bologna, Bologna, Italy; Maria Teresa Bersini, Cristina Cantù, Enrica Cattani, Carlotta Povesi: Pediatri di famiglia, AUSL Parma, Parma, Italy; Giacomo Biasucci: Unità di Pediatria e Neonatologia, Ospedale G. di Saliceto, Piacenza, Italy; Rosanna Cataldi, Valentina Allegri: Pediatri di famiglia, AUSL Piacenza, Piacenza, Italy; Ilaria Fontana, Sara Fornaciari, Irene Alberici: Unità di Pediatria, IRCCS-AUSL Reggio Emilia, Reggio Emilia, Italy; Mariassunta Torricelli, Simonetta Pistocchi, Ilaria D'Aquino, Annalisa Zini, Maria Luisa Villani, Maria Candida Tripodi, Fabio Guerrera, Stefano Colonna: Pediatri di famiglia, IRCCS-AUSL Reggio Emilia, Reggio Emilia, Italy; Lorenzo Iughetti, Maria Elena Guerzoni: Unità di Pediatria, Azienda Ospedaliera-Universitaria di Modena, Modena, Italy; Maria Chiara Molinari, Gianluca Iovine, Nicola Guaraldi, Simona Di Loreto, Rossella Berri, Dora Di Mauro, Alfredo Ferrari, Silvia Perrini: Pediatri di famiglia, AUSL Modena, Modena, Italy; Francesco Torcetta: Unità di Pediatria, Ospedale di Carpi, Carpi, Italy; Claudio Rota: Unità di Pediatria, Ospedale di Sassuolo, Sassuolo, Italy; Chiara Ghizzi: Unità di Pediatria, Ospedale Maggiore, AUSL Bologna, Bologna, Italy; Cristina Carboni, Ornella Parisini, Marco Parpanesi, Alessandro Fierro, Riccardo Congia, Federica Bellini, Giulia Brighi, Valeria Scialpi, Lanfranco Loretano, Veronica Conti, Lucia Rinaldi, Stefano Alboresi: Pediatri di famiglia, AUSL Bologna, Bologna, Italy; Laura Serra, Elisabetta Calamelli: UOC Pediatria, Ospedale di Imola, Imola, Italy; Enrico Valletta: Unità di Pediatria, Ospedale di Forlì, AUSL Romagna, Forlì, Italy; Anna Chiara Casadei, Lucia Boselli: Pediatri di famiglia, AUSL Romagna, Forlì, Italy; Marcello Stella: Unità di Pediatria e Terapia Intensiva Pediatrica, Ospedale di Cesena, AUSL Romagna, Cesena, Italy; Agnese Suppiej, Paola Gallo: Unità di Pediatria, Ospedale di Ferrara, Ferrara, Italy; Monica Malventano, Livia Manfredini, Lisa Pecorari: Pediatri di famiglia, AUSL Romagna, Ferrara, Italy; Simone Fontijn: Unità di Pediatria, Ospedale di Ravenna, AUSL Romagna, Ravenna, Italy; Mauro Baldini, Fabio Dal Monte, Elena Zamuner, Lucia Vignutelli: Pediatri di famiglia, AUSL Ravenna, Ravenna, Italy; Gianluca Vergine: Unità di Pediatria, Ospedale di Rimini, AUSL Romagna, Rimini, Italy; Carmelo Palmeri, Cecilia Argentina: Pediatri di famiglia, AUSL Romagna, Rimini, Italy; Margherita Marchiani: Associazione Respiro Libero Onlus, Parma, Parma, Italy.

Conflicts of Interest: The authors declare no conflict of interest.

References

1. Martinez, F.D.; Wright, A.L.; Taussig, L.M.; Holberg, C.J.; Halonen, M.; Morgan, W.J. Asthma and wheezing in the first six years of life. The Group Health Medical Associates. *N. Engl. J. Med.* **1995**, *332*, 133–138. [CrossRef] [PubMed]
2. Moorman, J.E.; Akinbami, L.J.; Bailey, C.M.; Zahran, H.S.; King, M.E.; Johnson, C.A.; Liu, X. National Surveillance of Asthma: United States, 2001–2010. *Vital Health Statistics. Ser. 3 Anal. Epidemiol. Stud.* **2012**, 1–58. Available online: https://europepmc.org/article/med/24252609 (accessed on 20 September 2022).
3. Paton, J. Paediatric Asthma 2015—British Thoracic Society. Audit-Reports. Available online: https://www.brit-thoracic.org.uk (accessed on 15 October 2022).
4. Principi, N.; Daleno, C.; Esposito, S. Human rhinoviruses and severe respiratory infections: Is it possible to identify at-risk patients early? *Expert Rev. Anti Infect. Ther.* **2014**, *12*, 423–430. [CrossRef] [PubMed]
5. Robinson, P.F.M.; Pattaroni, C.; Cook, J.; Gregory, L.; Alonso, A.M.; Fleming, L.J.; Lloyd, C.M.; Bush, A.; Marsland, B.J.; Saglani, S. Lower airway microbiota associates with inflammatory phenotype in severe preschool wheeze. *J. Allergy Clin. Immunol.* **2019**, *143*, 1607–1610.e3. [CrossRef] [PubMed]
6. Caffarelli, C.; Garrubba, M.; Greco, C.; Mastrorilli, C.; Dascola, C.P. Asthma and Food Allergy in Children: Is There a Connection or Interaction? *Front. Pediatr.* **2016**, *4*, 34. [CrossRef] [PubMed]

7. Deliu, M.; Fontanella, S.; Haider, S.; Sperrin, M.; Geifman, N.; Murray, C.; Simpson, A.; Custovic, A. Longitudinal trajectories of severe wheeze exacerbations from infancy to school age and their association with early-life risk factors and late asthma outcomes. *Clin. Exp. Allergy* **2020**, *50*, 315–324. [CrossRef] [PubMed]
8. Fainardi, V.; Caffarelli, C.; Bergamini, B.M.; Biserna, L.; Bottau, P.; Corinaldesi, E.; Dondi, A.; Fornaro, M.; Guidi, B.; Lombardi, F.; et al. Management of Children with Acute Asthma Attack: A RAND/UCLA Appropriateness Approach. *Int. J. Environ. Res. Public Health* **2021**, *18*, 12775. [CrossRef]
9. Brozek, J.L.; Akl, E.A.; Jaeschke, R.; Lang, D.M.; Bossuyt, P.; Glasziou, P.; Helfand, M.; Ueffing, E.; Alonso-Coello, P.; Meerpohl, J.; et al. Grading quality of evidence and strength of recommendations in clinical practice guidelines: Part 2 of 3. The GRADE approach to grading quality of evidence about diagnostic tests and strategies. *Allergy* **2009**, *64*, 1109–1116. [CrossRef]
10. Fainardi, V.; Caffarelli, C.; Deolmi, M.; Skenderaj, K.; Meoli, A.; Morini, R.; Bergamini, B.M.; Bertelli, L.; Biserna, L.; Bottau, P.; et al. Management of Preschool Wheezing: Guideline from the Emilia-Romagna Asthma (ERA) Study Group. *J. Clin. Med.* **2022**, *11*, 4763. [CrossRef]
11. Krzysztofiak, A.; Chiappini, E.; Venturini, E.; Gargiullo, L.; Roversi, M.; Montagnani, C.; Bozzola, E.; Chiurchiu, S.; Vecchio, D.; Castagnola, E.; et al. Italian consensus on the therapeutic management of uncomplicated acute hematogenous osteomyelitis in children. *Ital. J. Pediatr.* **2021**, *47*, 179. [CrossRef]
12. Andrews, J.C.; Schünemann, H.J.; Oxman, A.D.; Pottie, K.; Meerpohl, J.J.; Coello, P.A.; Rind, D.; Montori, V.M.; Brito, J.P.; Norris, S.; et al. GRADE guidelines: 15. Going from evidence to recommendation-determinants of a recommendation's direction and strength. *J. Clin. Epidemiol.* **2013**, *66*, 726–735. [CrossRef] [PubMed]
13. Lemanske, R.F., Jr.; Jackson, D.J.; Gangnon, R.E.; Evans, M.D.; Li, Z.; Shult, P.A.; Kirk, C.J.; Reisdorf, E.; Roberg, K.A.; Anderson, E.L.; et al. Rhinovirus illnesses during infancy predict subsequent childhood wheezing. *J. Allergy Clin. Immunol.* **2005**, *116*, 571–577. [CrossRef] [PubMed]
14. Fujitsuka, A.; Tsukagoshi, H.; Arakawa, M.; Goto-Sugai, K.; Ryo, A.; Okayama, Y.; Mizuta, K.; Nishina, A.; Yoshizumi, M.; Kaburagi, Y.; et al. A molecular epidemiological study of respiratory viruses detected in Japanese children with acute wheezing illness. *BMC Infect. Dis.* **2011**, *11*, 168. [CrossRef] [PubMed]
15. Takeyama, A.; Hashimoto, K.; Sato, M.; Sato, T.; Tomita, Y.; Maeda, R.; Ito, M.; Katayose, M.; Kawasaki, Y.; Hosoya, M. Clinical and epidemiologic factors related to subsequent wheezing after virus-induced lower respiratory tract infections in hospitalized pediatric patients younger than 3 years. *Eur. J. Pediatr.* **2014**, *173*, 959–966. [CrossRef]
16. Leino, A.; Lukkarinen, M.; Turunen, R.; Vuorinen, T.; Söderlund-Venermo, M.; Vahlberg, T.; Camargo, C.A., Jr.; Bochkov, Y.A.; Gern, J.E.; Jartti, T. Pulmonary function and bronchial reactivity 4 years after the first virus-induced wheezing. *Allergy* **2019**, *74*, 518–526. [CrossRef]
17. Stern, D.A.; Guerra, S.; Halonen, M.; Wright, A.L.; Martinez, F.D. Low IFN-gamma production in the first year of life as a predictor of wheeze during childhood. *J. Allergy Clin. Immunol.* **2007**, *120*, 835–841. [CrossRef]
18. Chawes, B.L.; Poorisrisak, P.; Johnston, S.L.; Bisgaard, H. Neonatal bronchial hyperresponsiveness precedes acute severe viral bronchiolitis in infants. *J. Allergy Clin. Immunol.* **2012**, *130*, 354–361.e3. [CrossRef]
19. Heymann, P.W.; Carper, H.T.; Murphy, D.D.; Platts-Mills, T.A.; Patrie, J.; McLaughlin, A.P.; Erwin, E.A.; Shaker, M.S.; Hellems, M.; Peerzada, J.; et al. Viral infections in relation to age, atopy, and season of admission among children hospitalized for wheezing. *J. Allergy Clin. Immunol.* **2004**, *114*, 239–247. [CrossRef]
20. De Winter, J.J.; Bont, L.; Wilbrink, B.; van der Ent, C.K.; Smit, H.A.; Houben, M.L. Rhinovirus wheezing illness in infancy is associated with medically attended third year wheezing in low risk infants: Results of a healthy birth cohort study. *Immun. Inflamm. Dis.* **2015**, *3*, 398–405. [CrossRef]
21. Van der Gugten, A.C.; van der Zalm, M.M.; Uiterwaal, C.S.; Wilbrink, B.; Rossen, J.W.; van der Ent, C.K. Human rhinovirus and wheezing: Short and long-term associations in children. *Pediatr. Infect. Dis. J.* **2013**, *32*, 827–833. [CrossRef]
22. Liu, L.; Pan, Y.; Zhu, Y.; Song, Y.; Su, X.; Yang, L.; Li, M. Association between rhinovirus wheezing illness and the development of childhood asthma: A meta-analysis. *BMJ Open* **2017**, *7*, e013034. [CrossRef]
23. Midulla, F.; Pierangeli, A.; Cangiano, G.; Bonci, E.; Salvadei, S.; Scagnolari, C.; Moretti, C.; Antonelli, G.; Ferro, V.; Papoff, P. Rhinovirus bronchiolitis and recurrent wheezing: 1-year follow-up. *Eur. Respir. J.* **2012**, *39*, 396–402. [CrossRef] [PubMed]
24. O'Callaghan-Gordo, C.; Bassat, Q.; Díez-Padrisa, N.; Morais, L.; Machevo, S.; Nhampossa, T.; Quintó, L.; Alonso, P.L.; Roca, A. Lower respiratory tract infections associated with rhinovirus during infancy and increased risk of wheezing during childhood. A cohort study. *PLoS ONE* **2013**, *8*, e69370. [CrossRef] [PubMed]
25. Midulla, F.; Nicolai, A.; Ferrara, M.; Gentile, F.; Pierangeli, A.; Bonci, E.; Scagnolari, C.; Moretti, C.; Antonelli, G.; Papoff, P. Recurrent wheezing 36 months after bronchiolitis is associated with rhinovirus infections and blood eosinophilia. *Acta Paediatr.* **2014**, *103*, 1094–1099. [CrossRef] [PubMed]
26. Rossi, G.A.; Colin, A.A. Infantile respiratory syncytial virus and human rhinovirus infections: Respective role in inception and persistence of wheezing. *Eur. Respir. J.* **2015**, *45*, 774–789. [CrossRef]
27. Feldman, A.S.; He, Y.; Moore, M.L.; Hershenson, M.B.; Hartert, T.V. Toward primary prevention of asthma. Reviewing the evidence for early-life respiratory viral infections as modifiable risk factors to prevent childhood asthma. *Am. J. Respir. Crit. Care Med.* **2015**, *191*, 34–44. [CrossRef]
28. Lee, W.M.; Lemanske, R.F., Jr.; Evans, M.D.; Vang, F.; Pappas, T.; Gangnon, R.; Jackson, D.J.; Gern, J.E. Human rhinovirus species and season of infection determine illness severity. *Am. J. Respir. Crit. Care Med.* **2012**, *186*, 886–891. [CrossRef]

29. Skevaki, C.L.; Psarras, S.; Volonaki, E.; Pratsinis, H.; Spyridaki, I.S.; Gaga, M.; Georgiou, V.; Vittorakis, S.; Telcian, A.G.; Maggina, P.; et al. Rhinovirus-induced basic fibroblast growth factor release mediates airway remodeling features. *Clin. Transl. Allergy* **2012**, *2*, 14. [CrossRef]
30. Legg, J.P.; Hussain, I.R.; Warner, J.A.; Johnston, S.L.; Warner, J.O. Type 1 and type 2 cytokine imbalance in acute respiratory syncytial virus bronchiolitis. *Am. J. Respir. Crit. Care Med.* **2003**, *168*, 633–639. [CrossRef]
31. Esposito, S.; Daleno, C.; Tagliabue, C.; Scala, A.; Tenconi, R.; Borzani, I.; Fossali, E.; Pelucchi, C.; Piralla, A.; Principi, N. Impact of rhinoviruses on pediatric community-acquired pneumonia. *Eur. J. Clin. Microbiol. Infect. Dis.* **2012**, *31*, 1637–1645. [CrossRef]
32. Ballarini, S.; Rossi, G.A.; Principi, N.; Esposito, S. Dysbiosis in Pediatrics Is Associated with Respiratory Infections: Is There a Place for Bacterial-Derived Products? *Microorganisms* **2021**, *9*, 448. [CrossRef] [PubMed]
33. Schwerk, N.; Brinkmann, F.; Soudah, B.; Kabesch, M.; Hansen, G. Wheeze in preschool age is associated with pulmonary bacterial infection and resolves after antibiotic therapy. *PLoS ONE* **2011**, *6*, e27913. [CrossRef] [PubMed]
34. Esposito, S.; Ballarini, S.; Argentiero, A.; Ruggiero, L.; Rossi, G.A.; Principi, N. Microbiota profiles in pre-school children with respiratory infections: Modifications induced by the oral bacterial lysate OM-85. *Front. Cell. Infect. Microbiol.* **2022**, *12*, 789436. [CrossRef] [PubMed]
35. De Schutter, I.; Dreesman, A.; Soetens, O.; De Waele, M.; Crokaert, F.; Verhaegen, J.; Piérard, D.; Malfroot, A. In young children, persistent wheezing is associated with bronchial bacterial infection: A retrospective analysis. *BMC Pediatr.* **2012**, *12*, 83. [CrossRef]
36. Teo, S.M.; Mok, D.; Pham, K.; Kusel, M.; Serralha, M.; Troy, N.; Holt, B.J.; Hales, B.J.; Walker, M.L.; Hollams, E.; et al. The infant nasopharyngeal microbiome impacts severity of lower respiratory infection and risk of asthma development. *Cell Host Microbe* **2015**, *17*, 704–715. [CrossRef]
37. Robinson, P.F.M.; Fontanella, S.; Ananth, S.; Alonso, A.M.; Cook, J.; Kaya-de Vries, D.; Polo Silveira, L.; Gregory, L.; Lloyd, C.; Fleming, L.; et al. Recurrent Severe Preschool Wheeze: From Prespecified Diagnostic Labels to Underlying Endotypes. *Am. J. Respir. Crit. Care Med.* **2021**, *204*, 523–535. [CrossRef]
38. Bacharier, L.B.; Guilbert, T.W.; Mauger, D.T.; Boehmer, S.; Beigelman, A.; Fitzpatrick, A.M.; Jackson, D.J.; Baxi, S.N.; Benson, M.; Burnham, C.D.; et al. Early Administration of Azithromycin and Prevention of Severe Lower Respiratory Tract Illnesses in Preschool Children with a History of Such Illnesses: A Randomized Clinical Trial. *JAMA* **2015**, *314*, 2034–2044, Erratum in *JAMA* **2016**, *315*, 204; Erratum in *JAMA* **2016**, *315*, 419. [CrossRef]
39. Stokholm, J.; Chawes, B.L.; Vissing, N.H.; Bjarnadóttir, E.; Pedersen, T.M.; Vinding, R.K.; Schoos, A.M.; Wolsk, H.M.; Thorsteinsdóttir, S.; Hallas, H.W.; et al. Azithromycin for episodes with asthma-like symptoms in young children aged 1–3 years: A randomised, double-blind, placebo-controlled trial. *Lancet Respir. Med.* **2016**, *4*, 19–26. [CrossRef]
40. Esposito, S.; Blasi, F.; Arosio, C.; Fioravanti, L.; Fagetti, L.; Droghetti, R.; Tarsia, P.; Allegra, L.; Principi, N. Importance of acute Mycoplasma pneumoniae and Chlamydia pneumoniae infections in children with wheezing. *Eur. Respir. J.* **2000**, *16*, 1142–1146. [CrossRef]
41. Esposito, S.; Droghetti, R.; Bosis, S.; Claut, L.; Marchisio, P.; Principi, N. Cytokine secretion in children with acute Mycoplasma pneumoniae infection and wheeze. *Pediatr. Pulmonol.* **2002**, *34*, 122–127. [CrossRef]
42. Liu, C.; Makrinioti, H.; Saglani, S.; Bowman, M.; Lin, L.L.; Camargo, C.A., Jr.; Hasegawa, K.; Zhu, Z. Microbial dysbiosis and childhood asthma development: Integrated role of the airway and gut microbiome, environmental exposures, and host metabolic and immune response. *Front. Immunol.* **2022**, *13*, 1028209. [CrossRef] [PubMed]
43. Zhu, Z.; Camargo, C.A., Jr.; Raita, Y.; Freishtat, R.J.; Fujiogi, M.; Hahn, A.; Mansbacj, J.M.; Spergel, J.M.; Pérez-Losada, M.; Hasegawa, K. Nasopharyngeal airway dual-transcriptome of infants with severe bronchiolitis and risk of childhood asthma: A multicenter prospective study. *J. Allergy Clin. Immunol.* **2022**, *150*, 806–816. [CrossRef] [PubMed]
44. Bosch, A.A.T.M.; de Steenhuijsen Piters, W.A.A.; van Houten, M.A.; Chu, M.L.J.N.; Biesbroek, G.; Kool, J.; Pernet, P.; de Groot, P.C.M.; Eijkemans, M.J.C.; Keijser, B.J.F.; et al. Maturation of the Infant Respiratory Microbiota, Environmental Drivers, and Health Consequences. A Prospective Cohort Study. *Am. J. Respir. Crit. Care Med.* **2017**, *196*, 1582–1590. [CrossRef] [PubMed]
45. Thavagnanam, S.; Williamson, G.; Ennis, M.; Heaney, L.G.; Shields, M.D. Does airway allergic inflammation pre-exist before late onset wheeze in children? *Pediatr. Allergy Immunol.* **2010**, *21*, 1002–1007. [CrossRef] [PubMed]
46. Lezmi, G.; Deschildre, A.; Abou Taam, R.; Fayon, M.; Blanchon, S.; Troussier, F.; Mallinger, P.; Mahut, B.; Gosset, P.; de Blic, J. Remodelling and inflammation in preschoolers with severe recurrent wheeze and asthma outcome at school age. *Clin. Exp. Allergy* **2018**, *48*, 806–813. [CrossRef]
47. Saglani, S.; Payne, D.N.; Zhu, J.; Wang, Z.; Nicholson, A.G.; Bush, A.; Jeffery, P.K. Early detection of airway wall remodeling and eosinophilic inflammation in preschool wheezers. *Am. J. Respir. Crit. Care Med.* **2007**, *176*, 858–864. [CrossRef]
48. Ferreira, M.A.; Vonk, J.W.; Baurecht, H.; Marenholz, I.; Tian, C.; Hoffman, J.D.; Helmer, Q.; Tillander, A.; Ullemar, V.; van Dongen, J.; et al. Shared genetic origin of asthma, hay fever and eczema elucidates allergic disease biology. *Nat. Genet.* **2017**, *49*, 1752–1757. [CrossRef]
49. Zhu, Z.; Lee, P.H.; Chaffin, M.D.; Chung, W.; Loh, P.O.; Lu, Q.; Christiani, D.C.; Liang, L. A genome-wide cross-trait analysis from UK Biobank highlights the shared genetic architecture of asthma and allergic diseases. *Nat. Genet.* **2018**, *50*, 857–864. [CrossRef]
50. Guiddir, T.; Saint-Pierre, P.; Purenne-Denis, E.; Lambert, N.; Laoudi, Y.; Couderc, R.; Gouvis-Echraghi, R.; Amat, F.; Just, J. Neutrophilic Steroid-Refractory Recurrent Wheeze and Eosinophilic Steroid-Refractory Asthma in Children. *J. Allergy Clin. Immunol. Pract.* **2017**, *5*, 1351–1361.e2. [CrossRef]

51. Turato, G.; Barbato, A.; Baraldo, S.; Zanin, M.E.; Bazzan, E.; Lokar-Oliani, K.; Calabrese, F.; Panizzolo, C.; Snijders, D.; Maestrelli, P.; et al. Nonatopic children with multitrigger wheezing have airway pathology comparable to atopic asthma. *Am. J. Respir. Crit. Care Med.* **2008**, *178*, 476–482. [CrossRef]
52. Just, J.; Nicoloyanis, N.; Chauvin, M.; Pribil, C.; Grimfeld, A.; Duru, G. Lack of eosinophilia can predict remission in wheezy infants? *Clin. Exp. Allergy* **2008**, *38*, 767–773. [CrossRef] [PubMed]
53. Fitzpatrick, A.M.; Jackson, D.J.; Mauger, D.T.; Boehmer, S.J.; Phipatanakul, W.; Sheehan, W.J.; Moy, J.N.; Paul, I.M.; Bacharier, L.B.; Cabana, M.D.; et al. Individualized therapy for persistent asthma in young children. *J. Allergy Clin. Immunol.* **2016**, *138*, 1608–1618.e12. [CrossRef] [PubMed]
54. Esposito, S.; Principi, N. Pharmacological approach to wheezing in preschool children. *Expert Opin. Pharmacother.* **2014**, *15*, 943–952. [CrossRef] [PubMed]
55. Shinohara, M.; Wakiguchi, H.; Saito, H.; Matsumoto, K. Presence of eosinophils in nasal secretion during acute respiratory tract infection in young children predicts subsequent wheezing within two months. *Allergol. Int.* **2008**, *57*, 359–365. [CrossRef]
56. Guo, Y.; Zou, Y.; Zhai, J.; Li, J.; Liu, J.; Ma, C.; Jin, X.; Zhao, L. Phenotypes of the inflammatory cells in the induced sputum from young children or infants with recurrent wheezing. *Pediatr. Res.* **2019**, *85*, 489–493. [CrossRef]
57. Ater, D.; Bar, B.E.; Fireman, N.; Fireman, E.; Shai, H.; Tasher, D.; Dalal, I.; Mandelberg, A. Asthma-predictive-index, bronchial-challenge, sputum eosinophils in acutely wheezing preschoolers. *Pediatr. Pulmonol.* **2014**, *49*, 952–959. [CrossRef]
58. De Sousa, R.B.; Medeiros, D.; Sarinho, E.; Rizzo, J.Â.; Silva, A.R.; Bianca, A.C. Risk factors for recurrent wheezing in infants: A case-control study. *Rev. Saude Publica* **2016**, *50*, 15. [CrossRef]
59. Quah, P.L.; Huang, C.H.; Shek, L.P.; Chua, K.Y.; Lee, B.W.; Kuo, I.C. Hyper-responsive T-cell cytokine profile in association with development of early childhood wheeze but not eczema at 2 years. *Asian Pac. J. Allergy Immunol.* **2014**, *32*, 84–92. [CrossRef]
60. Sly, P.D.; Boner, A.L.; Björksten, B.; Bush, A.; Custovic, A.; Eigenmann, P.A.; Gern, J.E.; Gerritsen, J.; Hamelmann, E.; Helms, P.J.; et al. Early identification of atopy in the prediction of persistent asthma in children. *Lancet* **2008**, *372*, 1100–1106. [CrossRef]
61. Lloyd, C.M.; Saglani, S. Development of allergic immunity in early life. *Immunol. Rev.* **2017**, *278*, 101–115. [CrossRef]
62. Lynch, S.V.; Wood, R.A.; Boushey, H.; Bacharier, L.B.; Bloomberg, G.R.; Kattan, M.; O'Connor, G.T.; Sandel, M.T.; Calatroni, A.; Matsui, E.; et al. Effects of early-life exposure to allergens and bacteria on recurrent wheeze and atopy in urban children. *J. Allergy Clin. Immunol.* **2014**, *134*, 593–601.e12. [CrossRef] [PubMed]
63. Henderson, J.; Granell, R.; Heron, J.; Sherriff, A.; Simpson, A.; Woodcock, A.; Strachan, D.P.; Shaheen, S.O.; Sterne, J.A. Associations of wheezing phenotypes in the first 6 years of life with atopy, lung function and airway responsiveness in mid-childhood. *Thorax* **2008**, *63*, 974–980. [CrossRef] [PubMed]
64. Just, J.; Belfar, S.; Wanin, S.; Pribil, C.; Grimfeld, A.; Duru, G. Impact of innate and environmental factors on wheezing persistence during childhood. *J. Asthma* **2010**, *47*, 412–416. [CrossRef]
65. Arshad, S.H.; Karmaus, W.; Raza, A.; Kurukulaaratchy, R.J.; Matthews, S.M.; Holloway, J.W.; Sadeghnejad, A.; Zhang, H.; Roberts, G.; Ewart, S.L. The effect of parental allergy on childhood allergic diseases depends on the sex of the child. *J. Allergy Clin. Immunol.* **2012**, *130*, 427–434.e6. [CrossRef] [PubMed]
66. Schmidt, F.; Hose, A.J.; Mueller-Rompa, S.; Brick, T.; Hämäläinen, A.M.; Peet, A.; Tillmann, V.; Niemelä, O.; Siljander, H.; Knip, M.; et al. Development of atopic sensitization in Finnish and Estonian children: A latent class analysis in a multicenter cohort. *J. Allergy Clin. Immunol.* **2019**, *143*, 1904–1913.e9. [CrossRef]
67. Donohue, K.M.; Al-alem, U.; Perzanowski, M.S.; Chew, G.L.; Johnson, A.; Divjan, A.; Kelvin, E.A.; Hoepner, L.A.; Perera, F.P.; Miller, R.L. Anti-cockroach and anti-mouse IgE are associated with early wheeze and atopy in an inner-city birth cohort. *J. Allergy Clin. Immunol.* **2008**, *122*, 914–920. [CrossRef] [PubMed]
68. Yu, C.L.; Huang, W.T.; Wang, C.M. Treatment of allergic rhinitis reduces acute asthma exacerbation risk among asthmatic children aged 2–18 years. *J. Microbiol. Immunol. Infect.* **2019**, *52*, 991–999. [CrossRef]
69. Von Kobyletzki, L.B.; Bornehag, C.G.; Hasselgren, M.; Larsson, M.; Lindström, C.B.; Svensson, Å. Eczema in early childhood is strongly associated with the development of asthma and rhinitis in a prospective cohort. *BMC Dermatol.* **2012**, *12*, 11. [CrossRef]
70. Saunes, M.; Øien, T.; Dotterud, C.K.; Romundstad, P.R.; Storrø, O.; Holmen, T.L.; Johnsen, R. Early eczema and the risk of childhood asthma: A prospective, population-based study. *BMC Pediatr.* **2012**, *12*, 168. [CrossRef]
71. Chiu, C.Y.; Yang, C.H.; Su, K.W.; Tsai, M.H.; Hua, M.C.; Liao, S.L.; Lai, S.H.; Chen, L.C.; Yeh, K.W.; Huang, J.L. Early-onset eczema is associated with increased milk sensitization and risk of rhinitis and asthma in early childhood. *J. Microbiol. Immunol. Infect.* **2020**, *53*, 1008–1013. [CrossRef]
72. Ekbäck, M.; Tedner, M.; Devenney, I.; Oldaeus, G.; Norrman, G.; Strömberg, L.; Fälth-Magnusson, K. Severe eczema in infancy can predict asthma development. A prospective study to the age of 10 years. *PLoS ONE* **2014**, *9*, e99609. [CrossRef] [PubMed]
73. Boersma, N.A.; Meijneke, R.W.H.; Kelder, J.C.; van der Ent, C.K.; Balemans, W.A.F. Sensitization predicts asthma development among wheezing toddlers in secondary healthcare. *Pediatr. Pulmonol.* **2017**, *52*, 729–736. [CrossRef] [PubMed]
74. Vermeulen, E.M.; Koplin, J.J.; Dharmage, S.C.; Gurrin, L.C.; Peters, R.L.; McWilliam, V.; Ponsonby, A.L.; Dwyer, T.; Lowe, A.J.; Tang, M.L.K.; et al. Food Allergy Is an Important Risk Factor for Childhood Asthma, Irrespective of Whether It Resolves. *J. Allergy Clin. Immunol. Pract.* **2018**, *6*, 1336–1341.e3. [CrossRef] [PubMed]
75. Illi, S.; von Mutius, E.; Lau, S.; Nickel, R.; Niggemann, B.; Sommerfeld, C.; Wahn, U.; Multicenter Allergy Study Group. The pattern of atopic sensitization is associated with the development of asthma in childhood. *J. Allergy Clin. Immunol.* **2001**, *108*, 709–714. [CrossRef]

76. Illi, S.; von Mutius, E.; Lau, S.; Niggemann, B.; Grüber, C.; Wahn, U.; Multicentre Allergy Study (MAS) Group. Perennial allergen sensitisation early in life and chronic asthma in children: A birth cohort study. *Lancet* **2006**, *368*, 763–770. [CrossRef]
77. Kenmoe, S.; Bowo-Ngandji, A.; Kengne-Nde, C.; Ebogo-Belobo, J.T.; Mbaga, D.S.; Mahamat, G.; Demeni Emoh, C.P.; Njouom, R. Association between early viral LRTI and subsequent wheezing development, a meta-analysis and sensitivity analyses for studies comparable for confounding factors. *PLoS ONE* **2021**, *16*, e0249831. [CrossRef]
78. Kovesi, T.A.; Cao, Z.; Osborne, G.; Egeland, G.M. Severe early lower respiratory tract infection is associated with subsequent respiratory morbidity in preschool Inuit children in Nunavut, Canada. *J. Asthma* **2011**, *48*, 241–247. [CrossRef]
79. Lin, H.W.; Lin, S.C. Environmental factors association between asthma and acute bronchiolitis in young children—A perspective cohort study. *Eur. J. Pediatr.* **2012**, *171*, 1645–1650. [CrossRef]
80. Mikalsen, I.B.; Halvorsen, T.; Eide, G.E.; Øymar, K. Severe bronchiolitis in infancy: Can asthma in adolescence be predicted? *Pediatr. Pulmonol.* **2013**, *48*, 538–544. [CrossRef]
81. Jeng, M.J.; Lee, Y.S.; Tsao, P.C.; Yang, C.F.; Soong, W.J. A longitudinal study on early hospitalized airway infections and subsequent childhood asthma. *PLoS ONE* **2015**, *10*, e0121906. [CrossRef]
82. Nicolai, A.; Frassanito, A.; Nenna, R.; Cangiano, G.; Petrarca, L.; Papoff, P.; Pierangeli, A.; Scagnolari, C.; Moretti, C.; Midulla, F. Risk Factors for Virus-Induced Acute Respiratory Tract Infections in Children Younger Than 3 Years and Recurrent Wheezing at 36 Months Follow-Up After Discharge. *Pediatr. Infect. Dis. J.* **2017**, *36*, 179–183. [CrossRef] [PubMed]
83. Díez-Domingo, J.; Pérez-Yarza, E.G.; Melero, J.A.; Sánchez-Luna, M.; Aguilar, M.D.; Blasco, A.J.; Alfaro, N.; Lázaro, P. Social, economic, and health impact of the respiratory syncytial virus: A systematic search. *BMC Infect. Dis.* **2014**, *14*, 544. [CrossRef]
84. Rinawi, F.; Kassis, I.; Tamir, R.; Kugelman, A.; Srugo, I.; Miron, D. Bronchiolitis in young infants: Is it a risk factor for recurrent wheezing in childhood? *World J. Pediatr.* **2017**, *13*, 41–48. [CrossRef] [PubMed]
85. Skirrow, H.; Wincott, T.; Cecil, E.; Bottle, A.; Costelloe, C.; Saxena, S. Preschool respiratory hospital admissions following infant bronchiolitis: A birth cohort study. *Arch. Dis. Child.* **2019**, *104*, 658–663. [CrossRef] [PubMed]
86. Dumas, O.; Hasegawa, K.; Mansbach, J.M.; Sullivan, A.F.; Piedra, P.A.; Camargo, C.A., Jr. Severe bronchiolitis profiles and risk of recurrent wheeze by age 3 years. *J. Allergy Clin. Immunol.* **2019**, *143*, 1371–1379.e7. [CrossRef]
87. Bacharier, L.B.; Cohen, R.; Schweiger, T.; Yin-Declue, H.; Christie, C.; Zheng, J.; Schechtman, K.B.; Strunk, R.C.; Castro, M. Determinants of asthma after severe respiratory syncytial virus bronchiolitis. *J. Allergy Clin. Immunol.* **2012**, *130*, 91–100.e3. [CrossRef]
88. Mansbach, J.M.; Hasegawa, K.; Geller, R.J.; Espinola, J.A.; Sullivan, A.F.; Camargo, C.A., Jr.; MARC-35 Investigators. Bronchiolitis severity is related to recurrent wheezing by age 3 years in a prospective, multicenter cohort. *Pediatr. Res.* **2020**, *87*, 428–430. [CrossRef]
89. Régnier, S.A.; Huels, J. Association between respiratory syncytial virus hospitalizations in infants and respiratory sequelae: Systematic review and meta-analysis. *Pediatr. Infect. Dis. J.* **2013**, *32*, 820–826. [CrossRef]
90. Coutts, J.; Fullarton, J.; Morris, C.; Grubb, E.; Buchan, S.; Rodgers-Gray, B.; Thwaites, R. Association between respiratory syncytial virus hospitalization in infancy and childhood asthma. *Pediatr. Pulmonol.* **2020**, *55*, 1104–1110. [CrossRef]
91. Nguyen-Van-Tam, J.; Wyffels, V.; Smulders, M.; Mazumder, D.; Tyagi, R.; Gupta, N.; Gavart, S.; Fleischhackl, R. Cumulative incidence of post-infection asthma or wheezing among young children clinically diagnosed with respiratory syncytial virus infection in the United States: A retrospective database analysis. *Influenza Other Respir. Viruses* **2020**, *14*, 730–738. [CrossRef]
92. Shi, T.; Ooi, Y.; Zaw, E.M.; Utjesanovic, N.; Campbell, H.; Cunningham, S.; Bont, L.; Nair, H.; RESCEU Investigators. Association Between Respiratory Syncytial Virus-Associated Acute Lower Respiratory Infection in Early Life and Recurrent Wheeze and Asthma in Later Childhood. *J. Infect. Dis.* **2020**, *222* (Suppl. 7), S628–S633. [CrossRef] [PubMed]
93. Romero, J.R.; Stewart, D.L.; Buysman, E.K.; Fernandes, A.W.; Jafri, H.S.; Mahadevia, P.J. Serious early childhood wheezing after respiratory syncytial virus lower respiratory tract illness in preterm infants. *Clin. Ther.* **2010**, *32*, 2422–2432. [CrossRef] [PubMed]
94. Escobar, G.J.; Masaquel, A.S.; Li, S.X.; Walsh, E.M.; Kipnis, P. Persistent recurring wheezing in the fifth year of life after laboratory-confirmed, medically attended respiratory syncytial virus infection in infancy. *BMC Pediatr.* **2013**, *13*, 97. [CrossRef] [PubMed]
95. Tan, S.; Szatkowski, L.; Moreton, W.; Fiaschi, L.; McKeever, T.; Gibson, J.; Sharkey, D. Early childhood respiratory morbidity and antibiotic use in ex-preterm infants: A primary care population-based cohort study. *Eur. Respir. J.* **2020**, *56*, 2000202. [CrossRef] [PubMed]
96. Van Wijhe, M.; Johannesen, C.K.; Simonsen, L.; Jørgensen, I.M.; RESCEU Investigators; Fischer, T.K. A retrospective cohort study on infant respiratory tract infection hospitalizations and recurrent wheeze and asthma risk: Impact of respiratory syncytial virus. *J. Infect. Dis.* **2022**, *226*, S55–S62. [CrossRef] [PubMed]
97. Brunwasser, S.M.; Snyder, B.M.; Driscoll, A.J.; Fell, D.B.; Savitz, D.A.; Feikin, D.R.; Skidmore, B.; Bhat, N.; Bont, L.J.; Dupont, W.D.; et al. Assessing the strength of evidence for a causal effect of respiratory syncytial virus lower respiratory tract infections on subsequent wheezing illness: A systematic review and meta-analysis. *Lancet Respir. Med.* **2020**, *8*, 795–806, Erratum in *Lancet Respir. Med.* **2021**, *9*, e10. [CrossRef]
98. Korppi, M.; Kotaniemi-Syrjänen, A.; Waris, M.; Vainionpää, R.; Reijonen, T.M. Rhinovirus-associated wheezing in infancy: Comparison with respiratory syncytial virus bronchiolitis. *Pediatr. Infect. Dis. J.* **2004**, *23*, 995–999. [CrossRef]
99. Jartti, T.; Gern, J.E. Rhinovirus-associated wheeze during infancy and asthma development. *Curr. Respir. Med. Rev.* **2011**, *7*, 160–166. [CrossRef]

100. Sun, H.; Sun, Q.; Jiang, W.; Chen, Z.; Huang, L.; Wang, M.; Ji, W.; Shao, X.; Yan, Y. Prevalence of rhinovirus in wheezing children: A comparison with respiratory syncytial virus wheezing. *Braz. J. Infect. Dis.* **2016**, *20*, 179–183. [CrossRef]
101. Cox, D.W.; Bizzintino, J.; Ferrari, G.; Khoo, S.K.; Zhang, G.; Whelan, S.; Lee, W.M.; Bochkov, Y.A.; Geelhoed, G.C.; Goldblatt, J.; et al. Human rhinovirus species C infection in young children with acute wheeze is associated with increased acute respiratory hospital admissions. *Am. J. Respir. Crit. Care Med.* **2013**, *188*, 1358–1364. [CrossRef]
102. Jartti, T.; Kuusipalo, H.; Vuorinen, T.; Söderlund-Venermo, M.; Allander, T.; Waris, M.; Hartiala, J.; Ruuskanen, O. Allergic sensitization is associated with rhinovirus-, but not other virus-, induced wheezing in children. *Pediatr. Allergy Immunol.* **2010**, *21*, 1008–1014. [CrossRef] [PubMed]
103. Hasegawa, K.; Mansbach, J.M.; Bochkov, Y.A.; Gern, J.E.; Piedra, P.A.; Bauer, C.S.; Teach, S.J.; Wu, S.; Sullivan, A.F.; Camargo, C.A., Jr. Association of Rhinovirus C Bronchiolitis and Immunoglobulin E Sensitization During Infancy with Development of Recurrent Wheeze. *JAMA Pediatr.* **2019**, *173*, 544–552. [CrossRef] [PubMed]
104. Reimerink, J.; Stelma, F.; Rockx, B.; Brouwer, D.; Stobberingh, E.; van Ree, R.; Dompeling, E.; Mommers, M.; Thijs, C.; Koopmans, M. Early-life rotavirus and norovirus infections in relation to development of atopic manifestation in infants. *Clin. Exp. Allergy* **2009**, *39*, 254–260. [CrossRef] [PubMed]
105. Li, S.; Williams, G.; Jalaludin, B.; Baker, P. Panel studies of air pollution on children's lung function and respiratory symptoms: A literature review. *J. Asthma* **2012**, *49*, 895–910. [CrossRef] [PubMed]
106. Nordling, E.; Berglind, N.; Melén, E.; Emenius, G.; Hallberg, J.; Nyberg, F.; Pershagen, G.; Svartengren, M.; Wickman, M.; Bellander, T. Traffic-related air pollution and childhood respiratory symptoms, function and allergies. *Epidemiology* **2008**, *19*, 401–408. [CrossRef] [PubMed]
107. Freid, R.D.; Qi, Y.S.; Espinola, J.A.; Cash, R.E.; Aryan, Z.; Sullivan, A.F.; Camargo, C.A., Jr. Proximity to Major Roads and Risks of Childhood Recurrent Wheeze and Asthma in a Severe Bronchiolitis Cohort. *Int. J. Environ. Res. Public Health* **2021**, *18*, 4197. [CrossRef] [PubMed]
108. Brunst, K.J.; Ryan, P.H.; Brokamp, C.; Bernstein, D.; Reponen, T.; Lockey, J.; Hershey, G.K.K.; Levin, L.; Grinshpun, S.A.; LeMasters, G. Timing and Duration of Traffic-related Air Pollution Exposure and the Risk for Childhood Wheeze and Asthma. *Am. J. Respir. Crit. Care Med.* **2015**, *192*, 421–427. [CrossRef]
109. Hasunuma, H.; Sato, T.; Iwata, T.; Kohno, Y.; Nitta, H.; Odajima, H.; Ohara, T.; Omori, T.; Ono, M.; Yamazaki, S.; et al. Association between traffic-related air pollution and asthma in preschool children in a national Japanese nested case-control study. *BMJ Open* **2016**, *6*, e010410. [CrossRef]
110. Esposito, S.; Galeone, C.; Lelii, M.; Longhi, B.; Ascolese, B.; Senatore, L.; Prada, E.; Montinaro, V.; Malerba, S.; Patria, M.F.; et al. Impact of air pollution on respiratory diseases in children with recurrent wheezing or asthma. *BMC Pulm. Med.* **2014**, *14*, 130. [CrossRef]
111. Bonato, M.; Gallo, E.; Turrin, M.; Bazzan, E.; Baraldi, F.; Saetta, M.; Gregori, D.; Papi, A.; Contoli, M.; Baraldo, S. Air Pollution Exposure Impairs Airway Epithelium IFN-β Expression in Pre-School Children. *Front. Immunol.* **2021**, *12*, 731968. [CrossRef]
112. Bonato, M.; Gallo, E.; Bazzan, E.; Marson, G.; Zagolin, L.; Cosio, M.G.; Barbato, A.; Saetta, M.; Gregori, D.; Baraldo, S. Air Pollution Relates to Airway Pathology in Children with Wheezing. *Ann. Am. Thorac. Soc.* **2021**, *18*, 2033–2040. [CrossRef] [PubMed]
113. Norbäck, D.; Lu, C.; Zhang, Y.; Li, B.; Zhao, Z.; Huang, C.; Zhang, X.; Qian, H.; Sun, Y.; Sundell, J.; et al. Onset and remission of childhood wheeze and rhinitis across China—Associations with early life indoor and outdoor air pollution. *Environ. Int.* **2019**, *123*, 61–69. [CrossRef] [PubMed]
114. Holst, G.J.; Pedersen, C.B.; Thygesen, M.; Brandt, J.; Geels, C.; Bønløkke, J.H.; Sigsgaard, T. Air pollution and family related determinants of asthma onset and persistent wheezing in children: Nationwide case-control study. *BMJ* **2020**, *370*, m2791. [CrossRef] [PubMed]
115. Zhang, Y.; Wei, J.; Shi, Y.; Quan, C.; Ho, H.C.; Song, Y.; Zhang, L. Early-life exposure to submicron particulate air pollution in relation to asthma development in Chinese preschool children. *J. Allergy Clin. Immunol.* **2021**, *148*, 771–782.e12. [CrossRef]
116. Brand, A.; McLean, K.E.; Henderson, S.B.; Fournier, M.; Liu, L.; Kosatsky, T.; Smargiassi, A. Respiratory hospital admissions in young children living near metal smelters, pulp mills and oil refineries in two Canadian provinces. *Environ. Int.* **2016**, *94*, 24–32. [CrossRef]
117. Makrinioti, H.; Camargo, C.A.; Zhu, Z.; Freishtat, R.J.; Hasegawa, K. Air pollution, bronchiolitis, and asthma: The role of nasal microRNAs. *Lancet Respir. Med.* **2022**, *10*, 733–734. [CrossRef]
118. Ji, H.; Myers, J.M.B.; Brandt, E.B.; Brokamp, C.; Ryan, P.H.; Hershey, G.K.K. Air pollution, epigenetics, and asthma. *Allergy Asthma Clin. Immunol.* **2016**, *12*, 51. [CrossRef]
119. Sharma, S.; Yang, I.V.; Schwartz, D.A. Epigenetic regulation of immune function in asthma. *J. Allergy Clin. Immunol.* **2022**, *150*, 259–265. [CrossRef]
120. Cai, J.; Li, B.; Yu, W.; Wang, H.; Du, C.; Zhang, Y.; Huang, C.; Zhao, Z.; Deng, Q.; Yang, X.; et al. Household dampness-related exposures in relation to childhood asthma and rhinitis in China: A multicentre observational study. *Environ. Int.* **2019**, *126*, 735–746. [CrossRef]
121. Saijo, Y.; Yoshioka, E.; Sato, Y.; Azuma, H.; Tanahashi, Y.; Ito, Y.; Kobayashi, S.; Minatoya, M.; Bamai, Y.A.; Yamazaki, K.; et al. Relations of mold, stove, and fragrance products on childhood wheezing and asthma: A prospective cohort study from the Japan Environment and Children's Study. *Indoor Air* **2022**, *32*, e12931. [CrossRef]

122. Mikeš, O.; Vrbová, M.; Klánová, J.; Čupr, P.; Švancara, J.; Pikhart, H. Early-life exposure to household chemicals and wheezing in children. *Sci. Total Environ.* **2019**, *663*, 418–425. [CrossRef]
123. Parks, J.; McCandless, L.; Dharma, C.; Brook, J.; Turvey, S.E.; Mandhane, P.; Becker, A.B.; Kozyrskyj, A.L.; Azad, M.B.; Moraes, T.J.; et al. Association of use of cleaning products with respiratory health in a Canadian birth cohort. *CMAJ* **2020**, *192*, E154–E161. [CrossRef] [PubMed]
124. Lin, S.C.; Lin, H.W. Urbanization factors associated with childhood asthma and prematurity: A population-based analysis aged from 0 to 5 years in Taiwan by using Cox regression within a hospital cluster model. *J. Asthma* **2015**, *52*, 273–278. [CrossRef] [PubMed]
125. Gascon, M.; Casas, M.; Morales, E.; Valvi, D.; Ballesteros-Gómez, A.; Luque, N.; Rubio, S.; Monfort, N.; Ventura, R.; Martínez, D.; et al. Prenatal exposure to bisphenol A and phthalates and childhood respiratory tract infections and allergy. *J. Allergy Clin. Immunol.* **2015**, *135*, 370–378. [CrossRef] [PubMed]
126. Bisgaard, H.; Bønnelykke, K.; Sleiman, P.M.; Brasholt, M.; Chawes, B.; Kreiner-Møller, E.; Stage, M.; Kim, C.; Tavendale, R.; Baty, F.; et al. Chromosome 17q21 gene variants are associated with asthma and exacerbations but not atopy in early childhood. *Am. J. Respir. Crit. Care Med.* **2009**, *179*, 179–185. [CrossRef]
127. Halapi, E.; Gudbjartsson, D.F.; Jonsdottir, G.M.; Bjornsdottir, U.S.; Thorleifsson, G.; Helgadottir, H.; Williams, C.; Koppelman, G.H.; Heinzmann, A.; Boezen, H.M.; et al. A sequence variant on 17q21 is associated with age at onset and severity of asthma. *Eur. J. Hum. Genet.* **2010**, *18*, 902–908. [CrossRef] [PubMed]
128. Koponen, P.; Nuolivirta, K.; Virta, M.; Helminen, M.; Hurme, M.; Korppi, M. Polymorphism of the rs1800896 IL10 promoter gene protects children from post-bronchiolitis asthma. *Pediatr. Pulmonol.* **2014**, *49*, 800–806. [CrossRef] [PubMed]
129. Amat, F.; Louha, M.; Benet, M.; Guiddir, T.; Bourgoin-Heck, M.; Saint-Pierre, P.; Paluel-Marmont, C.; Fontaine, C.; Lambert, N.; Couderc, R.; et al. The IL-4 rs2070874 polymorphism may be associated with the severity of recurrent viral-induced wheeze. *Pediatr. Pulmonol.* **2017**, *52*, 1435–1442. [CrossRef]
130. Korppi, M.; Teräsjärvi, J.; Lauhkonen, E.; Törmänen, S.; He, Q.; Nuolivirta, K. Interleukin-1 receptor-associated kinase-4 gene variation may increase post-bronchiolitis asthma risk. *Acta Paediatr.* **2021**, *110*, 952–958. [CrossRef]
131. Koponen, P.; Vuononvirta, J.; Nuolivirta, K.; Helminen, M.; He, Q.; Korppi, M. The association of genetic variants in toll-like receptor 2 subfamily with allergy and asthma after hospitalization for bronchiolitis in infancy. *Pediatr. Infect. Dis. J.* **2014**, *33*, 463–466. [CrossRef]
132. Törmänen, S.; Korppi, M.; Teräsjärvi, J.; Vuononvirta, J.; Koponen, P.; Helminen, M.; He, Q.; Nuolivirta, K. Polymorphism in the gene encoding toll-like receptor 10 may be associated with asthma after bronchiolitis. *Sci. Rep.* **2017**, *7*, 2956. [CrossRef] [PubMed]
133. Klaassen, E.M.; van de Kant, K.D.; Jöbsis, Q.; Penders, J.; van Schooten, F.J.; Quaak, M.; den Hartog, G.J.; Koppelman, G.H.; van Schayck, C.P.; van Eys, G.; et al. Integrative genomic analysis identifies a role for intercellular adhesion molecule 1 in childhood asthma. *Pediatr. Allergy Immunol.* **2014**, *25*, 166–172. [CrossRef] [PubMed]
134. Marenholz, I.; Kerscher, T.; Bauerfeind, A.; Esparza-Gordillo, J.; Nickel, R.; Keil, T.; Lau, S.; Rohde, K.; Wahn, U.; Lee, Y.A. An interaction between filaggrin mutations and early food sensitization improves the prediction of childhood asthma. *J. Allergy Clin. Immunol.* **2009**, *123*, 911–916. [CrossRef] [PubMed]
135. Dixon, A.E.; Peters, U. The effect of obesity on lung function. *Expert Rev. Respir. Med.* **2018**, *12*, 755–767. [CrossRef] [PubMed]
136. Lowe, J.; Kotecha, S.J.; Watkins, W.J.; Kotecha, S. Effect of fetal and infant growth on respiratory symptoms in preterm-born children. *Pediatr. Pulmonol.* **2018**, *53*, 189–196. [CrossRef]
137. Kotecha, S.J.; Lowe, J.; Granell, R.; Watkins, W.J.; Henderson, A.J.; Kotecha, S. The effect of catch-up growth in the first year of life on later wheezing phenotypes. *Eur. Respir. J.* **2020**, *56*, 2000884. [CrossRef]
138. Mensink-Bout, S.M.; Santos, S.; van Meel, E.R.; Oei, E.H.G.; de Jongste, J.C.; Jaddoe, V.W.V.; Duijts, L. General and Organ Fat Assessed by Magnetic Resonance Imaging and Respiratory Outcomes in Childhood. *Am. J. Respir. Crit. Care Med.* **2020**, *201*, 348–355. [CrossRef]
139. Sonnenschein-van der Voort, A.M.; Jaddoe, V.W.; Raat, H.; Moll, H.A.; Hofman, A.; de Jongste, J.C.; Duijts, L. Fetal and infant growth and asthma symptoms in preschool children: The Generation R Study. *Am. J. Respir. Crit. Care Med.* **2012**, *185*, 731–737. [CrossRef]
140. Pike, K.C.; Crozier, S.R.; Lucas, J.S.; Inskip, H.M.; Robinson, S.; Southampton Women's Survey Study Group; Roberts, G.; Godfrey, K.M. Patterns of fetal and infant growth are related to atopy and wheezing disorders at age 3 years. *Thorax* **2010**, *65*, 1099–1106. [CrossRef]
141. Zhang, Z.; Lai, H.J.; Roberg, K.A.; Gangnon, R.E.; Evans, M.D.; Anderson, E.L.; Pappas, T.E.; Dasilva, D.F.; Tisler, C.J.; Salazar, L.P.; et al. Early childhood weight status in relation to asthma development in high-risk children. *J. Allergy Clin. Immunol.* **2010**, *126*, 1157–1162. [CrossRef]
142. Murray, C.S.; Canoy, D.; Buchan, I.; Woodcock, A.; Simpson, A.; Custovic, A. Body mass index in young children and allergic disease: Gender differences in a longitudinal study. *Clin. Exp. Allergy* **2011**, *41*, 78–85. [CrossRef] [PubMed]
143. Rzehak, P.; Wijga, A.H.; Keil, T.; Eller, E.; Bindslev-Jensen, C.; Smit, H.A.; Weyler, J.; Dom, S.; Sunyer, J.; Mendez, M.; et al. Body mass index trajectory classes and incident asthma in childhood: Results from 8 European Birth Cohorts—A Global Allergy and Asthma European Network initiative. *J. Allergy Clin. Immunol.* **2013**, *131*, 1528–1536. [CrossRef] [PubMed]

144. Dai, R.; Miliku, K.; Gaddipati, S.; Choi, J.; Ambalavanan, A.; Tran, M.M.; Reyna, M.; Sbihi, H.; Lou, W.; Parvulescu, P.; et al. Wheeze trajectories: Determinants and outcomes in the CHILD Cohort Study. *J. Allergy Clin. Immunol.* **2022**, *149*, 2153–2165. [CrossRef]
145. Crump, C. Preterm birth and mortality in adulthood: A systematic review. *J. Perinatol.* **2020**, *40*, 833–843. [CrossRef] [PubMed]
146. Abe, K.; Shapiro-Mendoza, C.K.; Hall, L.R.; Satten, G.A. Late preterm birth and risk of developing asthma. *J. Pediatr.* **2010**, *157*, 74–78. [CrossRef] [PubMed]
147. Boyle, E.M.; Poulsen, G.; Field, D.J.; Kurinczuk, J.J.; Wolke, D.; Alfirevic, Z.; Quigley, M.A. Effects of gestational age at birth on health outcomes at 3 and 5 years of age: Population based cohort study. *BMJ* **2012**, *344*, e896. [CrossRef] [PubMed]
148. Been, J.V.; Lugtenberg, M.J.; Smets, E.; van Schayck, C.P.; Kramer, B.W.; Mommers, M.; Sheikh, A. Preterm birth and childhood wheezing disorders: A systematic review and meta-analysis. *PLoS Med.* **2014**, *11*, e1001596. [CrossRef]
149. Voge, G.A.; Katusic, S.K.; Qin, R.; Juhn, Y.J. Risk of Asthma in Late Preterm Infants: A Propensity Score Approach. *J. Allergy Clin. Immunol. Pract.* **2015**, *3*, 905–910. [CrossRef]
150. Leps, C.; Carson, C.; Quigley, M.A. Gestational age at birth and wheezing trajectories at 3–11 years. *Arch. Dis. Child.* **2018**, *103*, 1138–1144. [CrossRef]
151. Pike, K.C.; Lucas, J.S. Respiratory consequences of late preterm birth. *Paediatr. Respir. Rev.* **2015**, *16*, 182–188. [CrossRef]
152. Simões, M.C.R.D.S.; Inoue, Y.; Matsunaga, N.Y.; Carvalho, M.R.V.; Ribeiro, G.L.T.; Morais, E.O.; Ribeiro, M.A.G.O.; Morcillo, A.M.; Ribeiro, J.D.; Toro, A.A.D.C. Recurrent wheezing in preterm infants: Prevalence and risk factors. *J. Pediatr.* **2019**, *95*, 720–727. [CrossRef] [PubMed]
153. Algert, C.S.; Bowen, J.R.; Lain, S.L.; Allen, H.D.; Vivian-Taylor, J.M.; Roberts, C.L. Pregnancy exposures and risk of childhood asthma admission in a population birth cohort. *Pediatr. Allergy Immunol.* **2011**, *22*, 836–842. [CrossRef] [PubMed]
154. Kumar, R.; Yu, Y.; Story, R.E.; Pongracic, J.A.; Gupta, R.; Pearson, C.; Ortiz, K.; Bauchner, H.C.; Wang, X. Prematurity, chorioamnionitis, and the development of recurrent wheezing: A prospective birth cohort study. *J. Allergy Clin. Immunol.* **2008**, *121*, 878–884.e6. [CrossRef] [PubMed]
155. Yamamoto-Hanada, K.; Pak, K.; Saito-Abe, M.; Sato, M.; Ohya, Y.; Japan Environment and Children's Study (JECS) Group. Better maternal quality of life in pregnancy yields better offspring respiratory outcomes: A birth cohort. *Ann. Allergy Asthma Immunol.* **2021**, *126*, 713–721.e1. [CrossRef] [PubMed]
156. Liu, X.; Olsen, J.; Agerbo, E.; Yuan, W.; Sigsgaard, T.; Li, J. Prenatal stress and childhood asthma in the offspring: Role of age at onset. *Eur. J. Public Health* **2015**, *25*, 1042–1046. [CrossRef] [PubMed]
157. Smejda, K.; Polanska, K.; Merecz-Kot, D.; Krol, A.; Hanke, W.; Jerzynska, J.; Stelmach, W.; Majak, P.; Stelmach, I. Maternal Stress During Pregnancy and Allergic Diseases in Children During the First Year of Life. *Respir. Care* **2018**, *63*, 70–76. [CrossRef]
158. Stick, S.M.; Burton, P.R.; Gurrin, L.; Sly, P.D.; LeSouëf, P.N. Effects of maternal smoking during pregnancy and a family history of asthma on respiratory function in newborn infants. *Lancet* **1996**, *348*, 1060–1064. [CrossRef]
159. Lin, J.; Yuan, S.; Dong, B.; Zhang, J.; Zhang, L.; Wu, J.; Chen, J.; Tang, M.; Zhang, B.; Wang, H.; et al. The Associations of Caesarean Delivery with Risk of Wheezing Diseases and Changes of T Cells in Children. *Front. Immunol.* **2021**, *12*, 793762. [CrossRef]
160. Huang, L.; Chen, Q.; Zhao, Y.; Wang, W.; Fang, F.; Bao, Y. Is elective cesarean section associated with a higher risk of asthma? A meta-analysis. *J. Asthma* **2015**, *52*, 16–25. [CrossRef]
161. Abdullah, K.; Zhu, J.; Gershon, A.; Dell, S.; To, T. Effect of asthma exacerbation during pregnancy in women with asthma: A population-based cohort study. *Eur. Respir. J.* **2020**, *55*, 1901335. [CrossRef]
162. Gonçalves, D.M.M.; Wandalsen, G.F.; Scavacini, A.S.; Lanza, F.C.; Goulart, A.L.; Solé, D.; Dos Santos, A.M.N. Pulmonary function in former very low birth weight preterm infants in the first year of life. *Respir. Med.* **2018**, *136*, 83–87. [CrossRef] [PubMed]
163. Den Dekker, H.T.; Jaddoe, V.W.V.; Reiss, I.K.; de Jongste, J.C.; Duijts, L. Fetal and Infant Growth Patterns and Risk of Lower Lung Function and Asthma. The Generation R Study. *Am. J. Respir. Crit. Care Med.* **2018**, *197*, 183–192. [CrossRef] [PubMed]
164. Edwards, C.A.; Osman, L.M.; Godden, D.J.; Campbell, D.M.; Douglas, J.G. Relationship between birth weight and adult lung function: Controlling for maternal factors. *Thorax* **2003**, *58*, 1061–1065. [CrossRef] [PubMed]
165. Den Dekker, H.T.; Sonnenschein-van der Voort, A.M.M.; de Jongste, J.C.; Anessi-Maesano, I.; Arshad, S.H.; Barros, H.; Beardsmore, C.S.; Bisgaard, H.; Phar, S.C.; Craig, L.; et al. Early growth characteristics and the risk of reduced lung function and asthma: A meta-analysis of 25,000 children. *J. Allergy Clin. Immunol.* **2016**, *137*, 1026–1035. [CrossRef]
166. Principi, N.; Di Pietro, G.M.; Esposito, S. Bronchopulmonary dysplasia: Clinical aspects and preventive and therapeutic strategies. *J. Transl. Med.* **2018**, *16*, 36. [CrossRef]
167. Hollams, E.M.; de Klerk, N.H.; Holt, P.G.; Sly, P.D. Persistent effects of maternal smoking during pregnancy on lung function and asthma in adolescents. *Am. J. Respir. Crit. Care Med.* **2014**, *189*, 401–407. [CrossRef]
168. Gilliland, F.D.; Li, Y.F.; Peters, J.M. Effects of maternal smoking during pregnancy and environmental tobacco smoke on asthma and wheezing in children. *Am. J. Respir. Crit. Care Med.* **2001**, *163*, 429–436. [CrossRef]
169. Indinnimeo, L.; Porta, D.; Forastiere, F.; De Vittori, V.; De Castro, G.; Zicari, A.M.; Tancredi, G.; Melengu, T.; Duse, M. Prevalence and risk factors for atopic disease in a population of preschool children in Rome: Challenges to early intervention. *Int. J. Immunopathol. Pharmacol.* **2016**, *29*, 308–319. [CrossRef]
170. Selby, A.; Munro, A.; Grimshaw, K.E.; Cornelius, V.; Keil, T.; Grabenhenrich, L.; Clausen, M.; Dubakiene, R.; Fiocchi, A.; Kowalski, M.L.; et al. Prevalence estimates and risk factors for early childhood wheeze across Europe: The EuroPrevall birth cohort. *Thorax* **2018**, *73*, 1049–1061. [CrossRef]

171. Burke, H.; Leonardi-Bee, J.; Hashim, A.; Pine-Abata, H.; Chen, Y.; Cook, D.G.; Britton, J.R.; McKeever, T.M. Prenatal and passive smoke exposure and incidence of asthma and wheeze: Systematic review and meta-analysis. *Pediatrics* **2012**, *129*, 735–744. [CrossRef]
172. Vardavas, C.I.; Hohmann, C.; Patelarou, E.; Martinez, D.; Henderson, A.J.; Granell, R.; Sunyer, J.; Torrent, M.; Fantini, M.P.; Gori, D.; et al. The independent role of prenatal and postnatal exposure to active and passive smoking on the development of early wheeze in children. *Eur. Respir. J.* **2016**, *48*, 115–124. [CrossRef] [PubMed]
173. Collet, C.; Fayon, M.; Francis, F.; Galode, F.; Bui, S.; Debelleix, S. The First 1000 Days: Impact of Prenatal Tobacco Smoke Exposure on Hospitalization Due to Preschool Wheezing. *Healthcare* **2021**, *9*, 1089. [CrossRef] [PubMed]
174. Bolat, E.; Arikoglu, T.; Sungur, M.A.; Batmaz, S.B.; Kuyucu, S. Prevalence and risk factors for wheezing and allergic diseases in preschool children: A perspective from the Mediterranean coast of Turkey. *Allergol. Immunopathol.* **2017**, *45*, 362–368. [CrossRef] [PubMed]
175. Sahiner, U.M.; Buyuktiryaki, B.; Cavkaytar, O.; Yılmaz, E.A.; Soyer, O.; Sackesen, C.; Tuncer, A.; Sekerel, B.E. Recurrent wheezing in the first three years of life: Short-term prognosis and risk factors. *J. Asthma* **2013**, *50*, 370–375. [CrossRef]
176. Robison, R.G.; Kumar, R.; Arguelles, L.M.; Hong, X.; Wang, G.; Apollon, S.; Bonzagni, A.; Ortiz, K.; Pearson, C.; Pongracic, J.A.; et al. Maternal smoking during pregnancy, prematurity and recurrent wheezing in early childhood. *Pediatr. Pulmonol.* **2012**, *47*, 666–673. [CrossRef]
177. Lodge, C.J.; Zaloumis, S.; Lowe, A.J.; Gurrin, L.C.; Matheson, M.C.; Axelrad, C.; Bennett, C.M.; Hill, D.J.; Hosking, C.S.; Svanes, C.; et al. Early-life risk factors for childhood wheeze phenotypes in a high-risk birth cohort. *J. Pediatr.* **2014**, *164*, 289–294. [CrossRef]
178. Yilmaz, O.; Turkeli, A.; Onur, E.; Bilge, S.; Yuksel, H. Secondhand tobacco smoke and severity in wheezing children: Nasal oxidant stress and inflammation. *J. Asthma* **2018**, *55*, 477–482. [CrossRef]
179. Sadeghnejad, A.; Karmaus, W.; Arshad, S.H.; Kurukulaaratchy, R.; Huebner, M.; Ewart, S. IL13 gene polymorphisms modify the effect of exposure to tobacco smoke on persistent wheeze and asthma in childhood, a longitudinal study. *Respir. Res.* **2008**, *9*, 2. [CrossRef]
180. Bals, R.; Boyd, J.; Esposito, S.; Foronjy, R.; Hiemstra, P.S.; Jiménez-Ruiz, C.A.; Katsaounou, P.; Lindberg, A.; Metz, C.; Schober, W.; et al. Electronic cigarettes: A task force report from the European Respiratory Society. *Eur. Respir. J.* **2019**, *53*, 1801151. [CrossRef]
181. McCusker, C.; Upton, J.; Warrington, R. Primary immunodeficiency. *Allergy Asthma Clin. Immunol.* **2018**, *14* (Suppl. 2), 61. [CrossRef]
182. Ozbek, B.; Ayvaz, D.Ç.; Esenboga, S.; Halaçlı, S.O.; Aytekin, E.S.; Yaz, I.; Tan, Ç.; Tezcan, I. In case of recurrent wheezing and bronchiolitis: Think again, it may be a primary immunodeficiency. *Asian Pac. J. Allergy Immunol.* **2019**, *Online ahead of print*. [CrossRef]
183. Siriaksorn, S.; Suchaitanawanit, S.; Trakultivakorn, M. Allergic rhinitis and immunoglobulin deficiency in preschool children with frequent upper respiratory illness. *Asian Pac. J. Allergy Immunol.* **2011**, *29*, 73–77. [CrossRef] [PubMed]
184. Sandin, A.; Björkstén, B.; Böttcher, M.F.; Englund, E.; Jenmalm, M.C.; Bråbäck, L. High salivary secretory IgA antibody levels are associated with less late-onset wheezing in IgE-sensitized infants. *Pediatr. Allergy Immunol.* **2011**, *22*, 477–481. [CrossRef] [PubMed]
185. Papadopoulou, A.; Mermiri, D.; Taousani, S.; Triga, M.; Nicolaidou, P.; Priftis, K.N. Bronchial hyper-responsiveness in selective IgA deficiency. *Pediatr. Allergy Immunol.* **2005**, *16*, 495–500. [CrossRef]
186. Cinicola, B.L.; Pulvirenti, F.; Capponi, M.; Bonetti, M.; Brindisi, G.; Gori, A.; De Castro, G.; Anania, C.; Duse, M.; Zicari, A.M. Selective IgA Deficiency and Allergy: A Fresh Look to an Old Story. *Medicina* **2022**, *58*, 129. [CrossRef]
187. Vidarsson, G.; Dekkers, G.; Rispens, T. IgG subclasses and allotypes: From structure to effector functions. *Front. Immunol.* **2014**, *5*, 520. [CrossRef]
188. Kim, C.K.; Park, J.S.; Chu, S.Y.; Kwon, E.; Kim, H.; Callaway, Z. Low immunoglobulin G4 subclass level is associated with recurrent wheezing in young children. *Asia Pac. Allergy* **2020**, *10*, e43. [CrossRef]
189. Zaitsu, M.; Matsuo, M. Transient low IgG4 levels cause recurrent wheezing requiring multiple hospitalizations in infancy. *Pediatr. Pulmonol.* **2022**, *57*, 1631–1634. [CrossRef]
190. Prescott, S.L.; Björkstén, B. Probiotics for the prevention or treatment of allergic diseases. *J. Allergy Clin. Immunol.* **2007**, *120*, 255–262. [CrossRef]
191. Frati, F.; Salvatori, C.; Incorvaia, C.; Bellucci, A.; Di Cara, G.; Marcucci, F.; Esposito, S. The Role of the Microbiome in Asthma: The Gut-Lung Axis. *Int. J. Mol. Sci.* **2018**, *20*, 123. [CrossRef]
192. Azad, M.B.; Kozyrskyj, A.L. Perinatal programming of asthma: The role of gut microbiota. *Clin. Dev. Immunol.* **2012**, *2012*, 932072. [CrossRef] [PubMed]
193. Wang, M.; Karlsson, C.; Olsson, C.; Adlerberth, I.; Wold, A.E.; Strachan, D.P.; Martricardi, P.M.; Aberg, N.; Perkin, M.R.; Tripodi, S.; et al. Reduced diversity in the early fecal microbiota of infants with atopic eczema. *J. Allergy Clin. Immunol.* **2008**, *121*, 129–134. [CrossRef] [PubMed]
194. Abrahamsson, T.R.; Jakobsson, H.E.; Andersson, A.F.; Björkstén, B.; Engstrand, L.; Jenmalm, M.C. Low diversity of the gut microbiota in infants with atopic eczema. *J. Allergy Clin. Immunol.* **2012**, *129*, 434–440.e1-2. [CrossRef] [PubMed]
195. Zheng, T.; Yu, J.; Oh, M.H.; Zhu, Z. The atopic march: Progression from atopic dermatitis to allergic rhinitis and asthma. *Allergy Asthma Immunol. Res.* **2011**, *3*, 67–73. [CrossRef] [PubMed]

196. Li, L.; Wang, F.; Liu, Y.; Gu, F. Intestinal microbiota dysbiosis in children with recurrent respiratory tract infections. *Microb. Pathog.* **2019**, *136*, 103709. [CrossRef]
197. Stokholm, J.; Thorsen, J.; Blaser, M.J.; Rasmussen, M.A.; Hjelmsø, M.; Shah, S.; Christensen, E.D.; Chawes, B.L.; Bønnelykke, K.; Brix, S.; et al. Delivery mode and gut microbial changes correlate with an increased risk of childhood asthma. *Sci. Transl. Med.* **2020**, *12*, eaax9929. [CrossRef]
198. Arrieta, M.C.; Stiemsma, L.T.; Dimitriu, P.A.; Thorson, L.; Russell, S.; Yurist-Doutsch, S.; Kuzeljevic, B.; Gold, M.J.; Britton, H.M.; Lefebvre, D.L.; et al. Early infancy microbial and metabolic alterations affect risk of childhood asthma. *Sci. Transl. Med.* **2015**, *7*, 307ra152. [CrossRef]
199. Abrahamsson, T.R.; Jakobsson, H.E.; Andersson, A.F.; Björkstén, B.; Engstrand, L.; Jenmalm, M.C. Low gut microbiota diversity in early infancy precedes asthma at school age. *Clin. Exp. Allergy* **2014**, *44*, 842–850. [CrossRef]
200. Bannier, M.A.G.E.; van Best, N.; Bervoets, L.; Savelkoul, P.H.M.; Hornef, M.W.; van de Kant, K.D.G.; Jöbsis, Q.; Dompeling, E.; Penders, J. Gut microbiota in wheezing preschool children and the association with childhood asthma. *Allergy* **2020**, *75*, 1473–1476. [CrossRef]
201. Jensen, M.P.; Meldrum, S.; Taylor, A.L.; Dunstan, J.A.; Prescott, S.L. Early probiotic supplementation for allergy prevention: Long-term outcomes. *J. Allergy Clin. Immunol.* **2012**, *130*, 1209–1211.e5. [CrossRef]
202. Cabana, M.D.; McKean, M.; Caughey, A.B.; Fong, L.; Lynch, S.; Wong, A.; Leong, R.; Boushey, H.A.; Hilton, J.F. Early Probiotic Supplementation for Eczema and Asthma Prevention: A Randomized Controlled Trial. *Pediatrics* **2017**, *140*, e20163000. [CrossRef] [PubMed]
203. Canani, R.B.; Di Costanzo, M.; Bedogni, G.; Amoroso, A.; Cosenza, L.; Di Scala, C.; Granata, V.; Nocerino, R. Extensively hydrolyzed casein formula containing Lactobacillus rhamnosus GG reduces the occurrence of other allergic manifestations in children with cow's milk allergy: 3-year randomized controlled trial. *J. Allergy Clin. Immunol.* **2017**, *139*, 1906–1913.e4. [CrossRef] [PubMed]
204. Wei, X.; Jiang, P.; Liu, J.; Sun, R.; Zhu, L. Association between probiotic supplementation and asthma incidence in infants: A meta-analysis of randomized controlled trials. *J. Asthma* **2020**, *57*, 167–178. [CrossRef] [PubMed]
205. Cuello-Garcia, C.A.; Brożek, J.L.; Fiocchi, A.; Pawankar, R.; Yepes-Nuñez, J.J.; Terracciano, L.; Gandhi, S.; Agarwal, A.; Zhang, Y.; Schünemann, H.J. Probiotics for the prevention of allergy: A systematic review and meta-analysis of randomized controlled trials. *J. Allergy Clin. Immunol.* **2015**, *136*, 952–961. [CrossRef] [PubMed]
206. Azad, M.B.; Coneys, J.G.; Kozyrskyj, A.L.; Field, C.J.; Ramsey, C.D.; Becker, A.B.; Friesen, C.; Abou-Setta, A.M.; Zarychanski, R. Probiotic supplementation during pregnancy or infancy for the prevention of asthma and wheeze: Systematic review and meta-analysis. *BMJ* **2013**, *347*, f6471. [CrossRef]
207. Kuitunen, M.; Kukkonen, K.; Juntunen-Backman, K.; Korpela, R.; Poussa, T.; Tuure, T.; Haahtela, T.; Savilahti, E. Probiotics prevent IgE-associated allergy until age 5 years in cesarean-delivered children but not in the total cohort. *J. Allergy Clin. Immunol.* **2009**, *123*, 335–341. [CrossRef]
208. Lin, J.; Zhang, Y.; He, C.; Dai, J. Probiotics supplementation in children with asthma: A systematic review and meta-analysis. *J. Paediatr. Child. Health* **2018**, *54*, 953–961. [CrossRef]
209. Rose, M.A.; Stieglitz, F.; Köksal, A.; Schubert, R.; Schulze, J.; Zielen, S. Efficacy of probiotic Lactobacillus GG on allergic sensitization and asthma in infants at risk. *Clin. Exp. Allergy* **2010**, *40*, 1398–1405. [CrossRef]
210. Rose, M.A.; Schubert, R.; Schulze, J.; Zielen, S. Follow-up of probiotic Lactobacillus GG effects on allergic sensitization and asthma in infants at risk. *Clin. Exp. Allergy* **2011**, *41*, 1819–1821. [CrossRef]
211. Elazab, N.; Mendy, A.; Gasana, J.; Vieira, E.R.; Quizon, A.; Forno, E. Probiotic administration in early life, atopy, and asthma: A meta-analysis of clinical trials. *Pediatrics* **2013**, *132*, e666–e676. [CrossRef]
212. Esposito, S.; Lelii, M. Vitamin D and respiratory tract infections in childhood. *BMC Infect. Dis.* **2015**, *15*, 487. [CrossRef] [PubMed]
213. Pfeffer, P.E.; Hawrylowicz, C.M. Vitamin D in Asthma: Mechanisms of Action and Considerations for Clinical Trials. *Chest* **2018**, *153*, 1229–1239. [CrossRef] [PubMed]
214. Xystrakis, E.; Kusumakar, S.; Boswell, S.; Peek, E.; Urry, Z.; Richards, D.F.; Adikibi, T.; Pridgeon, C.; Dallman, M.; Loke, T.K.; et al. Reversing the defective induction of IL-10-secreting regulatory T cells in glucocorticoid-resistant asthma patients. *J. Clin. Investig.* **2006**, *116*, 146–155. [CrossRef] [PubMed]
215. Chambers, E.S.; Nanzer, A.M.; Pfeffer, P.E.; Richards, D.F.; Timms, P.M.; Martineau, A.R.; Griffiths, C.J.; Corrigan, C.J.; Hawrylowicz, C.M. Distinct endotypes of steroid-resistant asthma characterized by IL-17A(high) and IFN-γ(high) immunophenotypes: Potential benefits of calcitriol. *J. Allergy Clin. Immunol.* **2015**, *136*, 628–637.e4. [CrossRef] [PubMed]
216. Lan, N.; Luo, G.; Yang, X.; Cheng, Y.; Zhang, Y.; Wang, X.; Wang, X.; Xie, T.; Li, G.; Liu, Z.; et al. 25-Hydroxyvitamin D3-deficiency enhances oxidative stress and corticosteroid resistance in severe asthma exacerbation. *PLoS ONE* **2014**, *9*, e111599. [CrossRef]
217. Gupta, A.; Sjoukes, A.; Richards, D.; Banya, W.; Hawrylowicz, C.; Bush, A.; Saglani, S. Relationship between serum vitamin D, disease severity, and airway remodeling in children with asthma. *Am. J. Respir. Crit. Care Med.* **2011**, *184*, 1342–1349. [CrossRef]
218. Damera, G.; Fogle, H.W.; Lim, P.; Goncharova, E.A.; Zhao, H.; Banerjee, A.; Tliba, O.; Krymskaya, V.P.; Panettieri, R.A., Jr. Vitamin D inhibits growth of human airway smooth muscle cells through growth factor-induced phosphorylation of retinoblastoma protein and checkpoint kinase 1. *Br. J. Pharmacol.* **2009**, *158*, 1429–1441. [CrossRef]
219. Principi, N.; Bianchini, S.; Baggi, E.; Esposito, S. Implications of maternal vitamin D deficiency for the fetus, the neonate and the young infant. *Eur. J. Nutr.* **2013**, *52*, 859–867. [CrossRef]

220. Principi, N.; Esposito, S. Vitamin D Deficiency During Pregnancy and Autism Spectrum Disorders Development. *Front. Psychiatry* **2020**, *10*, 987. [CrossRef]
221. Lu, M.; Litonjua, A.A.; O'Connor, G.T.; Zeiger, R.S.; Bacharier, L.; Schatz, M.; Carey, V.J.; Weiss, S.T.; Mirzakhani, H. Effect of early and late prenatal vitamin D and maternal asthma status on offspring asthma or recurrent wheeze. *J. Allergy Clin. Immunol.* **2021**, *147*, 1234–1241.e3. [CrossRef]
222. Knihtilä, H.M.; Stubbs, B.J.; Carey, V.J.; Laranjo, N.; Chu, S.H.; Kelly, R.S.; Zeiger, R.S.; Bacharier, L.B.; O'Connor, G.T.; Lasky-Su, J.; et al. Low gestational vitamin D level and childhood asthma are related to impaired lung function in high-risk children. *J. Allergy Clin. Immunol.* **2021**, *148*, 110–119.e9. [CrossRef] [PubMed]
223. Li, W.; Qin, Z.; Gao, J.; Jiang, Z.; Chai, Y.; Guan, L.; Ge, Y.; Chen, Y. Vitamin D supplementation during pregnancy and the risk of wheezing in offspring: A systematic review and dose-response meta-analysis. *J. Asthma* **2019**, *56*, 1266–1273. [CrossRef] [PubMed]
224. Knihtilä, H.M.; Kelly, R.S.; Brustad, N.; Huang, M.; Kachroo, P.; Chawes, B.L.; Stokholm, J.; Bønnelykke, K.; Pedersen, C.T.; Bisgaard, H.; et al. Maternal 17q21 genotype influences prenatal vitamin D effects on offspring asthma/recurrent wheeze. *Eur. Respir. J.* **2021**, *58*, 2002012. [CrossRef] [PubMed]
225. Dogru, M.; Kirmizibekmez, H.; Yesiltepe Mutlu, R.G.; Aktas, A.; Ozturkmen, S. Clinical effects of vitamin D in children with asthma. *Int. Arch. Allergy Immunol.* **2014**, *164*, 319–325. [CrossRef] [PubMed]
226. Demirel, S.; Guner, S.N.; Celiksoy, M.H.; Sancak, R. Is vitamin D insufficiency to blame for recurrent wheezing? *Int. Forum Allergy Rhinol.* **2014**, *4*, 980–985. [CrossRef]
227. Beigelman, A.; Zeiger, R.S.; Mauger, D.; Strunk, R.C.; Jackson, D.J.; Martinez, F.D.; Morgan, W.J.; Covar, R.; Szefler, S.J.; Taussig, L.M.; et al. The association between vitamin D status and the rate of exacerbations requiring oral corticosteroids in preschool children with recurrent wheezing. *J. Allergy Clin. Immunol.* **2014**, *133*, 1489–1492.e1-3. [CrossRef]
228. Stenberg Hammar, K.; Hedlin, G.; Konradsen, J.R.; Nordlund, B.; Kull, I.; Giske, C.G.; Pedroletti, C.; Söderhäll, C.; Melén, E. Subnormal levels of vitamin D are associated with acute wheeze in young children. *Acta Paediatr.* **2014**, *103*, 856–861. [CrossRef]
229. Al-Zayadneh, E.; Alnawaiseh, N.A.; Ajarmeh, S.; Altarawneh, A.H.; Albataineh, E.M.; AlZayadneh, E.; Shatanawi, A.; Alzayadneh, E.M. Vitamin D deficiency in children with bronchial asthma in southern Jordan: A cross-sectional study. *J. Int. Med. Res.* **2020**, *48*, 300060520974242. [CrossRef]
230. Turkeli, A.; Ayaz, O.; Uncu, A.; Ozhan, B.; Bas, V.N.; Tufan, A.K.; Yilmaz, O.; Yuksel, H. Effects of vitamin D levels on asthma control and severity in pre-school children. *Eur. Rev. Med. Pharmacol. Sci.* **2016**, *20*, 26–36.
231. Urrutia-Pereira, M.; Solé, D. Is Vitamin D Deficiency a Marker of Severity of Wheezing in Children? A Cross-sectional Study. *J. Investig. Allergol. Clin. Immunol.* **2016**, *26*, 319–321. [CrossRef]
232. Omand, J.A.; To, T.; O'Connor, D.L.; Parkin, P.C.; Birken, C.S.; Thorpe, K.E.; Maguire, J.L. 25-hydroxyvitamin D and health service utilization for asthma in early childhood. *Pediatr. Pulmonol.* **2018**, *53*, 1018–1026. [CrossRef] [PubMed]
233. Adam-Bonci, T.I.; Chereches-Panta, P.; Bonci, E.A.; Man, S.C.; Cutas-Benedec, A.; Drugan, T.; Pop, R.M.; Irimie, A. Suboptimal Serum 25-Hydroxy-Vitamin D Is Associated with a History of Recent Disease Exacerbation in Pediatric Patients with Bronchial Asthma or Asthma-Suggestive Recurrent Wheezing. *Int. J. Environ. Res. Public Health* **2020**, *17*, 6545. [CrossRef] [PubMed]
234. Ducharme, F.M.; Jensen, M.; Mailhot, G.; Alos, N.; White, J.; Rousseau, E.; Tse, S.M.; Khamessan, A.; Vinet, B. Impact of two oral doses of 100,000 IU of vitamin D3 in preschoolers with viral-induced asthma: A pilot randomised controlled trial. *Trials* **2019**, *20*, 138. [CrossRef] [PubMed]
235. Rueter, K.; Jones, A.P.; Siafarikas, A.; Lim, E.M.; Prescott, S.L.; Palmer, D.J. In "High-Risk" Infants with Sufficient Vitamin D Status at Birth, Infant Vitamin D Supplementation Had No Effect on Allergy Outcomes: A Randomized Controlled Trial. *Nutrients* **2020**, *12*, 1747. [CrossRef] [PubMed]
236. Vlieg-Boerstra, B.; de Jong, N.; Meyer, R.; Agostoni, C.; De Cosmi, V.; Grimshaw, K.; Milani, G.P.; Muraro, A.; Oude Elberink, H.; Pali-Schöll, I.; et al. Nutrient supplementation for prevention of viral respiratory tract infections in healthy subjects: A systematic review and meta-analysis. *Allergy* **2022**, *77*, 1373–1388. [CrossRef]
237. Martineau, A.R.; Jolliffe, D.A.; Greenberg, L.; Aloia, J.F.; Bergman, P.; Dubnov-Raz, G.; Esposito, S.; Ganmaa, D.; Ginde, A.A.; Goodall, E.C.; et al. Vitamin D supplementation to prevent acute respiratory infections: Individual participant data meta-analysis. *Health Technol. Assess.* **2019**, *23*, 1–44. [CrossRef]
238. Jolliffe, D.A.; Camargo, C.A., Jr.; Sluyter, J.D.; Aglipay, M.; Aloia, J.F.; Ganmaa, D.; Bergman, P.; Bischoff-Ferrari, H.A.; Borzutzky, A.; Damsgaard, C.T.; et al. Vitamin D supplementation to prevent acute respiratory infections: A systematic review and meta-analysis of aggregate data from randomised controlled trials. *Lancet Diabetes Endocrinol.* **2021**, *9*, 276–292. [CrossRef]
239. Chen, Z.; Peng, C.; Mei, J.; Zhu, L.; Kong, H. Vitamin D can safely reduce asthma exacerbations among corticosteroid-using children and adults with asthma: A systematic review and meta-analysis of randomized controlled trials. *Nutr. Res.* **2021**, *92*, 49–61. [CrossRef]
240. Midodzi, W.K.; Rowe, B.H.; Majaesic, C.M.; Saunders, L.D.; Senthilselvan, A. Early life factors associated with incidence of physician-diagnosed asthma in preschool children: Results from the Canadian Early Childhood Development cohort study. *J. Asthma* **2010**, *47*, 7–13. [CrossRef]
241. Klopp, A.; Vehling, L.; Becker, A.B.; Subbarao, P.; Mandhane, P.J.; Turvey, S.E.; Lefebvre, D.L.; Sears, M.R.; CHILD Study Investigators; Azad, M.B. Modes of Infant Feeding and the Risk of Childhood Asthma: A Prospective Birth Cohort Study. *J. Pediatr.* **2017**, *190*, 192–199.e2. [CrossRef]

242. Leung, J.Y.; Kwok, M.K.; Leung, G.M.; Schooling, C.M. Breastfeeding and childhood hospitalizations for asthma and other wheezing disorders. *Ann. Epidemiol.* **2016**, *26*, 7.e1–e3. [CrossRef] [PubMed]
243. Xue, M.; Dehaas, E.; Chaudhary, N.; O'Byrne, P.; Satia, I.; Kurmi, O.P. Breastfeeding and risk of childhood asthma: A systematic review and meta-analysis. *ERJ Open Res.* **2021**, *7*, 00504-2021. [CrossRef] [PubMed]
244. Elliott, L.; Henderson, J.; Northstone, K.; Chiu, G.Y.; Dunson, D.; London, S.J. Prospective study of breast-feeding in relation to wheeze, atopy, and bronchial hyperresponsiveness in the Avon Longitudinal Study of Parents and Children (ALSPAC). *J. Allergy Clin. Immunol.* **2008**, *122*, 49–54.e3. [CrossRef]
245. Dogaru, C.M.; Nyffenegger, D.; Pescatore, A.M.; Spycher, B.D.; Kuehni, C.E. Breastfeeding and childhood asthma: Systematic review and meta-analysis. *Am. J. Epidemiol.* **2014**, *179*, 1153–1167. [CrossRef] [PubMed]
246. Patria, M.F.; Tenconi, R.; Esposito, S. Efficacy and safety of influenza vaccination in children with asthma. *Expert Rev. Vaccines* **2012**, *11*, 461–468. [CrossRef] [PubMed]
247. Grohskopf, L.A.; Sokolow, L.Z.; Broder, K.R.; Walter, E.B.; Fry, A.M.; Jernigan, D.B. Prevention and Control of Seasonal Influenza with Vaccines: Recommendations of the Advisory Committee on Immunization Practices-United States, 2018–2019 Influenza Season. *MMWR Recomm. Rep.* **2018**, *67*, 1–20. [CrossRef] [PubMed]
248. Bianchini, S.; Argentiero, A.; Camilloni, B.; Silvestri, E.; Alunno, A.; Esposito, S. Vaccination against Paediatric Respiratory Pathogens. *Vaccines* **2019**, *7*, 168. [CrossRef]
249. Bae, E.Y.; Choi, U.Y.; Kwon, H.J.; Jeong, D.C.; Rhim, J.W.; Ma, S.H.; Lee, K.I.; Kang, J.H. Immunogenicity and safety of an inactivated trivalent split influenza virus vaccine in young children with recurrent wheezing. *Clin. Vaccine Immunol.* **2013**, *20*, 811–817. [CrossRef]
250. Bergen, R.; Black, S.; Shinefield, H.; Lewis, E.; Ray, P.; Hansen, J.; Walker, R.; Hessel, C.; Cordova, J.; Mendelman, P.M. Safety of cold-adapted live attenuated influenza vaccine in a large cohort of children and adolescents. *Pediatr. Infect. Dis. J.* **2004**, *23*, 138–144. [CrossRef]
251. Miller, E.K.; Dumitrescu, L.; Cupp, C.; Dorris, S.; Taylor, S.; Sparks, R.; Fawkes, D.; Frontiero, V.; Rezendes, A.M.; Marchant, C.; et al. Atopy history and the genomics of wheezing after influenza vaccination in children 6–59 months of age. *Vaccine* **2011**, *29*, 3431–3437. [CrossRef]
252. Baxter, R.P.; Lewis, N.; Fireman, B.; Hansen, J.; Klein, N.P.; Ortiz, J.R. Live Attenuated Influenza Vaccination Before 3 Years of Age and Subsequent Development of Asthma: A 14-year Follow-up Study. *Pediatr. Infect. Dis. J.* **2018**, *37*, 383–386, Erratum in *Pediatr. Infect. Dis. J.* **2018**, *37*, 611. [CrossRef] [PubMed]
253. Gaglani, M.J.; Piedra, P.A.; Riggs, M.; Herschler, G.; Fewlass, C.; Glezen, W.P. Safety of the intranasal, trivalent, live attenuated influenza vaccine (LAIV) in children with intermittent wheezing in an open-label field trial. *Pediatr. Infect. Dis. J.* **2008**, *27*, 444–452. [CrossRef] [PubMed]
254. Sokolow, A.G.; Stallings, A.P.; Kercsmar, C.; Harrington, T.; Jimenez-Truque, N.; Zhu, Y.; Sokolow, K.; Moody, M.A.; Schlaudecker, E.P.; Walter, E.B.; et al. Safety of Live Attenuated Influenza Vaccine in Children With Asthma. *Pediatrics* **2022**, *149*, e2021055432. [CrossRef] [PubMed]
255. Turner, P.J.; Fleming, L.; Saglani, S.; Southern, J.; Andrews, N.J.; Miller, E.; SNIFFLE-4 Study Investigators. Safety of live attenuated influenza vaccine (LAIV) in children with moderate to severe asthma. *J. Allergy Clin. Immunol.* **2020**, *145*, 1157–1164.e6. [CrossRef] [PubMed]
256. Ambrose, C.S.; Wu, X.; Knuf, M.; Wutzler, P. The efficacy of intranasal live attenuated influenza vaccine in children 2 through 17 years of age: A meta-analysis of 8 randomized controlled studies. *Vaccine* **2012**, *30*, 886–892. [CrossRef]
257. Toivonen, L.; Karppinen, S.; Schuez-Havupalo, L.; Teros-Jaakkola, T.; Vuononvirta, J.; Mertsola, J.; He, Q.; Waris, M.; Peltola, V. Burden of Recurrent Respiratory Tract Infections in Children: A Prospective Cohort Study. *Pediatr. Infect. Dis. J.* **2016**, *35*, e362–e369. [CrossRef] [PubMed]
258. Principi, N.; Esposito, S.; Cavagna, R.; Bosis, S.; Droghetti, R.; Faelli, N.; Tosi, S.; Begliatti, E.; Snoopy Study Group. Recurrent respiratory tract infections in pediatric age: A population-based survey of the therapeutic role of macrolides. *J. Chemother.* **2003**, *15*, 53–59. [CrossRef]
259. Esposito, S.; Soto-Martinez, M.E.; Feleszko, W.; Jones, M.H.; Shen, K.L.; Schaad, U.B. Nonspecific immunomodulators for recurrent respiratory tract infections, wheezing and asthma in children: A systematic review of mechanistic and clinical evidence. *Curr. Opin. Allergy Clin. Immunol.* **2018**, *18*, 198–209. [CrossRef]
260. Esposito, S.; Bianchini, S.; Bosis, S.; Tagliabue, C.; Coro, I.; Argentiero, A.; Principi, N. A randomized, placebo-controlled, double-blinded, single-centre, phase IV trial to assess the efficacy and safety of OM-85 in children suffering from recurrent respiratory tract infections. *J. Transl. Med.* **2019**, *17*, 284. [CrossRef]
261. Cao, C.; Wang, J.; Li, Y.; Li, Y.; Ma, L.; Abdelrahim, M.E.A.; Zhu, Y. Efficacy and safety of OM-85 in paediatric recurrent respiratory tract infections which could have a possible protective effect on COVID-19 pandemic: A meta-analysis. *Int. J. Clin. Pract.* **2021**, *75*, e13981. [CrossRef]
262. Yin, J.; Xu, B.; Zeng, X.; Shen, K. Broncho-Vaxom in pediatric recurrent respiratory tract infections: A systematic review and meta-analysis. *Int. Immunopharmacol.* **2018**, *54*, 198–209. [CrossRef] [PubMed]
263. Schaad, U.B. OM-85 BV, an immunostimulant in pediatric recurrent respiratory tract infections: A systematic review. *World J. Pediatr.* **2010**, *6*, 5–12. [CrossRef] [PubMed]

264. Esposito, S.; Musio, A. Immunostimulants and prevention of recurrent respiratory tract infections. *J. Biol. Regul. Homeost. Agents* **2013**, *27*, 627–636. [PubMed]
265. Razi, C.H.; Harmancı, K.; Abacı, A.; Özdemir, O.; Hızlı, S.; Renda, R.; Keskin, F. The immunostimulant OM-85 BV prevents wheezing attacks in preschool children. *J. Allergy Clin. Immunol.* **2010**, *126*, 763–769. [CrossRef] [PubMed]

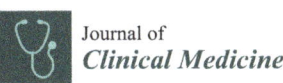

Review

Challenges in DICER1-Associated Lung Disease

Kamal Masarweh [1], Oz Mordechai [2,3], Michal Gur [1,3], Ronen Bar-Yoseph [1,3], Lea Bentur [1,3] and Anat Ilivitzki [3,4,*]

1. Pediatric Pulmonary Institute, Ruth Rappaport Children's Hospital, Rambam Health Care Campus, Haifa 3109601, Israel
2. Pediatric Hematology and Oncology Department, Ruth Rappaport Children's Hospital, Rambam Health Care Campus, Haifa 3109601, Israel
3. Rappaport Faculty of Medicine, Technion–Israel Institute of Technology, Haifa 3200003, Israel
4. Radiology Department, Rambam Health Care Campus, Haifa 3109601, Israel
* Correspondence: a_ilivitzki@rambam.health.gov.il; Tel.: +972-52-6330-032

Abstract: Pleuropulmonary blastoma (PPB) is a tumor occurring almost exclusively in infants and young children. This is the most common primary-lung malignancy in childhood. There is age-associated progression through a distinctive sequence of pathologic changes, from a purely multicystic lesion type I to a high-grade sarcoma type II and III. While complete resection is the cornerstone treatment for type I PPB, aggressive chemotherapy with a less favorable prognosis is associated with type II and III. DICER1 germline mutation is positive in 70% of children with PPB. Diagnosis is challenging, as it resembles congenital pulmonary airway malformation (CPAM) in imaging. Although PPB is an extremely rare malignancy, over the past five years we have encountered several children diagnosed with PPB in our medical center. Herein, we present some of these children and discuss diagnostic, ethical, and therapeutic challenges.

Keywords: pleuropulmonary blastoma; DICER1; lung cyst

1. Introduction

Pleuropulmonary blastoma (PPB) the most common primary lung malignancy in childhood [1]. First recognized in 1988, it is considered a dysembryonic equivalent to embryonal malignancies of childhood such as neuroblastoma, hepatoblastoma and other organ-based solid malignancies of childhood [2]. PPB is a rare tumor, occurring almost exclusively in infants and young children under 6 years of age, similar to other embryonal malignancies [3].

PPB is unique among developmental malignancies of childhood in its age-associated progression through a distinctive sequence of pathologic changes from a purely multicystic lesion to a high-grade sarcoma. Type I PPB is composed of air-filled cysts with primitive mesenchymal cells beneath an intact, benign-appearing epithelium. These cysts can progress into type II PPB, in which the mesenchymal cells overgrow the septa, producing a cystic and solid neoplasm. Type III PPB is an exclusively solid sarcomatous neoplasm [2,3].

There is strong evidence for progression from type I to type II and type III PPB. Type Ir (regressed) PPB is a purely cystic lesion, microscopically devoid of subepithelial septal primitive cells, and it is considered to have a lower risk for neoplastic progression [4,5]. The pathological progression in the PPB types correlates with both age at diagnosis and clinical outcome [5]. Type I and type Ir present at a younger age, and the prognosis is favorable, with a 5-year survival of 98% and 100% of patients, respectively. Type II and type III PPB are typically diagnosed in older children, with 5-year-overall-survival estimates of 75% and 53%, respectively [6].

Type I PPB may present with respiratory symptoms such as cough, dyspnea, chest pain or abdominal pain. Chest X-rays may show signs of pneumonia, and some cases may present with difficulty in breathing, from a pneumothorax or a large lung cyst, or

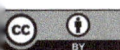

a PPB can also present as an incidental radiologic finding of a lung cyst. The purely cystic type I PPB can be easily mistaken for other congenital lung malformations such as congenital pulmonary airway malformation (CPAM), as CPAM origins can be from the acinar structures of the lungs, thus creating a multiseptated cystic lesion similar to type I PPB. The diagnosis of type I PPB should be considered in the evaluation of any multicystic specimen of peripheral lung from young children. The final diagnosis requires meticulous pathological examination.

Given the rarity and clinical heterogeneity, it is still unclear what is the optimal therapeutic approach. The treatment for type I and type Ir PPB evolved over time; most cases are treated with surgical resection alone, while in some cases adjuvant chemotherapy is added. Most type Ir PPBs are followed clinically after complete surgical resection, due to the low risk of tumor progression. Cases of type I PPB are treated with oncologic surgery alone. In cases of suspected incomplete resection or unresectable lesion, chemotherapy is added [7]. A recent study found that adjuvant chemotherapy in cases of complete resection in type I PPB was found to be protective, with lower rate of recurrence of progression compared to surgery alone [8]. Type II and type III PPB have a more aggressive clinical behavior, requiring both surgery and chemotherapy [9].

PPB may be associated with other unique malignant syndromes. An important discovery was the identification of the pathogenic germline *DICER1* variants as the first known genetic causes of PPB familial syndrome [10], and these variants are found in 70% of patients with all types of PPB. DICER1 is inherited in an autosomal dominant condition with variable penetrance. In addition to PPB, DICER1 syndrome includes, among others, Wilms' tumor, cystic nephroma, clear cell sarcoma, ovarian Sertoli-Leydig cell and granulosa cell tumors, testicular Sertoli-Leydig cell tumors, medulloblastoma, neuroblastoma, seminoma germ cell tumors, pituitary blastoma, pineoblastoma, ciliary body medulloepithelioma, thyroid nodular hyperplasia, papillary and follicular thyroid carcinomas, rhabdomyosarcoma, fibrosarcoma, Ewing sarcoma, osteosarcoma, hepatoblastoma and hepatocellular carcinoma cancer and pineoblastoma [11]. Germline DICER1 mutations are also associated with non-neoplastic conditions, including macrocephaly, retinal abnormalities, renal anomalies, dental perturbations, and GLOW syndrome (global developmental delay, lung cysts, overgrowth and Wilms' tumor) [12]. DICER1 is an important gene, located on chromosome 14q32.13 in the biogenesis of microRNAs, a class of small RNA molecules essential in organ development and suppression of neoplasia [13]. Deficient microRNA suppression can lead to oncogenic transformation [14]. In contrast to loss-of-function germline *DICER1* mutations, missense mutations in the RNase IIIb domain of *DICER1* are found as 'second hits' in tumors associated with germline mutations [15].

The International PPB/DICER1 Registry (IPPBR) was founded in 1987 to advance research and improve outcomes for children with PPB and DICER1 syndrome. The registry allows free central-pathology review in questionable cases, review of records in a standardized method, longitudinal follow-up and worldwide collaboration. Since its inception, more than 800 patients from 47 countries have enrolled in the registry [9]. The registry's research includes efforts to define optimal therapy regimens for PPB and DICER1-related cancers and to discover new therapies for DICER1-related cancers, develop new ways to diagnose children with DICER1-related cancers and present surveillance guidelines for patients with germline DICER1 mutations [16]. Based on information collected from the registry, a study by Hill et al. identified germline loss-of-function DICER1 mutations affecting the RNase IIIb domain in affected families with PPB and a spectrum of other tumors in the DICER1 syndrome [10].

Although PPB is considered a rare malignancy, several children have been diagnosed with PPB in our medical center in the last 5 years. We present some of these cases, clinical, radiological, pathology and genetic-testing findings, and discuss challenging questions that were raised regarding diagnosis, optimal management and treatment.

1.1. Patient No 1

A 6-day-old term girl presented with severe respiratory distress and a large pneumothorax on the right side, requiring chest drainage and a prolonged course of treatment, including intubation (Figure 1a). Chest computed tomography (CT) showed a pneumothorax and a cystic mass on the right upper lobe (Figure 1b). Although lobectomy was recommended, she underwent segmentectomy on day 11 of life. The pathologic diagnosis was CPAM type 4. Due to the early pneumothorax and normal prenatal ultrasound, pleuropulmonary blastoma was suspected. Genetic counseling revealed *DICER1* germline mutation. We consulted the IPPBR, and they revised the pathologic specimen. Based on the cellularity and hyperchromasia of spindle cells within the cyst walls, a diagnosis of type I PPB was confirmed (Figure 2). Completion lobectomy, chemotherapy or close follow-up were suggested as treatment options. The parents chose a follow-up regimen. Nine months later, a new bullous lesion (6 mm) appeared in the right upper lobe (RUL) (Figure 1c). Consequently, a completion RUL lobectomy was performed. The patient received no chemotherapy. Currently she is under close monitoring in our pediatric pulmonology and haemato-oncology units, with the periodic evaluations of a *DICER1*-positive patient, including chest CT scans. She is now 5-year PPB-event free, and thriving.

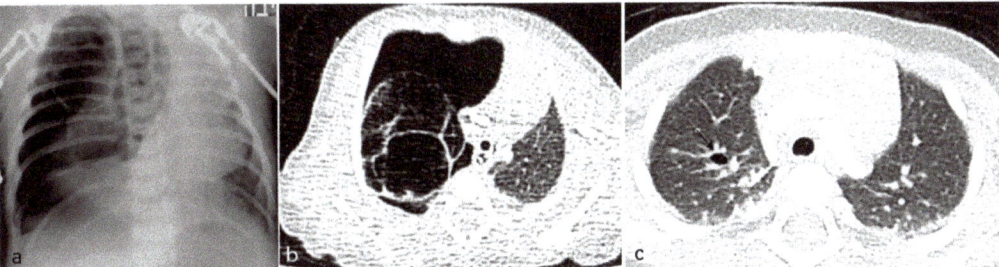

Figure 1. Six-day-old infant with respiratory distress. (**a**) Chest X-ray on day two of life: cystic lesion and tension pneumothorax on the right. (**b**) Chest CT without IV contrast performed on the same day, axial image: multicystic lesion and adjacent pneumothorax on the right hemithorax. (**c**) Chest CT performed 9 months later, with tiny cystic lesion on the right (arrow).

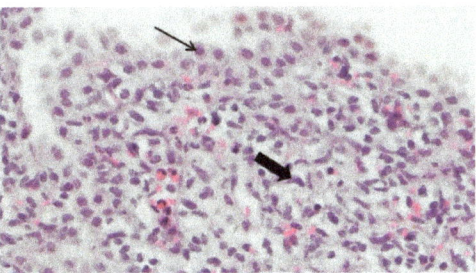

Figure 2. Pathology specimen of the cystic lung lesion in case number 1 (H&E). Alveolar cell (thin black arrow) and spindle cell (thick black arrow).

1.2. Patient No 2

A 2-day-old term girl presented with severe respiratory distress. Chest X-ray showed large multicystic lesion on the left hemithorax with compressive atelectasis of the lung, small pneumothorax and mediastinal shift to the right (Figure 3a). Prenatal follow-up was normal. An urgent thoracoscopy and positioning of chest tube was performed, followed by CT angiography (CTA) that better delineated the same findings, suggestive of type 1 PPB (Figure 3b). Under left thoracotomy she underwent left lower-lobe lobectomy with complete resection of the mass. The pathologic diagnosis was type 1 PPB, positive *DICER1* in the specimen (using PCR amplification with full exonic coverage, followed by NGS sequencing), but negative *DICER1* germline. More than a year later, she is well.

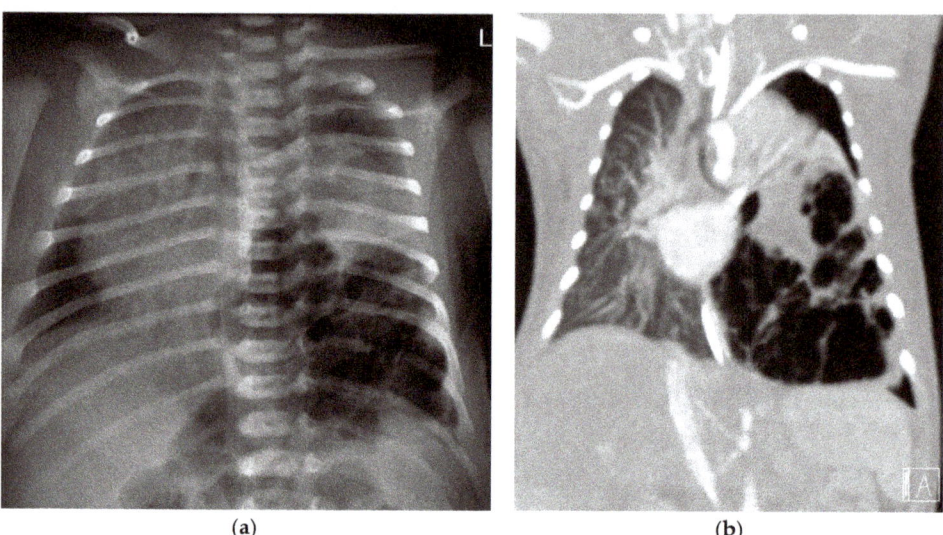

(a) (b)

Figure 3. Two-day-old infant with respiratory distress. (**a**) Chest X-ray and (**b**) Coronal image of CTA: Large multilocular cystic lesion in the right lower hemithorax, with mediastinal shift to the right. There is an atelectasis of the left upper lung and apical pneumothorax.

1.3. Patient No 3

A 3-year-old healthy boy experienced increasing weakness and shortness of breath several weeks after a febrile upper-respiratory disease. He lost 1 kg of weight. A chest X-ray performed in the community showed complete opacification of the right hemithorax (Figure 4a), and he was referred to the hospital. A chest CTA revealed a large tumor occupying most of the right hemithorax, without any aeration of the lung (Figure 4b). Most of the tumor was solid hypodense tissue, with some cysts on the periphery. An ultrasound study was able to better delineate the multicystic hemorrhagic nature of the tumor (Figure 4c). A biopsy was taken under sonographic guidance and the pathologic diagnosis was type II PPB with foci of RMS (rhabdomyosarcoma). The *DICER1* germline was positive, and staging with FDG PET-CT (2-[(18)F]-fluoro-2-deoxy-d-glucose positron emission tomography-computed tomography showed no metastases (Figure 5). The tumor was unresectable, and the patient received neoadjuvant chemotherapy with IVADo (Ifosfamide, vincristine, actinomycin-D, and doxorubicin) followed by resection of the tumor, which was pleural based. He received completion chemotherapy of up to 12 courses. There was 80% tumor necrosis in the final specimen. After 3 years of follow up, both clinical and with CTA, there is no recurrence (Figure 4d). The *DICER1* germline mutation was positive in the patient's father and in his three siblings. The siblings were all asymptomatic. They all underwent CTA of the chest, with the following findings:

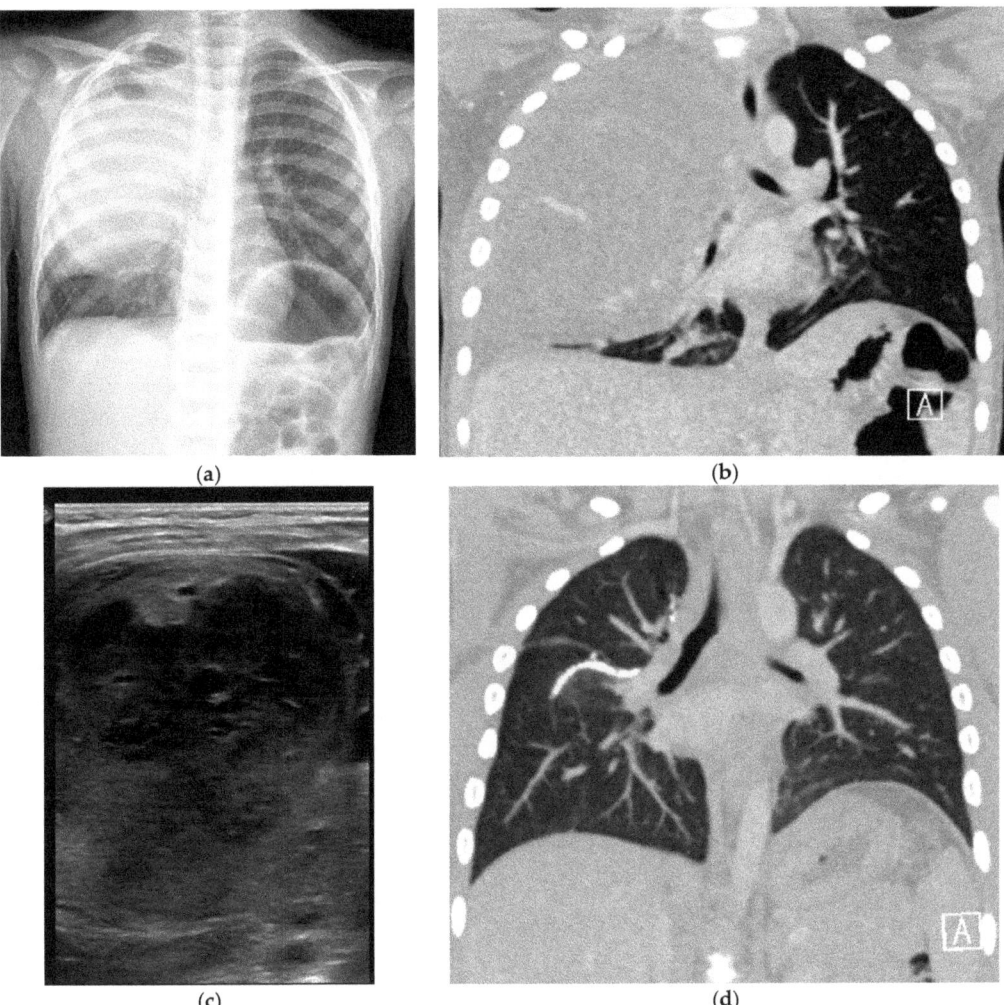

Figure 4. Six-year-old boy with progressive shortness of breath, fatigue and weight loss. (**a**) Chest X-ray: Opacification of the upper two thirds of the right upper hemithorax by a pleural-based lesion. There is a slight shift of the trachea to the left, and a caudal shift of the right diaphragm. (**b**) Coronal image of CTA showing large aberrant vessels within the lesion. (**c**) Sonographic gray-scale high-resolution image of the lesion (linear array transducer) shows the cystic/solid nature of the lesion. (**d**) Coronal image of CTA at the end of treatment, showing no evidence of recurrent disease.

1.4. Patient No 4

Nine-year-old girl (the older sister of patient no 3): complex cystic lesion with aberrant vessels within the cyst septa located in the right upper lobe (Figure 6a). We suspected that this lesion might be PPB, and consulted the International Pleuropulmonary Blastoma registry team. They agreed, and suggested lobectomy.

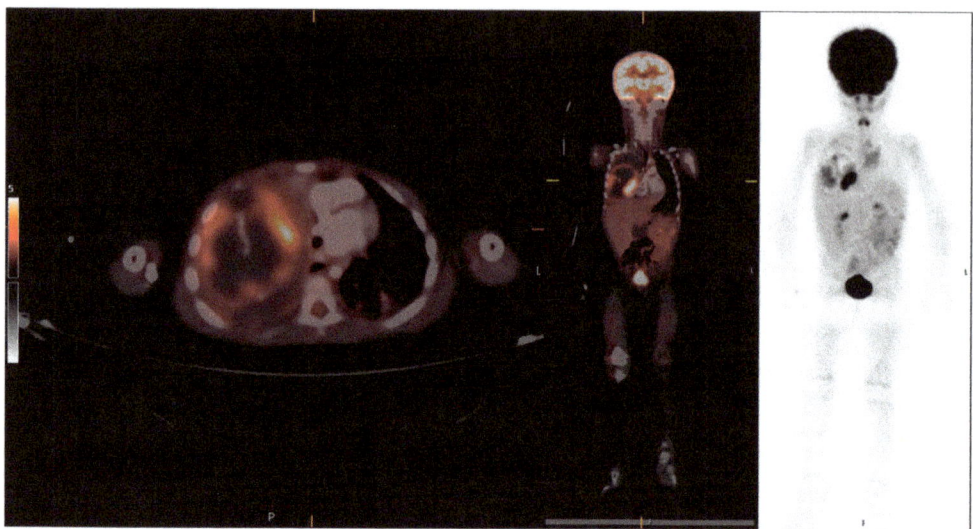

Figure 5. The same patient as in image 4. FDG PET-CT in the axial and coronal hybrid images and coronal PET image show peripheral uptake in the lung lesion. No metastases seen.

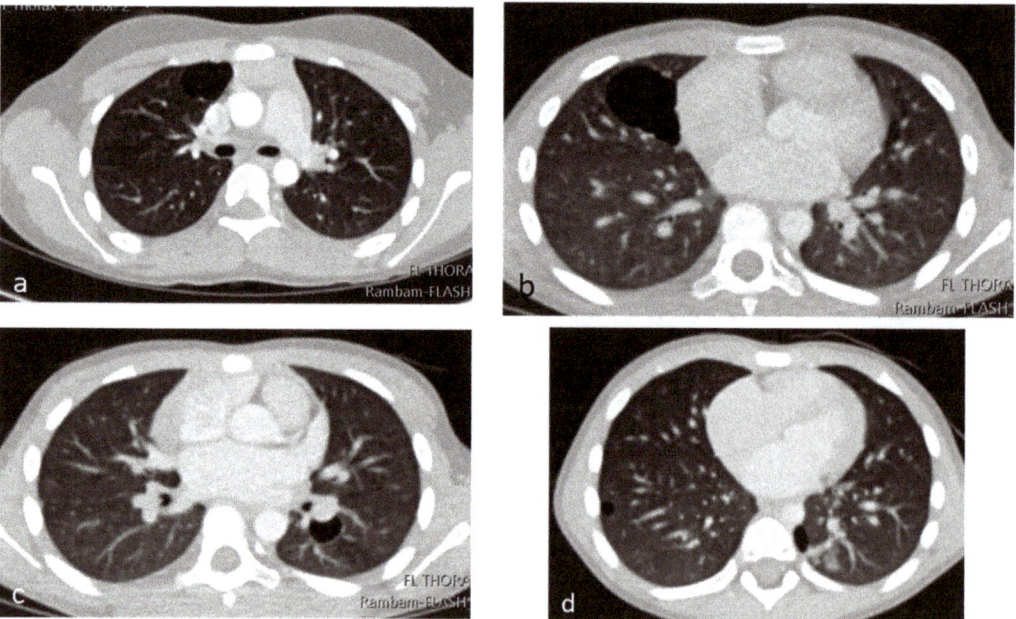

Figure 6. Asymptomatic *DICER1*-germline-positive siblings of index patient number 3. Axial images of Chest CTA: (**a**) Nine-year-old girl with RUL anterior multiseptated cystic lesion. (**b**,**c**) Six-year-old boy with right and left cystic lesion. (**d**) Fifteen-month-old boy with bilateral, small cystic lesions.

1.5. Patient No 5

Six-year-old boy (older brother of patient no 3): two purely cystic lesions, one in the right middle lobe (diameter of 4 cm) and a smaller cyst in the left lower lobe (Figure 6b,c).

1.6. Patient No 6

Fifteen-month-old boy (younger brother of patient no 3): two purely cystic lesions, one in the right lower lobe (diameter of 0.6 cm) and a second cyst (diameter of 1 cm) in the left lower lobe (Figure 6d).

We consulted the IPPBR team about the other three siblings as well; they considered the lesions to be a type I PPB, and resection was suggested.

The parents were given the complete information about the findings and the consultations. They decided to proceed with a more conservative approach, with clinical and radiological follow up only. Two years later, the children are healthy, and the radiological findings are stable.

2. Discussion

We presented six children with either proven PPB or DICER1-related cystic lung disease suspected to be PPB, all treated in our hospital within the last 5 years. This cluster of patients raised our awareness about this rare tumor and the diagnostic and management challenges it brings. Timely diagnosis and resection of type I PPB is crucial, but this entity is elusive, masquerading as a lung malformation, or growing silently in *DICER1*-germline-positive patients. We summarize some of the challenges we dealt with while treating these patients.

2.1. Challenge No 1

Can we differentiate CPAM from type 1 PPB, based on clinical aspects and imaging?

Differentiating the entities may influence management. There are different approaches for the management of CPAM. Some centers advocate an aggressive approach by resection of all lesions, in fear of future progression to malignant PPB. Others choose to follow up, advocating that PPB is a rare entity and CPAM 1–3 are benign lesions that will not progress to PPB [17]. The real concern is CPAM type 4 that might progress to type I PPB, so defining clues for diagnosis will allow for more judgmental choice of management.

Imaging alone cannot differentiate CPAM type 4 from type I PPB [5,17,18]. In a recent retrospective study by Engwall-Gill et al., nine pediatric radiologists reviewed the CT scans of patients with postnatal cystic lesions, and could not find any specific imaging characteristics that could safely differentiate type I PPB from congenital lung malformation. The sensitivity for diagnosis of PPB was 58%, with a specificity of 83%, with poor interrater reliability ($\kappa = 0.36$; $p < 0.01$) [19].

What are the differences between CPAM type 4 and type I PPB? Dehner et al. stated that CPAM type 4 and type I PPB are in fact synonymous, and, due to the concern of progression from type I PPB to the malignant type II and III PPB, it would be wiser to define these lesions as type I PPB rather than CPAM 4, and thus promote a more aggressive approach toward oncologic resection and genetic counselling [20].

In Feinberg A. et al., the IPPBR team summarized their experience with the goal of answering this question. Overall, 112 cases of type I PPB gathered in the registry between 2002 and 2013 and 103 cases of CPAM that were resected in the same institution during the same period were reviewed. Features favoring CPAM were prenatal diagnosis, and CTA findings of a systemic feeding vessel and hyperinflated lung. Features that raised the suspicion of PPB were multi-segmental or bilateral lesions and the absence of prenatal ultrasonography findings [18].

In our first two patients, the suspicion of type I PPB was high, due to the early symptomatic cystic lung lesion and normal prenatal follow up. In the recent IPPBR report, 85% of type I PPB cases were symptomatic at presentation, 32% with pneumothorax [18]. The positive-*DICER1* germline mutation further confirmed our concern. We consulted the IPPBR, which supported our diagnosis of type I PPB. In the family with four children with DICER1 (patients 3–6), two of the three asymptomatic siblings have bilateral cystic lesions, and thus they are highly likely to having type I PPB.

2.2. Challenge No 2

What are the indications for *DICER1* germline testing? Any congenital cystic lesion? Only in cases that are highly suspicious? Only in pathology-determined PPB?

In 2016, the IPPBR convened an international DICER1 symposium and published a consensus paper on the indications for testing and the surveillance advised for DICER1-positive children [16]. The paper presents recommendations for genetic testing, prenatal management and suggested signs and symptoms and imaging-surveillance strategies for DICER1-associated conditions including pulmonary, renal, gynecologic, thyroid, ophthalmologic, otolaryngologic, central nervous system tumors and gastrointestinal polyps [16]. Any clinical pathology that might be related to DICER1 was considered as a criterion. Pathology-confirmed PPB is considered a major criterion, as well as any lung cyst in childhood. Based on this consensus, any major criterion, two minor criteria (such as cystic lung disease in adulthood and renal cysts), or a first-degree relative with positive-germline DICER1 should be tested.

Recommendation for screening in *DICER1*-germline-positive children are age based, with at least one chest CT performed in all cases [16]. These indications for testing and screening elevated the awareness about PPB among pediatric caregivers, and increased the diagnosis of type I PPB and type Ir PPB.

Based on the IPPBR recommendations, we tested and diagnosed the siblings of patient number 3, who presented with malignant PPB: all three siblings had CT findings suggestive of PPB. The family decided to continue with clinical and radiological follow up instead of resecting all lesions. This family evoked an ethical question regarding the indications for testing an asymptomatic sibling. The parents of patient no 3 stated during the follow up, post factum, that they preferred not to know the child's DICER1 status. With increased awareness of the advantages of early detection of type I PPB, and the possible prevention of progression through early intervention, more families will eventually choose to know the DICER1 status. These four DICER1 siblings bring us to the next challenge.

2.3. Challenge No 3

When can we safely say that a type I PPB lesion has regressed to Type Ir PPB?

We know that pathology alone can provide the final discrimination between type I and Ir PPB, but in our DICER1 family, pathology was not available for the three siblings of patient no 3. The children differ in age and appearance of the lesions. The oldest sibling was 9 years old when diagnosed, and had a multiseptated single cyst, while the two younger brothers had multifocal simple cysts. Over 2 years of CT follow up, we saw no change in the appearance of the lesions in all three children (patients Nos. 4–6). Does it give us any reassurance? We know that the median age for diagnosis of type I PPB is 7 months, for type II PPB 35 months and for type Ir PPB 2.6 years [4,5,8], and that after the age of 3 years, type Ir PPB is considerably more common than type I [8]. Were they all type Ir PPB at presentation? Can type Ir PPB progress to a malignant PPB?

The IPPBR reported two cases of progression in type Ir PPB, both occurring within 2 years. They suggested 2 years of follow up for resected type Ir PPB. In type I PPB recurrence occurred more frequently and within 63 months, so they advised a longer follow up for type I PPB, of at least 6 years [8]. We intend to continue the follow-up of the DICER1 family for at least 6 years. This family is registered in the IPPB registry, and this follow-up may shed additional light on type I PPB DICER1-related tumor.

2.4. Challenge No 4

Multifocal cystic lesions in a *DICER1*-germline-positive, asymptomatic child. Oncologic resection versus close radiologic and clinical follow-up: pros and cons.

Multifocal cysts are more difficult to manage. On the one hand, multifocal cysts have an increased risk of progression compared to a single cyst, while on the other hand multiple surgeries might increase surgical complications and decrease lung function. In the last IPPBR report [8], 25% of cases of type I PPB I were multifocal, and many of them had multiple surgeries at an early age. Some cysts were not resected, due to their location. Only one child had a serious complication of pulmonary artery stenosis. At the moment, the IPPRB's recommendation in multifocal cystic PPB is to individualize management, as additional studies are needed [8].

2.5. Challenge No 5

The role of chemotherapy in cases of suspected incomplete resection of type 1 PPB.

PPB Ttpes II and III are aggressive malignant diseases and chemotherapy is mandatory. The primary treatment for type I and Ir PPB is surgery with complete resection. The reasoning for adjuvant chemotherapy in type IPPB and even type Ir PPB is to prevent recurrence or progression of any residual disease (microscopic or macroscopic) to the more aggressive tumor type II and type III PPB. In the recent report by the IPPBR [8], the group summarized their experience with type I PPB and type Ir PPB cases treated between 2006 and 2022. Altogether, they had 118 cases of type I PPB and 87 cases of type Ir PPB. In the PPB cases, chemotherapy (VAC, VA or IVADo) was given to 39% of the cases after surgery and in one case prior to surgery. In this study, chemotherapy proved protective, as none of the cases that received adjuvant chemotherapy progressed. For the cases that were not treated with chemotherapy, two factors were found to correlate with recurrent disease or progression: inadequate surgery, meaning less than complete resection, and multicentric disease [8]. A prior publication by the same group did not find any benefit from chemotherapy for type I PPB [6]. In patient 1, the first surgery was inadequate, and a local recurrence occurred. Following completion of the lobectomy, we consulted the IPPBR, and they suggested adding adjuvant chemotherapy. A close follow-up was decided upon, and no chemotherapy was given.

2.6. Challenge No 6

Is the prevalence of Type I PPB increasing in recent years, or have we misdiagnosed some of them as CPAM?

Within five years we diagnosed six patients with DICER1 due to high level of suspicion, five of them were diagnosed with type I PPB. We consulted the IPPBR team in all our cases and learnt that there is a need for a high level of suspicion and experienced teamwork in order not to miss the type I PPB patients and to be able to treat them accordingly. It is possible that the prevalence of type I PPB is on the rise, due to the fact we might have misread some of our previous cases as CPAM. In fact, to emphasize the importance of a central pathology review for rare tumors such as PPB, it was reported that almost 20% of the pathology specimens submitted for review by IPPBR had another initial diagnosis. Thus, it may be challenging to identify a lesion as PPB, even for experienced pathologists [6].

3. Conclusions

PPB is a rare tumor, with predicted progression from the benign type I PPB to malignant tumor. Timely diagnosis and complete resection of type I PPB correlates with the best prognosis. Symptomatic cystic lung lesion in infants, unidentified during pregnancy, especially when septated or multifocal, should raise the suspicion of type I PPB rather than CPAM, and induce testing for DICERI mutation and early complete resection. The management of multifocal cysts, the role of chemotherapy and management of older asymptomatic DICER1 children is complicated, and should sometimes be individualized. Consultation with the IPPBR team is recommended.

Author Contributions: K.M.—literature review, analysis of data, manuscript draft preparation; O.M., M.G., R.B.-Y.—analysis of data and manuscript review and editing; L.B.—conceptualization, literature review, analysis of data and editing. A.I.—conceptualization, literature review, analysis of data and images, manuscript preparation and final review. All authors have read and agreed to the published version of the manuscript.

Funding: This research received no external funding.

Institutional Review Board Statement: Ethical review and approval were waived by the local institutional review board for this study.

Informed Consent Statement: Informed consent was obtained from all subjects involved in the study.

Data Availability Statement: The data presented in this study are available on request from the corresponding author.

Acknowledgments: The authors would like to acknowledge the PBB/DICER1 registry team, especially Ann K Schultz, for their ongoing support in the diagnosis and treatment of these patients. The authors would also like to thank the patients' parents for giving permission for presentation.

Conflicts of Interest: The authors declare no conflict of interest.

References

1. Dishop, M.K.; Kuruvilla, S. Primary and Metastatic Lung Tumors in the Pediatric Population: A Review and 25-Year Experience at a Large Children's Hospital. *Arch. Pathol. Lab. Med.* **2008**, *132*, 1079–1103. [CrossRef] [PubMed]
2. Dehner, L.P. Pleuropulmonary blastoma is THE pulmonary blastoma of childhood. *Semin. Diagn. Pathol.* **1994**, *11*, 144–151. [PubMed]
3. Hill, D.A.; Jarzembowski, J.A.; Priest, J.R.; Williams, G.; Schoettler, P.; Dehner, L.P. Type I Pleuropulmonary Blastoma: Pathology and Biology Study of 51 Cases From the International Pleuropulmonary Blastoma Registry. *Am. J. Surg. Pathol.* **2008**, *32*, 282–295. [CrossRef] [PubMed]
4. Priest, J.R.; McDermott, M.B.; Bhatia, S.; Watterson, J.; Manivel, J.C.; Dehner, L.P. Pleuropulmonary blastoma: A clinicopathologic study of 50 cases. *Cancer* **1997**, *80*, 147–161. [CrossRef]
5. Priest, J.R.; Williams, G.M.; Hill, D.A.; Dehner, L.P.; Jaffé, A. Pulmonary cysts in early childhood and the risk of malignancy. *Pediatr. Pulmonol.* **2009**, *44*, 14–30. [CrossRef] [PubMed]
6. Messinger, Y.H.; Stewart, D.R.; Priest, J.R.; Williams, G.M.; Harris, A.K.; Schultz KA, P.; Yang, J.; Doros, L.; Rosenberg, P.S.; Hill, D.A.; et al. Pleuropulmonary blastoma: A report on 350 central pathology-confirmed pleuropulmonary blastoma cases by the international pleuropulmonary blastoma registry. *Cancer* **2015**, *121*, 276–285. [CrossRef] [PubMed]
7. Priest, J.R.; Hill, D.A.; Williams, G.M.; Moertel, C.L.; Messinger, Y.; Finkelstein, M.J.; Dehner, L.P. Type I pleuropulmonary blastoma: A report from the international pleuropulmonary blastoma registry. *J. Clin. Oncol.* **2006**, *24*, 4492–4498. [CrossRef] [PubMed]
8. Nelson, A.T.; Harris, A.K.; Watson, D.; Miniati, D.; Finch, M.; Kamihara, J.; Mitchell, S.G.; Wilson, D.B.; Gettinger, K.; Rangaswami, A.A.; et al. Type I and Ir pleuropulmonary blastoma (PPB): A report from the International PPB/DICER1 Registry. *Cancer* **2022**, *129*, 600–613. [CrossRef] [PubMed]
9. Schultz, K.A.P.; Harris, A.K.; Nelson, A.T.; Watson, D.; Lucas, J.T., Jr.; Miniati, D.; Stewart, D.R.; Hagedorn, K.N.; Mize, W.; Kamihara, J.; et al. Outcomes for Children With Type II and Type III Pleuropulmonary Blastoma Following Chemotherapy: A Report From the International PPB/DICER1 Registry. *J. Clin. Oncol.* **2023**, *41*, 778–789. [CrossRef] [PubMed]
10. Hill, D.A.; Ivanovich, J.; Priest, J.R.; Gurnett, C.A.; Dehner, L.P.; Desruisseau, D.; Jarzembowski, J.A.; Wikenheiser-Brokamp, K.A.; Suarez, B.K.; Whelan, A.J.; et al. DICER1 mutations in familial pleuropulmonary blastoma. *Science* **2009**, *325*, 965. [CrossRef] [PubMed]
11. Slade, I.; Bacchelli, C.; Davies, H.; Murray, A.; Abbaszadeh, F.; Hanks, S.; Barfoot, R.; Burke, A.; Chisholm, J.; Hewitt, M.; et al. DICER1 syndrome: Clarifying the diagnosis, clinical features and management implications of a pleiotropic tumour predisposition syndrome. *J. Med. Genet.* **2011**, *48*, 273–278. [CrossRef] [PubMed]
12. González, I.A.; Stewart, D.R.; Schultz, K.A.P.; Field, A.P.; Hill, D.A.; Dehner, L.P. DICER1 tumor predis-position syndrome: An evolving story initiated with the pleuropulmonary blastoma. *Mod Pathol.* **2022**, *35*, 4–22. [CrossRef] [PubMed]
13. Bartel, D.P. MicroRNAs: Genomics, biogenesis, mechanism, and function. *Cell* **2004**, *116*, 281–297. [CrossRef] [PubMed]
14. Harfe, B.D.; McManus, M.T.; Mansfield, J.H.; Hornstein, E.; Tabin, C.J. The RNaseIII enzyme Dicer is required for morphogenesis but not patterning of the vertebrate limb. *Proc. Natl. Acad. Sci. USA* **2005**, *102*, 10898–10903. [CrossRef] [PubMed]
15. Foulkes, W.D.; Priest, J.R.; Duchaine, T.F. DICER1: Mutations, microRNAs and mechanisms. *Nat. Rev. Cancer* **2014**, *14*, 662–672. [CrossRef] [PubMed]
16. Schultz, K.A.P.; Williams, G.M.; Kamihara, J.; Stewart, D.R.; Harris, A.K.; Bauer, A.J.; Turner, J.; Shah, R.; Schneider, K.; Schneider, K.W.; et al. Dicer1 and associated conditions: Identification of at-risk individuals and recommended surveillance strategies. *Clin. Cancer Res.* **2018**, *24*, 2251–2261. [CrossRef] [PubMed]
17. Oliveira, C.; Himidan, S.; Pastor, A.C.; Nasr, A.; Manson, D.; Taylor, G.; Yanchar, N.L.; Brisseau, G.; Kim, P.C.W. Discriminating Preoperative Features of Pleuropulmonary Blastomas (PPB) from Congenital Cystic Adenomatoid Malformations (CCAM): A Retrospective, Age-Matched Study. *Eur. J. Pediatr. Surg.* **2011**, *21*, 2–7. [CrossRef] [PubMed]
18. Feinberg, A.; Hall, N.J.; Williams, G.M.; Schultz, K.A.P.; Miniati, D.; Hill, D.A.; Dehner, L.P.; Messinger, Y.H.; Langer, J.C. Can congenital pulmonary airway malformation be distinguished from Type i pleuropulmonary blastoma based on clinical and radiological features? *J. Pediatr. Surg.* **2016**, *51*, 33–37. [CrossRef] [PubMed]

19. Engwall-Gill, A.J.; Chan, S.S.; Boyd, K.P.; Saito, J.M.; Fallat, M.E.; Peter, S.D.S.; Bolger-Theut, S.; Crotty, E.J.; Green, J.R.; Bowling, R.L.H.; et al. Accuracy of Chest Computed Tomography in Distinguishing Cystic Pleuropulmonary Blastoma from Benign Congenital Lung Malformations in Children. *JAMA Netw. Open.* **2022**, *5*, E2219814. [CrossRef] [PubMed]
20. Dehner, L.P.; Messinger, Y.H.; Williams, G.M.; Stewart, D.R.; Harney, L.A.; Schultz, K.A.; Hill, D.A. Type i Pleuropulmonary Blastoma versus Congenital Pulmonary Airway Malformation Type IV. *Neonatology* **2016**, *111*, 76. [CrossRef] [PubMed]

Disclaimer/Publisher's Note: The statements, opinions and data contained in all publications are solely those of the individual author(s) and contributor(s) and not of MDPI and/or the editor(s). MDPI and/or the editor(s) disclaim responsibility for any injury to people or property resulting from any ideas, methods, instructions or products referred to in the content.

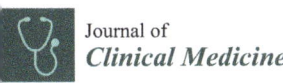

Review

Pregnancy in Cystic Fibrosis—Past, Present, and Future

Michal Gur [1,2,*,†], Mordechai Pollak [1,2,†], Ronen Bar-Yoseph [1,2] and Lea Bentur [1,2]

1. Pediatric Pulmonary Institute and CF Center, Rappaport Children's Hospital, Rambam Health Care Campus, Haifa 3109601, Israel
2. Rappaport Faculty of Medicine, Technion–Israel Institute of Technology, Haifa 3525422, Israel
* Correspondence: m_gur@rambam.health.gov.il; Tel.: +972-4-7774360; Fax: +972-4-7774395
† These authors contributed equally to this work.

Abstract: The introduction of mutation-specific therapy led to a revolution in cystic fibrosis (CF) care. These advances in CF therapies have changed the disease profile from a severe incurable disease with limited survival to a treatable disease with improved quality of life and survival into adulthood. CF patients are now able to plan their future, including marriage and parenthood. Side by side with the optimism, new issues and concerns are arising, including fertility and preparation for pregnancy, maternal and fetal care during pregnancy, and post-partum care. While cystic fibrosis transmembrane regulator (CFTR) modulators show promising results for improving CF lung disease, data on their safety in pregnancy are still limited. We performed a literature review on pregnancy in CF from the past, with the first described pregnancy in 1960, through the current fascinating changes in the era of CFTR modulators, to ongoing studies and future directions. Current advances in knowledge give hope for improved outcomes of pregnancy, towards the best possible prognosis for the mother and for the baby.

Keywords: cystic fibrosis; pregnancy; CFTR modulators

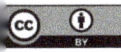

1. Introduction

Advances in the care of cystic fibrosis (CF) led to improved life expectancy. Thus, CF patients have been able to reach adulthood; consequently, issues like marriage and pregnancy became relevant. Clinicians are now required to address new challenges, such as fertility, family planning, pregnancy, and post-partum care [1].

The first pregnancy in CF was described in 1960, but unfortunately the mother deceased shortly after giving birth [2]. Thereafter, an increasing number of successful pregnancies were reported in the literature. According to the United States (US) CF patient registry, the yearly number of pregnancies increased from 230 in 2009 to 310 in 2019 [3]. This number nearly doubled in 2020, with a total of 619 pregnancies reported [4]. While in the past a cut-off of forced expiratory volume in one second (FEV1) > 60% was considered necessary to undergo a successful pregnancy, more recent studies report positive outcomes, even in women with advanced pulmonary disease. However, these women are at increased risk of premature delivery, and should be followed more closely [5].

In 2008, Edenborough et al. published guidelines for the management of pregnancy in women with CF. The authors addressed several important aspects, from the pre-conceptual until the post-partum period [6]. A few years later, the introduction of cystic fibrosis transmembrane regulator (CFTR) modulators opened new horizons for CF patients. Currently, approximately 90% of CF patients are eligible for this treatment, while the remaining 10% are still waiting for a novel precise medicine to address their molecular defect. The introduction of a new triple combination therapy of elexacaftor/tezacaftor/ivacaftor (ETI) in 2019 has been a significant game changer for eligible patients. Even in patients that were previously candidates for lung transplantation, the introduction of CFTR modulators resulted in such impressive improvement, that pregnancy has become feasible. In this context, new issues arise, such as the effect of CFTR modulators on fertility, and their safety during pregnancy [7]. It should be noted that mutation-specific therapy is still not available and funded for all eligible patients.

The European Respiratory Society (ERS)/Thoracic Society of Australia and New Zealand (TSANZ) published a consensus statement about the management of pregnancy in CF, as well as other chronic airway diseases [8]. More recently, a multidisciplinary panel of women with CF and CF clinicians published recommendations on pre-conception, intrapartum, and post-partum care for people with CF [9].

Herein we performed a literature review on pregnancy in CF going over a longitudinal timeline: from the past—before the era of CFTR modulators; through present—current knowledge about factors affecting pregnancy outcomes, including the use of CFTR modulators in pregnancy; to the future—on-going studies and future directions for the care of pregnancy in women with CF.

2. Pregnancy before the Era of CFTR Modulators

2.1. Preparation for Pregnancy

In CF, as in other chronic diseases, there is utmost importance for optimization of pre-conception health; thus, discussion about fertility and family planning should begin during adolescent years and continue into adulthood [9]. One of the fundamental aspects of CF care is the multidisciplinary clinic. To prepare for pregnancy, all team members should be involved, targeting medical and psychological aspects, and optimizing chronic therapies, including inhalations of mucolytics and antibiotics, and chest physiotherapy [8]. In addition, it is important to hold a realistic discussion about the patient's current health status, and the potential impact of pregnancy on maternal health and fetal outcomes, as well as short- and long-term morbidity [9,10].

2.1.1. Infertility and Subfertility

Almost all adult men with CF are infertile due to failure of normal development of the vas deferens; although, there are functioning sperm in their testicles. Obliteration of the vas deferens by retained secretions in utero leads to congenital bilateral absence of vas deference (CBAVD) and azoospermia. Notably, CBAVD may be the sole manifestation of CF [3,11].

In women with CF, subfertility was first described in the 1970s. CFTR was found to be expressed in the cervical epithelium; thus, deficient CFTR led to thick cervical mucus and reduced sperm permeability [3,12]. In addition, malabsorption and chronic inflammatory state lead to impaired growth, and delays in puberty and menarche. After reaching menarche, anovulatory cycles have been an important cause of impaired fertility [12]. Girls with CF were found to have delays in achieving pubertal levels of insulin-like growth factor-I (IGF-I), follicle-stimulating hormone (FSH), and luteinizing hormone (LH) [13]; low levels of anti-Mullerian hormone (AMH), considered to be a marker of ovarian reserve, were found in women with CF [14].

In a retrospective study from 11 centers, a higher rate of subfertility was found in 605 CF woman (35%, compared to 5–15% in the general population). In a multivariate analysis, pancreatic insufficiency (PI) and older age were associated with subfertility, while lung function, body mass index (BMI), CF-related diabetes (CFRD), and number of exacerbations in the previous year were not associated. CFRD was present in 16% of women with normal fertility and 23% of sub-fertile women ($p = 0.02$) [15]. Similarly, a French registry study found a slightly higher rate of assisted conception in women with pre-gestational diabetes (53.8% vs. 34.5%, $p = 0.06$) [16]. In another study, a questionnaire was sent to women with CF, of whom 46 sought pregnancies; 17 (37%) had no spontaneous pregnancy, from whom 13 had infertility treatment and 11 were successful.

2.1.2. Genetic Testing

Women with CF who desire to get pregnant should undergo genotype analysis, if previously unknown. In addition, carrier screening should be offered for partners. As there are more than 300 disease-causing mutations in the CFTR gene, a limited panel of the 25 most common mutations may miss up to 30% of cases, especially in non-Caucasians. Thus, next-generation sequencing is the preferred method [12,17]. If the partner is found to carry a CF disease-causing mutation, pre-implantation genetic diagnosis may be offered [8]. While many developed and developing countries have implemented newborn screening for CF as routine, prenatal genetic screening tests are not broadly used. However, when there is family history of CF, and there is high suspicion that parents might be carriers, parental screening would be suggested. Ideally, genetic screening should be utilized for the suspected carrier and if a mutation is found, then the partner should be screened as well. These tests should be performed prior to conception in order to allow, for families that are interested, the possibility of pre-implantation genetic diagnosis (PGD). In our country, a unique population carrier screening (PCS) has been available since 1999, and universally subsidized since 2008. Stafler et al. assessed the impact of this screening program and showed a dramatic reduction in CF birth rates with a shift towards milder mutations [18].

2.1.3. Risk Factors for Poor Outcome of Pregnancy in CF

Several factors related to maternal health have been found to contribute to outcomes of pregnancy in CF. These include pancreatic insufficiency (PI) and nutritional status, CFRD, pulmonary and cardiac function, and bacterial burden [17].

Nutrition should be optimized through diet, fat-soluble vitamins, and pancreatic enzyme replacement therapy (PERT). Poor nutritional status has been found to be related to poor outcomes, including prematurity and low birth weight [17]. A BMI of 22 kg/m^2 is considered the goal prior to pregnancy [9]. Historically, weight gain of 11 kg (kg) in pregnancy was recommended; recent recommendations depend on pre-pregnancy BMI, with higher weight gain expected for women with low BMI [17].

CFRD was also found to be a risk factor for poor outcome of pregnancy. Adequate glucose control should be achieved prior to and during pregnancy, with a goal of hemoglobin A1c (HbA1c) of <6.5% at the time of conception and <6.0% during pregnancy. Gestational diabetes is more common in women with CF, occurring in 10–36% of pregnancies [9]. Guidelines for CFRD in pregnancy recommend an oral glucose tolerance test (OGTT) at 12–16 weeks and at 24–28 weeks of pregnancy to detect the development of gestational diabetes [19].

In patients with low pre-conception BMI, or poor weight gain during pregnancy, enteral feeding should be considered. However, enteral tube feeding may unmask diabetes, thus closer follow up and blood glucose monitoring are warranted [10].

Several studies suggest that cor pulmonale and pulmonary hypertension are absolute contraindications for pregnancy in CF women. Increased right ventricular pressure can cause right ventricular dysfunction, tricuspid regurgitation, and, in severe cases, death. The mortality in parturient with pulmonary hypertension is reported to be around 30%. Thus, screening patients with CF with an echocardiogram during prenatal care is very important [20].

2.2. Therapies during Pregnancy

The treatment regimen for CF patients is often complex, and includes PERT, antibiotics (inhaled or oral), mucolytics, and anti-inflammatory medications [12]. During pregnancy, the therapeutic benefits for the mother, possible adverse effects on the fetus, and the risks of cessation of therapies, all should be considered [9,21]. Because pregnancy is almost always an exclusion criterion in clinical trials of new therapies, much of the available data are based on animal models rather than human studies [9]. This illustrates the importance of an individualized approach in optimizing CF care during pregnancy, specifically for those with more compromised lung function. During the first six months of pregnancy, the woman should be seen frequently in clinic, perhaps monthly and two-weekly in the final trimester or more frequently as progress dictates. At each visit, physical examination, measurement of oxygen saturation and pulmonary function, and weight should be performed, and sputum should be obtained [6].

To ensure adequate nutritional status and normal vitamin levels, PERT and vitamin supplementation should continue during pregnancy [8]. PERT appears to pose no significant risk during pregnancy. Vitamin A should be given in doses of less than 10,000 IU daily; higher doses in early pregnancy have been found to be associated with neural crest defects [12,17]. Folate supplementation is recommended as in non-CF pregnancy guidelines [9].

The two most common inhaled mucolytics are dornase alfa and hypertonic saline; both are used as chronic maintenance therapies. Both are considered safe to use in pregnancy, as the systemic absorption is minimal [9].

Airway clearance therapy (ACT) and physical activity should be established as routine before pregnancy and continued through pregnancy. As reflux may be increased during pregnancy, adjustment of physiotherapy may be necessary; timing of physiotherapy before meals, as well as upright sitting during ACT, may aid in minimizing reflux [8]. In severely ill patients, supplemental oxygen or even non-invasive assisted ventilatory support may be required during physiotherapy. If oxygen saturation falls to below 90% during ACT or physical exercise, supplemental oxygen should be administered to maintain oxygen saturations at around 92%. Overnight pulse-oximetry should be considered to check for nocturnal desaturation [6].

Inhaled antibiotics (AB) are recommended for patients chronically colonized with Pseudomonas aeruginosa (PSA). Tobramycin, aztreonam, and colistimethate sodium are most used. As in mucolytics, the inhaled route is considered safe due to minimal systemic absorption [9].

Azithromycin is a macrolide oral AB used as maintenance therapy due to its immunomodulatory effects. The drug is considered "probably safe" to continue during pregnancy; while women should be informed about a very small potential risk for the fetus, it is important to note that the risk of cessation of treatment is unknown [9,17]. It should be noted that treatment with azithromycin in the neonatal period was found to be associated with pyloric stenosis [22].

Treatment of Pulmonary Exacerbations (PEx)

The general approach for treating PEx in CF includes optimizing ACT, as well as the use or oral or intravenous (IV) AB, targeting the most recent cultured respiratory pathogens. Mild PEx usually is treated by oral AB, while moderate to severe exacerbations require IV treatment. Systemic AB use in pregnancy may be challenging due to placental transfer and potential risk of teratogenesis of some antibiotics [9].

Staphylococcus aureus (S. aureus) and PSA are the two most prevalent pathogens in the airways of CF patients. For the treatment of S. aureus, penicillins and cephalosporins are considered safe to use throughout pregnancy [9,12]. Trimethoprim-sulfamethoxazole use in the first and third trimesters has been associated with neural tube defects and hemolytic anemia, respectively. Therefore, their use should be avoided during the first and third trimesters, and at delivery [9,23].

Treatment of methicillin-resistant *S. aureus* (MRSA) in non-pregnant CF patients includes trimethoprim/sulfamethoxazole, vancomycin, or linezolid. Human studies of vancomycin are limited to first trimester, but no teratogenic effect has been found. Thus, vancomycin is considered "probably safe". Regarding linezolid, animal models have not shown a teratogenic effect, but data in humans are limited to case reports. Thus, it should be used if allergies or intolerance prevent the use of vancomycin, and only if benefit outweighs the risk [9].

For the treatment of PSA, the fluoroquinolones (levofloxacin and ciprofloxacin) are the oral AB of choice. Due to concerns for cartilage damage in animal models, their use has been typically avoided in pregnancy. However, recent evidence in human studies suggests low risk of teratogenesis, and they are considered "possibly safe" [8,9]. If a fluoroquinolone is indicated, ciprofloxacin is probably the preferred choice [6]. Antipseudomonas beta-lactam antibiotics (ceftazidime, ticarcillin) are considered safe during pregnancy. IV aminoglycosides can potentially cause fetal nephrotoxicity and ototoxicity, and their use should be limited to critically ill patients. If given during pregnancy, the once-daily dosing is preferable, with monitoring of drug levels [9,10,23]. Meropenem is considered "possibly safe" during the first trimester and "probably safe" during the remainder of pregnancy. However, women with CF have been found to be at increased risk of pre-eclampsia, and carbapenems lower the seizure threshold [9].

Table 1 summarizes the recommendations for CF therapies during pregnancy.

Table 1. Summary of recommendations for CF therapies during pregnancy.

Drug	Use in Pregnancy	Remarks
PERT	Probably safe	
DEKAs	Probably safe	Vitamin A doses < 10,000 IU
Dornase alfa	Probably safe	Inhaled route—minimal systemic absorption
Hypertonic saline	Probably safe	
ACT	Continue during pregnancy	Adjust to minimize reflux
Antibiotics		
Inhaled AB	Probably safe	Minimal systemic absorption
Inhaled levofloxacin	Probably safe	Minimal systemic absorption
Azithromycin	Probably safe	Minimal possible risk for fetus
Penicillins and cephalosporins *	Probably safe	
TMX/SMZ	Avoid 1st and 3rd trimester and delivery	Neural tube defects, hem. anemia
Vancomycin	Probably safe	
Linezolid	No harm in animal models	Limited human data
Ciprofloxacin	Possibly safe	Concern of cartilage damage
Levofloxacin	Possibly safe	Ciprofloxacin is preferrable
Aminoglycosides *	Save for critically ill	Nephrotoxicity & ototoxicity
Meropenem *	Possibly safe in 1st trimester	Lowers seizure threshold

PERT = pancreatic enzyme replacement therapy; DEKAs = vitamin D, E, K, A (fat-soluble vitamins); AB = antibiotics; ACT = airway clearance therapy; TMX/SMZ = trimethoprim-sulfamethoxazole; * = intravenous (IV).

2.3. Outcome of Pregnancy

CF team, obstetricians, anesthesiologists, and the patient should be prepared for the delivery. Most CF women can have a spontaneous delivery with careful hemodynamic monitoring. Cesarean delivery should be reserved for usual obstetric indications. The increased cardiac output during delivery (about 50%) poses an acute risk of heart failure in women with pulmonary hypertension or core pulmonale. Regional analgesia may be beneficial for women with CF as it provides ability to rest and increased pain control [17].

In most studies, approximately two-thirds of births to women with CF are by vaginal delivery. Previous studies found an increased rate of cesarean section (CS) in preterm deliveries and in women with lower pulmonary function or CFRD. In cases of CS for maternal or fetal indications, spinal anesthesia is preferred over general anesthesia. After delivery, adapted analgesia is important to reduce pain, fatigue, and anxiety, and to allow re-initiation of airway clearance soon after delivery [3].

The use of extracorporeal membrane oxygenation (ECMO) during pregnancy is described in an interesting systemic review by Naoum et al. Some of the reported patients were diagnosed with pulmonary hypertension [24]. However, data on use of ECMO for the obstetric population with CF are extremely limited. One unique case of perioperative management and preemptive ECMO cannulation in a parturient with CF undergoing CS was reported by Dos Santos et al. and highlights individualized approach for CF pregnancy and delivery [20].

Most CF pregnancies result in live births, ranging from 67% to 85% in series from the United States, Canada, United Kingdom, and France [12]. As already mentioned, poor nutritional status and CFRD are considered as risk factors for poor pregnancy outcomes. Low baseline weight is associated with prematurity and low birth weight. Pre-conception hyperglycemia is associated with a higher risk of fetal malformations, while hyperglycemia during pregnancy is associated with fetal macrosomia and increased risk of caesarean section (CS) [9].

Pre-pregnancy lung function is often considered as the most important factor for predicting pregnancy, both for the mother and the baby. Women with poorer lung function at the beginning of pregnancy have a higher risk for prematurity or small-for-gestational age (SGA) baby [17,25]. Case series have shown increased risk of miscarriages, both early and mid-pregnancy, especially in mothers with worse lung function. Thus, some authors have suggested that a pre-pregnancy FEV1 >60% predicted should be present before pregnancy is undertaken [8]; however, there are reports of successful pregnancies, even in advanced lung disease. In general, Cheng et al. found that birth weight was lower with maternal FEV1 < 50% [26]. In a French survey, 61/77 (79%) pregnancies resulted in live births, with 19% and 16% of premature deliveries and low birth weight, respectively; the rate of CS was 16% [27]. In a small Scandinavian series, the rate of preterm delivery was 24%; low maternal weight and poor maternal lung function before pregnancy increased the risk of preterm delivery [28]. More recently, Reynaud et al. found that in women with FEV1 < 50%, the rate of CS was higher and birth weight was lower, but rate of prematurity was similar [5]. Similarly, the Toronto CF database reported a low rate of prematurity, with similar rates in those with FEV1 above and below 50% [29]. In a population-based UK study, 69/71 (97.2%) pregnancies were live births. Similar to previous findings, maternal FEV1 correlated with gestational age and birth weight [25]. Recently, in a multicenter-retrospective cohort study, moderate–severe disease (FEV1 $\leq$ 60% and/or BMI $\leq$ 21 kg/m^2 prior to pregnancy) was associated with prematurity, while pancreatic insufficiency (PI) increased the risk for SGA infants [30].

Effect of Pregnancy on Lung Disease and Overall Survival

In 1995, Edenborough et al. followed 22 pregnancies in 20 women and found a 13% decrease in FEV1 during pregnancy [31]. A few years later, they performed a multi-center study with 72 pregnancies in 55 patients, and 65% of them required IV AB treatment during pregnancy [32]. Data from a French registry found even worse outcomes: 77.5% of women required IV AB treatment. Maternal mortality within one year after birth was 15% for those with FEV1 < 50% and 3% for those with FEV1 > 50% [33]. Nevertheless, other studies reported better outcomes. In the Toronto database mentioned earlier, pregnancy did not result in a greater decrease in FEV1 on follow up of 11 years. Nineteen percent of women died: FEV1 < 50%, colonization with Burkholderia cepacia, and PI were associated with decreased survival [29]. It should be noted that these studies followed pregnancies more than 20 years ago. The French registry data are from 1980–1999, and the Toronto database is from 1961–1998. Some authors even found that pregnancy was not associated with decreased lung function or shortened survival [1,34].

Data from the CF Epidemiologic Study demonstrated increased AB use during pregnancy, as well as increased outpatient and inpatient hospital visits [35]. Similarly, in the retrospective study mentioned earlier, patients with FEV1 $\leq$ 60% and/or low BMI $\leq$ 21 kg/m^2 experienced more disease related complications during and after pregnancy; but on the other hand, FEV1 and BMI did not decline more rapidly after pregnancy [30].

In a large cohort study, women who reported pregnancy (n = 680) were more likely to have better baseline FEV1. Using Kaplan–Meier survival curves, the 10-year survival rate in pregnant women was higher than in those women who did not become pregnant (77% (95% confidence interval (CI), 71 to 82%) compared to 58% (95% CI, 55 to 62%), respectively). The pregnant cohort also had better survival among specific high-risk subgroups, FEV1 < 40% (p < 0.001) and CFRD (p = 0.02). The authors postulated that closer follow up during preparation for pregnancy resulted in improved compliance and better baseline health status [34].

Pregnancy was also found to increase the risk of diabetes. The number of women receiving diabetes therapy more than doubled during pregnancy, and half of them required long-term therapy [1]. In the French study mentioned earlier, there was no difference in FEV1 and BMI decline following pregnancy between those with and without CFRD [16].

2.4. Pregnancy after Lung Transplantation (LTX)

In 2006, Gyi et al. described 10 pregnancies in lung transplant recipients, and demonstrated that pregnancy after LTX is feasible. There were nine live births, five of them premature. Three women developed rejection during pregnancy, and four died within 38 months after delivery [36].

In a registry analysis from the US National Transplantation Pregnancy Registry, 12/30 patients had CF. There were 60% preterm births, with 11 infant complications and two neonatal deaths. The rate of rejection was higher in CF patients (25% vs. 11%), and mean birth weight was lower [37].

Some lung transplant centers recommend avoiding pregnancy all together; others recommend waiting for 2–3 years after LTX. Patients with a history of acute or chronic rejection should be advised against pregnancy [12,36].

Caution should be also taken with immunosuppressive medication use during pregnancy. Therapies such as cyclosporine and tacrolimus require frequent monitoring, and dose adjustment with weight changes. Mycophenolate mofetil is teratogenic and should be avoided. Safety data on other immunosuppressants, such as prednisone, azathioprine, and calcineurin inhibitors, remains limited [17].

Overall, pregnancy post lung transplantation is still considered high risk. Patients should be carefully counselled about the potential risks to graft function and overall health.

Figure 1 summarizes the considerations and recommendations before pregnancy, during pregnancy, and in the post-partum period, including after LTX.

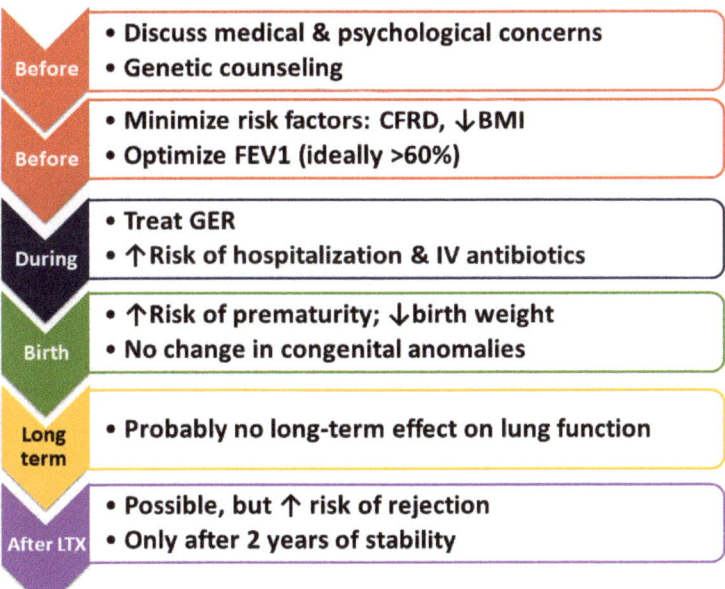

Figure 1. Summary of recommendations pre-conception, during pregnancy, and post-partum. CFRD = cystic fibrosis-related diabetes; BMI = body mass index; FEV1 = forced expiratory volume in one second; GER = gastro-esophageal reflux; IV = intravenous; LTX = lung transplantation.

3. Pregnancy in the Era of CFTR Modulators

3.1. Introduction

Three decades after the discovery of the CFTR gene [38], mutation specific therapy is now available for most CF patients. Ivacaftor was the first mutation-specific therapy approved for clinical use and improved FEV1 by an average of 10.6% for those with the G551D gating mutation [39,40]. Shortly after, two modulator combinations were shown to modestly improve FEV1 and decrease pulmonary exacerbations [41–43]. Finally, in 2019, trikafta, a new triple combination therapy of elexacaftor/tezacaftor/ivacaftor (ETI) showed extraordinary results. ETI improved FEV1 by an average of 13.8% in eligible patients [44,45]. This combination therapy has changed the lives of patients who are eligible for it, which is estimated to be 90% of CF patients. As mentioned earlier, one of the most exciting consequences of the new CF era is that people that were previously preoccupied with health and survival issues are now healthy enough and emotionally ready to consider planning families and children of their own. In this section we will focus on the impact of CFTR mutation-specific therapy on reproductive health in CF.

3.2. Effects of CFTR Modulators on Fertility

Since development of the vas deferens is already disturbed in utero, eventually leading to obstructive azoospermia, it is unlikely that CFTR modulators will have a significant impact on this aspect once fetal development is completed. However, an interesting study found that in CF ferrets homozygous for the gating mutation G551D, treatment with ivacaftor during pregnancy led to development of the vas deferens and epididymis [46]. Whether it is possible to rescue the formation of vas deferens following in utero exposure to highly efficient modulators such as ETI, and whether it is safe, is still unknown. Additionally, males with CF are known to have smaller volume of ejaculate than healthy men. There is a possibility that CFTR modulators can lead to increased ejaculate volume by acting on CFTR channels present in the male reproductive tract [47]. Perhaps related to that, some cases of acute testicular pain in men with CF have been reported following initiation of ETI therapy. The pain onset occurred within two weeks of ETI initiation and in all cases but one, the symptom resolved within one week [48]. While the mechanism of this side effect is still unknown, it can be speculated that restoration of CFTR function in the male reproductive tract had a role in this side effect.

As mentioned earlier, the reproductive anatomy in women with CF is not different than healthy women, but several factors contribute to subfertility. Mutation-specific therapy may potentially increase fertility rates, both by directly affecting the female reproductive tract, and indirectly by improving nutrition and health status.

Although it is early to appreciate the impact of ETI on fertility fully and accurately, experience with ivacaftor showed improved fertility in women that were previously considered infertile. In the phase 3 study of ivacaftor, despite the fact that women agreed to use contraceptives while on the study, 2% of the women became pregnant, thus illustrating the importance of proper guidance for women starting use of CFTR modulators [39,49,50]. The exact mechanism of improved fertility is not yet known, but the CFTR modulators are thought to decrease viscosity and increase pH in cervical mucous secretions, promoting a more fertile environment [49].

3.3. Use and Safety of CFTR Modulators in Pregnancy

Placental transfer of CFTR modulators has been observed in animal models and in humans [51,52]. When tested in three women using ETI during pregnancy, ETI was found in high concentrations in cord blood, suggesting that concentrations in utero are within therapeutic range. Although in lower levels, detectable concentrations of ETI were also seen in breast milk [21]. In line with that, an astonishing case report described a CF patient homozygous for F508del mutation, treated with ETI before and during pregnancy. The fetus was found to have echogenic bowel on week 20 and was found to be F508del homozygous as well. The mother chose to continue ETI despite the lack of sufficient safety data. At week 32, the fetal bowel was reported to be normal. Finally, the baby was delivered at term, with no meconium ileus. Surprisingly, the baby had normal immunoreactive trypsinogen (IRT) levels, leading to a false negative newborn screening for CF. Moreover, despite having typical CF, he did not suffer from PI. Repeated tests showed normal fecal elastase (>200 µg/g), and therefore PERT was stopped [21]. In another similar case, a F508del carrier was pregnant with a F508del homozygous fetus. The fetus was diagnosed with meconium ileus at 23 weeks of gestation; thus, the mother began ETI at 32 weeks with intent to treat fetal meconium ileus. A female infant was delivered at 36 weeks with no complications. Fecal elastase at age two weeks was 240 mcg/g and maternal and infant liver enzymes were within normal levels [53].

In terms of safety, when tested on animal models, elexacaftor and ivacaftor given at high doses that are toxic to humans, caused impaired fertility in male and female rats. However, CFTR modulators did not show adverse impact on fertility or show teratogenicity when given at normal human doses [54]. Another area of concern is the development of bilateral cataracts. Toxicity studies of ivacaftor in rats demonstrated infant cataracts, but until recently this was not reported in human infants. Recently, Jain et al. described three cases of infants exposed to ETI in utero and while breastfeeding, who were found to have bilateral congenital cataracts within six months of birth. Importantly, none of these infants had significant visual impairment [55].

3.4. Pregnancy Outcomes with CFTR Modulators

Currently, there is a lack of high-quality data to properly assess the maternal and fetal effects of CFTR modulators given during pregnancy. Until today, some case reports and surveys have been published, giving first signs of optimism in this area.

In a recent review by Taylor-Cousar, several case reports of women using ivacaftor or lumacaftor/ivacaftor were summarized. Out of 11 cases described, no adverse impacts on the infants were reported (other than prematurity that was attributed to significant maternal lung disease). One infant was reported to have mild hyperbilirubinemia that resolved spontaneously. In four cases, a formal ophthalmologic exam was carried out to the fetus, and all exams were normal [54]. Interestingly, there have also been reports of patients that stopped CFTR modulators due to concerns about the unknown safety to their fetus, and eventually re-introduced therapy due to declining lung function [56].

On a larger scale, two international surveys were reported on the outcomes of pregnancies for women treated with CFTR modulators. Their results are summarized in Table 2. The first survey focused on outcomes of pregnancies prior to ETI. A total of 64 pregnancies in 61 women were reported. Of these, 31 pregnancies were exposed to ivacaftor, 26 to lumacaftor/ivacaftor, and 7 to tezacaftor/ivacaftor. The physicians were asked to report their opinions about whether the complications were related to treatment. Only two complications were reported as being related to modulator use—one pulmonary exacerbation, and a case of acute myelocytic leukemia (AML). Notably, no other reports have shown a connection between leukemia with use of CFTR modulators. On the other hand, in those choosing to stop therapy due to unknown risks to the fetus, nine women experienced a decline in lung function leading to re-introducing modulator use during pregnancy [57].

A similar, more recent survey, using the same methodology, focused on outcomes of pregnancies for those treated with ETI [58]. In this survey, 47 pregnancies in 46 women were reported. Forty-one women were on ETI at the time of diagnosis of pregnancy and six elected to discontinue after pregnancy was diagnosed. Four women decided to begin ETI in the second or third trimester. Twenty-three women continued ETI throughout all trimesters. There were four miscarriages reported in the first trimester (8.9%); none was classified as related to ETI therapy (in one, the relation was deemed unknown, and the rest non-related). As reported in older CFTR modulators and perhaps to a larger extent, five women that elected to stop ETI, experienced a deterioration in lung function or increased symptoms; one patient experienced a severe deterioration including massive hemoptysis and significant fall in lung function. In terms of maternal outcomes, 28 events were deemed unrelated to therapy, one event was thought to be related to therapy (cholecystitis requiring cholecystectomy), and two with unknown relationship to ETI (cholestasis). Results of formal cataract inspections were not available in this report. At last, two cases were reported of unintended pregnancies shortly after delivery, and eventually were terminated [58]. The current limited data call for careful consideration of the beneficial versus the toxic effects of mutation specific therapy during pregnancy and lactation and continuing data collection and analysis.

Table 2. Use of CFTR modulators in pregnancy according to international surveys.

Modulator	Pregnancies/Modulator Used throughout Preg, (n)	Miscarriage	Prematurity	Fetal Complications Related to Modulator *	Fetal Complications Unknown/Not Related	Maternal Complications Related to Modulator *	Maternal Complications Unknown/Not Related
IVA	31/15	2	-	0	3	0	16
LUM/IVA	26/16	0	4	0	8	2	17
TEZ/IVA	7/5	1	-	0	2	0	5
ETI **	47/23	4	5	0	20 [a]	1	30 [b]

IVA = ivacaftor; LUM = lumacaftor; TEZ = tezacaftor; ETI = elexacaftor + tezacaftor + ivacaftor; preg. = pregnancy; n = number. * Determined by a CF specialist responding to the survey. [a] None of the fetal complications were considered related to ETI. The most common complication was cesarean section (n = 4) as a result of infant factors (large for gestational age, n = 2; abnormal presentation, n = 2). Three infants were born with mild congenital malformations, for whom the relatedness was considered unknown; two of them were born to mothers with poorly controlled diabetes. One fetus had multiple anomalies (considered unrelated to ETI) and pregnancy was terminated. One patient had trisomy 16. [b] Events that occurred in more than one woman—gestational diabetes (n = 2), preeclampsia (n = 2), pre-term labor (n = 2), and need for Cesarean section (C-section) for maternal reasons (n = 4); two seizures occurred in a woman with a history of seizures. All these were considered unrelated to ETI. There were three events of cholestasis—one cholecystitis considered related to ETI, one episode in a woman with previous obstetric was considered unrelated, and one was considered with unknown relatedness. ** Recently, Jain et al. described three cases of infants exposed to ETI in utero and while breastfeeding: bilateral congenital cataracts were found, with no significant visual impairment [55]. Nash et al. for IVA, LUM/IVA and TEZ/IVA [54], Taylor-Cousar et al. for ETI [55].

According to the US prescribing information (USPI) of ETI, there are limited and incomplete human data from clinical trials on the use of ETI or its individual components in pregnant women to inform a drug-associated risk [59]. Therefore, there is no assigned FDA risk category [60]. According to the European drug information, as a precautionary measure, it is preferable to avoid the use of ETI during pregnancy [61].

For infants exposed to ETI during pregnancy or breastfeeding, it is recommended to perform ophthalmologic screening examinations for neonatal cataract evaluation and liver function testing [9].

4. Conclusions and Future Directions

In conclusion, optimizing pre-conception medical and emotional status, addressing specific risk factors that are associated with poor outcome; integrated multi-disciplinary care during pregnancy, taking in account the risk-benefit ratio of additional treatments; and close follow up in the post-partum period, are all necessary for the best outcomes of pregnancy in CF patients, both for the mother and the newborn.

As detailed above, at this point, data on the safety of CFTR modulators in pregnancy are limited. There is some evidence, however, that cessation of therapy may lead to declining lung function or increasing symptoms. On the other hand, there is no evidence for significant teratogenicity or severe side effects related to pregnancy. Accordingly, a European Respiratory Society/Thoracic Society of Australia and New Zealand statement concerning the management of reproduction and pregnancy in women with airway diseases, considered CFTR modulators to be "probably safe", and that maternal benefit may outweigh potential risk during pregnancy and/or breastfeeding [8].

As discussed, modulators have been proven to cross the placenta efficiently, and limited evidence shows that maternal treatment can potentially rescue some of the irreversible damage that occurs in utero. Additional safety and efficacy data are still needed, but perhaps the dream may come into reality in the near future. Prenatally treating a fetus that is known to have CF may change the course of CF; we may postulate with caution, that even areas previously considered untreatable, such as pancreatic function and male fertility, may be reversible.

Currently, the "Maternal and Fetal Outcomes in the Era of Modulators" (MAYFLOW-ERS) study sponsored by the CF Foundation and CF Therapeutics Development Network, is taking place in 40 CF care centers across the United States. CF women on CFTR modulators are enrolled during the first trimester of pregnancy to assess maternal and fetal outcomes during and after pregnancy [62].

Until additional information is available and specific guidelines are published, the decisions should be individualized and a risk–benefit approach should be discussed to ensure the best combined maternal and fetal health.

Author Contributions: M.G. and M.P.—equal contribution—literature review, analysis of data, manuscript preparation; R.B.-Y.—manuscript draft preparation; L.B.—responsible for analysis of data, manuscript preparation, and review. All authors have read and agreed to the published version of the manuscript.

Funding: This research received no external funding.

Data Availability Statement: The data presented in this study are available on request from the corresponding author.

Conflicts of Interest: The authors declare no conflict of interest.

References

1. McMullen, A.H.; Pasta, D.J.; Frederick, P.D.; Konstan, M.W.; Morgan, W.J.; Schechter, M.S.; Wagener, J.S. Impact of pregnancy on women with cystic fibrosis. *Chest* **2006**, *129*, 706–711. [CrossRef] [PubMed]
2. Siegel, B.; Siegel, S. Pregnancy and Delivery in a Patient with Cystic Fibrosis of the Pancreas: Report of a case. *Obstet. Gynecol.* **1960**, *16*, 438–440.
3. Shteinberg, M.; Taylor-Cousar, J.L.; Durieu, I.; Cohen-Cymberknoh, M. Fertility and Pregnancy in Cystic Fibrosis. *Chest* **2021**, *160*, 2051–2060. [CrossRef]
4. Cystic Fibrosis Foundation. *Patient Registry 2020 Annual Data Report*; Cystic Fibrosis Foundation: Bethesda, MD, USA, 2021.
5. Reynaud, Q.; Rousset Jablonski, C.; Poupon-Bourdy, S.; Denis, A.; Rabilloud, M.; Lemonnier, L.; Nove-Josserand, R.; Durupt, S.; Touzet, S.; Durieu, I. Pregnancy outcome in women with cystic fibrosis and poor pulmonary function. *J. Cyst. Fibros.* **2020**, *19*, 80–83. [CrossRef] [PubMed]
6. Edenborough, F.P.; Borgo, G.; Knoop, C.; Lannefors, L.; Mackenzie, W.E.; Madge, S.; Morton, A.M.; Oxley, H.C.; Touw, D.J.; Benham, M.; et al. Guidelines for the management of pregnancy in women with cystic fibrosis. *J. Cyst. Fibros.* **2008**, *7*, S2–S32. [CrossRef]
7. Heltshe, S.L.; Godfrey, E.M.; Josephy, T.; Aitken, M.L.; Taylor-Cousar, J.L. Pregnancy among cystic fibrosis women in the era of CFTR modulators. *J. Cyst. Fibros.* **2017**, *16*, 687–694. Available online: https://pubmed-ncbi-nlm-nih-gov.ezlibrary.technion.ac.il/28190780/ (accessed on 21 November 2022). [CrossRef] [PubMed]
8. Middleton, P.G.; Gade, E.J.; Aguilera, C.; MacKillop, L.; Button, B.M.; Coleman, C.; Johnson, B.; Albrechtsen, C.; Edenborough, F.; Rigau, D.; et al. ERS/TSANZ Task Force Statement on the management of reproduction and pregnancy in women with airways diseases. *Eur. Respir. J.* **2020**, *55*, 1901208. [CrossRef]
9. Montemayor, K.; Tullis, E.; Jain, R.; Taylor-Cousar, J.L. Management of pregnancy in cystic fibrosis. *Breathe* **2022**, *18*, 220005. [CrossRef]
10. Lau, E.M.T.; Moriarty, C.; Ogle, R.; Bye, P.T. Pregnancy and cystic fibrosis. *Paediatr. Respir. Rev.* **2010**, *11*, 90–94. Available online: https://pubmed-ncbi-nlm-nih-gov.ezlibrary.technion.ac.il/20416544/ (accessed on 27 November 2022). [CrossRef]
11. Kaplan, E.; Shwachman, H.; Perlmutter, A.D.; Rule, A.; Khaw, K.-T.; Holsclaw, D.S. Reproductive Failure in Males with Cystic Fibrosis. *N. Engl. J. Med.* **1968**, *279*, 65–69. [CrossRef]
12. Mcardle, J.R. Pregnancy in Cystic Fibrosis. *Clin. Chest Med.* **2011**, *32*, 111–120. [CrossRef]
13. Goldsweig, B.; Kaminski, B.; Sidhaye, A.; Blackman, S.M.; Kelly, A. Puberty in cystic fibrosis. *J. Cyst. Fibros.* **2019**, *18*, S88–S94. [CrossRef]
14. Schram, C.A.; Stephenson, A.L.; Hannam, T.G.; Tullis, E. Cystic fibrosis (cf) and ovarian reserve: A cross-sectional study examining serum anti-mullerian hormone (amh) in young women. *J. Cyst. Fibros.* **2015**, *14*, 398–402. Available online: https://pubmed-ncbi-nlm-nih-gov.ezlibrary.technion.ac.il/25280785/ (accessed on 9 December 2022). [CrossRef] [PubMed]
15. Shteinberg, M.; Lulu, A.B.; Downey, D.G.; Blumenfeld, Z.; Rousset-Jablonski, C.; Perceval, M.; Colombo, A.; Stein, N.; Livnat, G.; Gur, M.; et al. Failure to conceive in women with CF is associated with pancreatic insufficiency and advancing age. *J. Cyst. Fibros.* **2019**, *18*, 525–529. [CrossRef]

16. Reynaud, Q.; Poupon-Bourdy, S.; Rabilloud, M.; Al Mufti, L.; Rousset Jablonski, C.; Lemonnier, L.; Nove-Josserand, R.; Touzet, S.; Durieu, I. Pregnancy outcome in women with cystic fibrosis-related diabetes. *Acta Obstet. Gynecol. Scand.* **2017**, *96*, 1223–1227. [CrossRef]
17. Jain, R.; Kazmerski, T.M.; Zuckerwise, L.C.; West, N.E.; Montemayor, K.; Aitken, M.L.; Cheng, E.; Roe, A.H.; Wilson, A.; Mann, C.; et al. Pregnancy in cystic fibrosis : Review of the literature and expert recommendations. *J. Cyst. Fibros.* **2022**, *21*, 387–395. [CrossRef] [PubMed]
18. Stafler, P.; Mei-Zahav, M.; Wilschanski, M.; Mussaffi, H.; Efrati, O.; Lavie, M.; Shoseyov, D.; Cohen-Cymberknoh, M.; Gur, M.; Bentur, L.; et al. The impact of a national population carrier screening program on cystic fibrosis birth rate and age at diagnosis: Implications for newborn screening. *J. Cyst. Fibros.* **2016**, *15*, 460–466. Available online: https://pubmed-ncbi-nlm-nih-gov.ezlibrary.technion.ac.il/26386752/ (accessed on 7 February 2023). [CrossRef]
19. Moran, A.; Brunzell, C.; Cohen, R.C.; Katz, M.; Marshall, B.C.; Onady, G.; Robinson, K.A.; Sabadosa, K.A.; Stecenko, A.; Slovis, B.; et al. Clinical care guidelines for cystic fibrosis-related diabetes: A position statement of the American Diabetes Association and a clinical practice guideline of the Cystic Fibrosis Foundation, endorsed by the Pediatric Endocrine Society. *Diabetes Care* **2010**, *33*, 2697–2708. Available online: https://pubmed-ncbi-nlm-nih-gov.ezlibrary.technion.ac.il/21115772/ (accessed on 9 December 2022). [CrossRef]
20. Dos Santos, T.F.; Rabassa, A.; Aljure, O.; Zbeidy, R. Perioperative Management and Preemptive ECMO Cannulation of a Parturient with Cystic Fibrosis Undergoing Cesarean Delivery. *Case Rep. Anesthesiol.* **2020**, *2020*, 8814729. Available online: https://pubmed-ncbi-nlm-nih-gov.ezlibrary.technion.ac.il/33457018/ (accessed on 7 February 2023).
21. Collins, B.; Fortner, C.; Cotey, A.; Esther, C.R.; Trimble, A. Drug exposure to infants born to mothers taking Elexacaftor, Tezacaftor, and Ivacaftor. *J. Cyst. Fibros.* **2022**, *21*, 725–727. Available online: https://pubmed.ncbi.nlm.nih.gov/34952795/ (accessed on 6 December 2022). [CrossRef]
22. Zeng, L.; Xu, P.; Choonara, I.; Bo, Z.; Pan, X.; Li, W.; Ni, X.; Xiong, T.; Chen, C.; Huang, L.; et al. Safety of azithromycin in pediatrics: A systematic review and meta-analysis. *Eur. J. Clin. Pharmacol.* **2020**, *76*, 1709–1721. Available online: https://pubmed-ncbi-nlm-nih-gov.ezlibrary.technion.ac.il/32681202/ (accessed on 18 December 2022). [CrossRef] [PubMed]
23. Kroon, M.A.G.M.; Akkerman-Nijland, A.M.; Rottier, B.L.; Koppelman, G.H.; Akkerman, O.W.; Touw, D.J. Drugs during pregnancy and breast feeding in women diagnosed with Cystic Fibrosis—An update. *J. Cyst. Fibros.* **2018**, *17*, 17–25. [CrossRef] [PubMed]
24. Naoum, E.E.; Chalupka, A.; Haft, J.; Maceachern, M.; Vandeven, C.J.M.; Easter, S.R.; Maile, M.; Bateman, B.T.; Bauer, M.E. Extracorporeal Life Support in Pregnancy: A Systematic Review. *J. Am. Heart Assoc.* **2020**, *9*, e016072. Available online: https://pubmed-ncbi-nlm-nih-gov.ezlibrary.technion.ac.il/32578471/ (accessed on 7 February 2023). [CrossRef] [PubMed]
25. Ashcroft, A.; Chapman, S.J.; Mackillop, L. The outcome of pregnancy in women with cystic fibrosis: A UK population-based descriptive study. *BJOG Int. J. Obstet. Gynaecol.* **2020**, *127*, 1696–1703. [CrossRef]
26. Cheng, E.Y.; Goss, C.H.; McKone, E.F.; Galic, V.; Debley, C.K.; Tonelli, M.R.; Aitken, M.L. Aggressive prenatal care results in successful fetal outcomes in CF women. *J. Cyst. Fibros.* **2006**, *5*, 85–91. Available online: https://pubmed-ncbi-nlm-nih-gov.ezlibrary.technion.ac.il/16650742/ (accessed on 11 December 2022). [CrossRef]
27. Tournier, A.; Murris, M.; Prevotat, A.; Fanton, A.; Bettiol, C.; Parinaud, J. Fertility of women with cystic fibrosis: A French survey. *Reprod. Biomed. Online* **2019**, *39*, 492–495. [CrossRef] [PubMed]
28. Ødegaard, I.; Stray-Pedersen, B.; Hallberg, K.; Haanaes, O.C.; Storrøsten, O.T.J.M. Maternal and fetal morbidity in pregnancies of Norwegian and Swedish women with cystic fibrosis. *Acta Obs. Gynecol. Scand.* **2002**, *81*, 698–705. Available online: https://pubmed-ncbi-nlm-nih-gov.ezlibrary.technion.ac.il/12174152/ (accessed on 11 December 2022).
29. Gilljam, M.; Antoniou, M.; Shin, J.; Dupuis, A.; Corey, M.; Tullis, D.E. Pregnancy in cystic fibrosis. Fetal and maternal outcome. *Chest* **2000**, *118*, 85–91. Available online: https://pubmed-ncbi-nlm-nih-gov.ezlibrary.technion.ac.il/10893364/ (accessed on 11 December 2022). [CrossRef]
30. Cohen-Cymberknoh, M.; Gindi Reiss, B.; Reiter, J.; Lechtzin, N.; Melo, J.; Pérez, G.; Blau, H.; Mussaffi, H.; Levine, H.; Bentur, L.; et al. Baseline Cystic fibrosis disease severity has an adverse impact on pregnancy and infant outcomes, but does not impact disease progression. *J. Cyst. Fibros.* **2021**, *20*, 388–394. Available online: https://pubmed-ncbi-nlm-nih-gov.ezlibrary.technion.ac.il/32917549/ (accessed on 18 November 2022). [CrossRef]
31. Edenborough, F.P.; Stableforth, D.E.; Mackenzie, W.E. Pregnancy in women with cystic fibrosis. *Thorax* **1995**, *311*, 170–174. [CrossRef]
32. Edenborough, F.P.; Mackenzie, W.E.; Stableforth, D.E. The outcome of 72 pregnancies in 55 women with cystic fibrosis in the United Kingdom 1977–1996. *BJOG Int. J. Obstet. Gynaecol.* **2000**, *107*, 254–261. Available online: https://onlinelibrary-wiley-com.ezlibrary.technion.ac.il/doi/full/10.1111/j.1471-0528.2000.tb11697.x (accessed on 11 December 2022). [CrossRef] [PubMed]
33. Gillet, D.; de Braekeleer, M.; Bellis, G.; Durieu, I. Cystic fibrosis and pregnancy. Report from French data (1980–1999). *BJOG Int. J. Obstet. Gynaecol.* **2002**, *109*, 912–918. Available online: https://onlinelibrary-wiley-com.ezlibrary.technion.ac.il/doi/full/10.1111/j.1471-0528.2002.01511.x (accessed on 11 December 2022).
34. Goss, C.H.; Rubenfeld, G.D.; Otto, K.; Aitken, M.L. The Effect of Pregnancy on Survival in Women with Cystic Fibrosis. *Chest* **2003**, *124*, 1460–1468. [CrossRef] [PubMed]
35. Schechter, M.S.; Quittner, A.L.; Konstan, M.W.; Millar, S.J.; Pasta, D.J.; McMullen, A. Long-term effects of pregnancy and motherhood on disease outcomes of women with cystic fibrosis. *Ann. Am. Thorac. Soc.* **2013**, *10*, 213–219. Available online: https://pubmed-ncbi-nlm-nih-gov.ezlibrary.technion.ac.il/23802817/ (accessed on 21 November 2022). [CrossRef]

36. Gyi, K.M.; Hodson, M.E.; Yacoub, M.Y. Pregnancy in cystic fibrosis lung transplant recipients: Case series and review. *J. Cyst. Fibros.* **2006**, *5*, 171–175. [CrossRef]
37. Shaner, J.; Coscia, L.A.; Constantinescu, S.; McGrory, C.H.; Doria, C.; Moritz, M.J.; Armenti, V.T.; Cowan, S.W. Pregnancy after lung transplant. *Prog. Transplant.* **2012**, *22*, 134–140. Available online: https://pubmed-ncbi-nlm-nih-gov.ezlibrary.technion.ac.il/22878069/ (accessed on 11 December 2022). [CrossRef] [PubMed]
38. Kerem, B.-S.; Rommens, J.M.; Buchanan, J.A.; Markiewicz, D.; Cox, T.K.; Chakravarti, A.; Buchwald, M.; Tsui, L.-C. Identification of the Cystic Fibrosis Gene: Genetic Analysis. *Science* **1989**, *245*, 1073–1080. [CrossRef]
39. Ramsey, B.W.; Davies, J.; McElvaney, N.G.; Tullis, E.; Bell, S.C.; Dřevínek, P.; Griese, M.; McKone, E.F.; Wainwright, C.E.; Konstan, M.W.; et al. A CFTR Potentiator in Patients with Cystic Fibrosis and the *G551D* Mutation. *N. Engl. J. Med.* **2011**, *365*, 1663–1672. [CrossRef]
40. Accurso, F.J.; Rowe, S.M.; Clancy, J.P.; Boyle, M.P.; Dunitz, J.M.; Durie, P.R.; Sagel, S.D.; Hornick, D.B.; Konstan, M.W.; Donaldson, S.H.; et al. Effect of VX-770 in persons with cystic fibrosis and the G551D-CFTR mutation. *N. Engl. J. Med.* **2010**, *363*, 1991–2003. [CrossRef]
41. Rowe, S.M.; Daines, C.; Ringshausen, F.C.; Kerem, E.; Wilson, J.; Tullis, E.; Nair, N.; Simard, C.; Han, L.; Ingenito, E.P.; et al. Tezacaftor–Ivacaftor in Residual-Function Heterozygotes with Cystic Fibrosis. *N. Engl. J. Med.* **2017**, *377*, 2024–2035. [CrossRef]
42. Taylor-Cousar, J.L.; Munck, A.; McKone, E.F.; van der Ent, C.K.; Moeller, A.; Simard, C.; Wang, L.T.; Ingenito, E.P.; McKee, C.; Lu, Y.; et al. Tezacaftor–Ivacaftor in Patients with Cystic Fibrosis Homozygous for Phe508del. *N. Engl. J. Med.* **2017**, *377*, 2013–2023. [CrossRef] [PubMed]
43. Wainwright, C.E.; Elborn, J.S.; Ramsey, B.W.; Marigowda, G.; Huang, X.; Cipolli, M.; Colombo, C.; Davies, J.C.; De Boeck, K.; Flume, P.A.; et al. Lumacaftor–Ivacaftor in Patients with Cystic Fibrosis Homozygous for Phe508del *CFTR*. *N. Engl. J. Med.* **2015**, *373*, 220–231. [CrossRef]
44. Middleton, P.G.; Mall, M.A.; Dřevínek, P.; Lands, L.C.; McKone, E.F.; Polineni, D.; Ramsey, B.W.; Taylor-Cousar, J.L.; Tullis, E.; Vermeulen, F.; et al. Elexacaftor–Tezacaftor–Ivacaftor for Cystic Fibrosis with a Single Phe508del Allele. *N. Engl. J. Med.* **2019**, *381*, 1809–1819. [CrossRef] [PubMed]
45. Heijerman, H.G.M.; McKone, E.F.; Downey, D.G.; Van Braeckel, E.; Rowe, S.M.; Tullis, E.; Mall, M.A.; Welter, J.J.; Ramsey, B.W.; McKee, C.M.; et al. Efficacy and safety of the elexacaftor plus tezacaftor plus ivacaftor combination regimen in people with cystic fibrosis homozygous for the F508del mutation: A double-blind, randomised, phase 3 trial. *Lancet* **2019**, *394*, 1940–1948. [CrossRef] [PubMed]
46. Sun, X.; Yi, Y.; Yan, Z.; Rosen, B.H.; Liang, B.; Winter, M.C.; Evans, T.I.A.; Rotti, P.G.; Yang, Y.; Gray, J.S.; et al. In utero and postnatal VX-770 administration rescues multiorgan disease in a ferret model of cystic fibrosis. *Sci. Transl. Med.* **2019**, *11*, eaau7531. [CrossRef]
47. West, N.E.; Kazmerski, T.M.; Taylor-Cousar, J.L.; Tangpricha, V.; Pearson, K.; Aitken, M.L.; Jain, R. Optimizing sexual and reproductive health across the lifespan in people with cystic fibrosis. *Pediatr. Pulmonol.* **2022**, *57*, S89–S100. [CrossRef]
48. Rotolo, S.M.; Duehlmeyer, S.; Slack, S.M.; Jacobs, H.R.; Heckman, B. Testicular pain following initiation of elexacaftor/tezacaftor/ivacaftor in males with cystic fibrosis. *J. Cyst. Fibros.* **2020**, *19*, e39–e41. [CrossRef]
49. Jones, G.H.; Walshaw, M.J. Potential impact on fertility of new systemic therapies for cystic fibrosis. *Paediatr. Respir. Rev.* **2015**, *16*, 25–27. [CrossRef]
50. Ladores, S.; Bray, L.A.; Brown, J. Two Unanticipated Pregnancies While on Cystic Fibrosis Gene-Specific Drug Therapy. *J. Patient Exp.* **2020**, *7*, 4–7. [CrossRef]
51. Qiu, F.; Habgood, M.D.; Huang, Y.; Dziegielewska, K.M.; Toll, S.; Schneider-Futschik, E.K. Entry of cystic fibrosis transmembrane conductance potentiator ivacaftor into the developing brain and lung. *J. Cyst. Fibros.* **2021**, *20*, 857–864. Available online: https://pubmed.ncbi.nlm.nih.gov/34193363/ (accessed on 4 December 2022). [CrossRef] [PubMed]
52. Trimble, A.; McKinzie, C.; Terrell, M.; Stringer, E.; Esther, C.R. Measured fetal and neonatal exposure to Lumacaftor and Ivacaftor during pregnancy and while breastfeeding. *J. Cyst. Fibros.* **2018**, *17*, 779–782. [CrossRef] [PubMed]
53. Szentpetery, S.; Foil, K.; Hendrix, S.; Gray, S.; Mingora, C.; Head, B.; Johnson, D.; Flume, P.A. A case report of CFTR modulator administration via carrier mother to treat meconium ileus in a F508del homozygous fetus. *J. Cyst. Fibros.* **2022**, *21*, 721–724. Available online: https://pubmed.ncbi.nlm.nih.gov/35422395/ (accessed on 6 December 2022). [CrossRef] [PubMed]
54. Taylor-Cousar, J.L. CFTR Modulators: Impact on Fertility, Pregnancy, and Lactation in Women with Cystic Fibrosis. *J. Clin. Med.* **2020**, *9*, 2706. [CrossRef] [PubMed]
55. Jain, R.; Wolf, A.; Molad, M.; Taylor-Cousar, J.L.; Esther, C.R., Jr.; Shteinberg, M. Congenital bilateral cataracts in newborns exposed to elexacaftor-tezacaftor-ivacaftor in utero and while breast feeding. *J. Cyst. Fibros.* **2022**, *21*, 1074–1076. [CrossRef]
56. Vekaria, S.; Popowicz, N.; White, S.W.; Mulrennan, S. To be or not to be on CFTR modulators during pregnancy: Risks to be considered. *J. Cyst. Fibros.* **2020**, *19*, e7–e8. [CrossRef]
57. Nash, E.F.; Middleton, P.G.; Taylor-Cousar, J.L. Outcomes of pregnancy in women with cystic fibrosis (CF) taking CFTR modulators—An international survey. *J. Cyst. Fibros.* **2020**, *19*, 521–526. [CrossRef]
58. Taylor-Cousar, J.L.; Jain, R. Maternal and fetal outcomes following elexacaftor-tezacaftor-ivacaftor use during pregnancy and lactation. *J. Cyst. Fibros.* **2021**, *20*, 402–406. [CrossRef] [PubMed]
59. Trikafta (Elexacaftor/Tezacaftor/Ivacaftor) [Package Insert]. Vertex, Pharmaceuticals Inc.: Boston, MA, USA, 2019. Available online: https://www.accessdata.fda.gov/drugsatfda_docs/label/2019/212273s000lbl.pdf (accessed on 2 December 2021).

60. Elexacaftor/Ivacaftor/Tezacaftor (Trikafta) Use During Pregnancy. Available online: https://www.drugs.com/pregnancy/elexacaftor-ivacaftor-tezacaftor.html (accessed on 7 February 2023).
61. Kaftrio ANNEX I—Summary of Product Characteristics:1–47. Available online: https://www.ema.europa.eu/en/documents/product-information/kaftrio-epar-product-information_en.pdf (accessed on 2 December 2021).
62. MAYFLOWERS: Study of Pregnancy in Women with Cystic Fibrosis (MAYFLOWERS-OB-20)—Search Results—PubMed. Available online: https://pubmed-ncbi-nlm-nih-gov.ezlibrary.technion.ac.il/?term=MAYFLOWERS%3A+Study+of+pregnancy+in+women+with+cystic+fibrosis+%28MAYFLOWERS-OB-20%29 (accessed on 12 December 2022).

Disclaimer/Publisher's Note: The statements, opinions and data contained in all publications are solely those of the individual author(s) and contributor(s) and not of MDPI and/or the editor(s). MDPI and/or the editor(s) disclaim responsibility for any injury to people or property resulting from any ideas, methods, instructions or products referred to in the content.

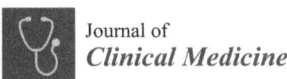

Journal of
Clinical Medicine

Commentary

A Review, Update, and Commentary for the Cough without a Cause: Facts and Factoids of the Habit Cough

Miles Weinberger [1,2,*], Dennis Buettner [3] and Ran D. Anbar [4]

1. Rady Children's Hospital, University of California San Diego, San Diego, CA 92123, USA
2. University of Iowa, Iowa City, IA 50011, USA
3. Habit Cough Association, Severna Park, MD 21146, USA
4. Center Point Medicine, La Jolla, CA 92037, USA
* Correspondence: miles-weinberger@uiowa.edu; Tel.: +1-760-487-5531

Abstract: Background: A habitual cough, persisting after the cause is gone, was described in a 1694 medical book. Successful treatment of this disorder known as habit cough was reported in 1966 by the "art of suggestion". The purpose of this article is to provide the current basis for diagnosis and treatment of the Habit Cough Syndrome. Method: The epidemiology and clinical course of habit cough were reviewed; original data were obtained from three sources. Results: Unique clinical presentation was the basis for diagnosis of habit cough. Diagnosis was made 140 times with increasing frequency over 20 years at the University of Iowa clinic and 55 times over 6 years at a London clinic. Suggestion therapy provided more frequent cessation of cough than just reassurance. A Mayo Clinic archive of chronic involuntary cough found 16 of 60 still coughing 5.9 years after initial evaluation. Ninety-one parents of children with habit cough and 20 adults reported cessation of coughing from viewing a publicly available video of successful suggestion therapy. Conclusions: Habit cough is recognizable from the clinical presentation. It is effectively treated in most children by suggestion therapy in clinics, by remote video conferencing, and by proxy from viewing a video of effective suggestion therapy.

Keywords: cough; chronic cough; habit cough; suggestion therapy; hypnosis; behavioral therapy; clinical education

1. Introduction

"The morbidity, cost, and impact of somatoform (functional) pediatric respiratory syndromes are far more impactful than that experienced by most of our severe asthmatics and CF patients. These conditions are NOT trivial, 'just in your head' conditions. A confident diagnostic approach and an optimistic therapeutic regimen are critically important."
(George Mallory MD)

Physician education focuses on anatomical, physiological, and organic disorders that cause illness. Emphasis is on identifying what is wrong with the body that is causing the patient's symptoms. When the cause is not identified, medication typically is provided in an attempt to relieve the symptoms. But some symptoms are not caused by corporal dysfunction and do not respond to usual pharmacotherapy. The medical term for those is functional. Among the clinically important functional respiratory disorders is the habit cough [1]. Habit cough has a long history in the medical literature. Unfortunately, habit cough currently often has been associated with inadequate recognition and alternative diagnoses.

The purpose of this article is to promote increased awareness among physicians regarding this often misdiagnosed and overtreated disorder. Habit cough is not influenced by any pharmacotherapy but does respond, with rare exceptions, to a simple behavioral measure. This narrative of the history, current status, and barriers to physician education regarding habit cough includes the encounters and accumulated data from the three authors who

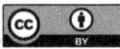

have an extraordinary amount of exposure to this disorder. We will review the chronology, epidemiology, etiology, treatment, and educational efforts to increase the understanding of this disorder. We will also describe the efforts to increase the knowledge and clinical skills of physicians likely to encounter this disorder. However, we cannot discuss habit cough without also examining the prevailing controversies and misinformation regarding this functional disorder, the cough without a cause.

2. Methods

Three present sources of data were used to characterize habit cough: (1) The University of Iowa Pediatric Allergy and Pulmonary Clinic from 1994 to 2014 provided epidemiologic data not previously published. (2) Over 200 remote contacts from February 2019 to September 2022 provided insights and aspects of outcome beyond what could be derived from clinic patients. (3) Selected patients from a private practice of author RA provided observational and treatment data about children with recalcitrant habit cough. Data from these sources will be contrasted with guidelines for cough management from authoritative committees.

The three sources of habit cough used for this publication provide data on the successes and limitations of suggestion therapy for habit cough as direct treatment, indirect treatment by remote video conferencing, and treatment by proxy where a video of a child receiving suggestion therapy is the source of successful therapy in others. From these data sources, epidemiology, outcome, and phenotypical variations of habit cough can be extracted.

Recognizing the relative deficiency of knowledge about habit cough and its treatment outside of those of us with extensive exposure, present physician care of habit cough also was available from almost 4 years of remote contact. Phenotypical variations of intractable habit cough and their treatment were available from the hypnosis and counseling practice of author RA.

3. Results

3.1. Chronology of Habit Cough

We found medical books from the 17th and 19th centuries with descriptions of specific examples of chronic cough that are consistent with current observations of habit cough. A medical textbook from 1685 by Thomas Willis (1621–1675) [2] described an adult woman with *"a violent dry cough following her day and night, unless she was fallen asleep"*, a description that would fit the habit cough diagnosis today. Franciscus Mercurios (1614–1699), a Flemish physician, alchemist, kabbalist, and writer, in a 1694 medical book, *The Spirit of Diseases*, described, " . . . *Habitual Cough, which often continues after the first cough, which was caused by the cold, is gone . . . and the Habitual Cough often proceed*" [3]. Charles Creighton (1847–1927), a British physician and medical author, in an 1886 medical book, *Illustrations of Unconscious Memory in Disease*, described, " . . . *a habit cough—a reflex effect persisting after the cause is gone . . . or an acquired habit . . .* " He went on to state, " . . . *the treatment of it is to break the habit . . .* " [4]. This was insightful reasoning on the part of Dr. Creighton.

Breaking the habit was essentially what Dr. Bernard Berman, a Boston allergist, reported in a 1966 publication [5]. He described six children seen in his practice over a 5-year period, three boys and three girls between the ages of 9 and 13 years. They all had daily barking coughing for the prior 3–6 months with absence of cough when asleep. He concluded that they were *"afflicted with habit cough"*; Dr. Berman stopped the coughing by what he called *"a simple modality of therapy"* that required an *"understanding and experience in the art of suggestion"*. Being aware that this repetitive cough had been considered a tic by some and as psychogenic by others, Dr. Berman considered those diagnostic terms for the disorder. However, he commented that he observed no motor or vocal tics and no evidence of concerning emotional problems in those children. He reasoned that the ease of stopping the cough with a simple behavioral technique justified the term, habit cough. To this day, there is no reasoned justification for considering habit cough as a tic disorder, a tic cough, or psychogenic cough, terms that have been used by some without any basis.

A 1991 publication reported three boys and six girls, median age 11 years, who had been previously seen at the University of Iowa Pediatric Allergy and Pulmonary Clinic with histories of 2–5 months of a harsh barking nonproductive repetitive cough during all waking hours but absent when sleeping [6]. Coughing occurred in spasms and with unusual frequency. Medications prescribed by the referring physicians had been ineffective. The coughing was stopped within 15 min using an adaptation of Berman's "art of suggestion". Sustained benefit was documented by telephone contact a median of 3.6 years (ranging up to 9.4 years) after the clinic visit. Psychopathology was not apparent from a standardized psychological questionnaire. On the basis of that experience, suggestion therapy continued as the standard of care at the University of Iowa.

3.2. Clinical Characteristics of Habit Cough

Thus, habit cough is not a new disorder despite the frequent lack of awareness regarding this disorder among much of the medical community. Just as described in the 1694 and subsequent publications, a respiratory illness is often an initiating factor at the onset of the repetitive cough [2]. Multiple case and series reports of children have since described a repetitive, daily nonproductive cough that is absent during sleep [5–11]. Habit cough is a distinctive syndrome recognizable and diagnosable by its unique clinical presentation. While the cough is most commonly described as barking or honking, home videos provided by parents demonstrate variability in the sound and frequency of the cough (https://youtu.be/U7p2B_Zt6AM, accessed 1 November 2022) Data from the University of Iowa clinic reported about 10% of the children having softer, throat-clearing type coughs [11].

While habit cough may not be recognized by a patient's primary care doctor, parents generally readily recognize that their child's cough is different from usual coughs with colds. A common comment from parents is that their child had a cold with a cough, and then after 1 or 2 weeks, the cough changed in sound and frequency. Routine spirometry and a chest X-ray provide sufficient reassurance that there is no physical basis for the cough. Further testing and therapeutic trials of medication result only in an iatrogenic component to the morbidity. The diagnosis is based on the uniqueness of the cough, its sound, frequency, nonproductive, and absence during sleep [11,12].

Occasionally, a child with successfully treated habit cough has a recurrence. While that data had not been systematically reported, our remote contact information included several parents reporting a recurrence of habit cough as much as a year later. Typically, it's another viral respiratory infection that is followed by the recurrence of the habit cough. Children with recurrences self-managed their cough when reminded that they knew how to control the cough from their prior experience. One younger child, who had a return of habit cough a year later, required repeat suggestion therapy to stop the returned cough because she could not remember what she had previously done.

3.3. Epidemiology of Habit Cough

In 2016, the diagnosis of habit cough was identified at the University of Iowa 140 times over a 20-year period from 1995 to 2014 based on information from the electronic medical record [11]. The average age was 10 years; 85% were between 8 and 13 years of age. The diagnosis was made by the frequent repetitive dry (nonproductive) cough that was absent once asleep. The absence once asleep despite a severe daily cough is a *sine qua non* for this disorder. A seasonal pattern with late spring and midsummer decreases in the frequency of diagnosis approximates the seasonal pattern of common viral respiratory infections.

Using the same criteria for diagnosis of habit cough, a repetitive dry cough that was absent during sleep, Brompton Hospital in London, England reported the diagnosis of 55 children during a 6-year period, an average of nine per year [12]. Approximately the same frequency occurred at the Iowa clinic during the 12-year period from 2003 to 2014. The median age was 10 years at both institutions. For most of the children seen at these two institutions, cough had been present for periods from about a month to greater than 12 months prior to being seen. An increased frequency of habit cough diagnosis from 2.2 to 4.5 cases per year was attributed to a period of financial stress in Greece [13]. However, year-to-year variation of that magnitude also was seen during the 20 years at the University of Iowa (Figure 1).

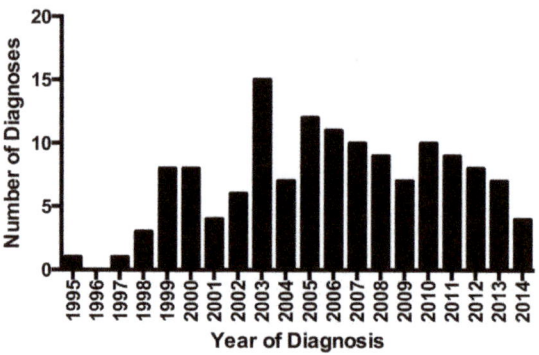

Figure 1. Annual diagnoses of habit cough by the faculty of the University of Iowa Allergy and Pulmonary Clinic from 1995 to 2014.

More data on the prevalence of habit cough were a systemic evaluation of 346 children brought to centers in Australia, specifically for chronic cough. Protracted bacterial bronchitis, a cause of chronic cough primarily in infants, was present in 142 of the 346. Asthma was diagnosed in 55, and 48 had spontaneous resolution of the cough. Of the 101 other cases, 15 were diagnosed as "habitual" cough [14]. These data on the frequency of diagnosing habit cough among those presenting with chronic cough and the frequency with which habit cough is diagnosed at two major referral centers provide the best information we have regarding the prevalence of this functional disorder. A few physicians, predominantly pediatric pulmonologists, in 14 states in the U.S. and 10 other countries currently have indicated that they are diagnosing and treating habit cough in a manner similar to that described here.

The COVID-19 pandemic was associated with some community physicians indicating to us that they were seeing more children with habit cough. From the 11 children reported to us with characteristic habit cough post-COVID-19, it did not appear that habit cough post-COVID-19 differed from habit cough triggered by other viral respiratory infections. COVID-19 can cause an acute cough, but a chronic dry cough is reported to follow recovery that can last for months. This is described in an extensively referenced review [15]. The post-COVID-19 prolonged cough may or may not be accompanied by other long COVID-19 symptoms. Data in publications of respiratory post-COVID-19 follow-up in children are insufficient to ascertain the frequency with which some have the characteristics of habit cough [16,17].

3.4. Etiology of Habit Cough

The cause of habit cough is an enigma. Why does it start? Why does it happen in some but not others? Why does it persist for months and even years? Cough hypersensitivity has been proposed as a hypothesis for the persistence of idiopathic or refractory chronic cough [18]. However, evidence suggests that cough hypersensitivity may be both a cause and consequence of persistent coughing.

Mucosal biopsies obtained by bronchoscopy in adults with no medical explanation for their chronic cough showed inflammation [19]. Increased nerve density was reported in bronchial mucosal biopsies from adults with chronic unexplained cough [20]. The investigators of both of those studies suggested that the sustained daily coughing could be the cause of their findings. Thus, this neuropathic inflammation could be the cause of cough hypersensitivity and could be the stimulus for chronic daily cough. Essentially, this suggests a vicious cycle where repetitive daily coughing causes the mucosal pathology that is the nidus for the cough.

Clinical support for this explanation of persistent coughing is the common patient awareness of a "sensation" (sometimes called a tickle) in their airway that triggers their repetitive cough. Many patients have told us that the feeling that had been stimulating the repetitive cough only gradually fades over weeks even after cessation of cough. Thus, many patients continue to struggle with the stimulus to cough even after they have learned how to resist that urge. An analogy to which patients can relate is a mosquito bite that itches; the more you scratch it, the more it itches. It does not heal until the scratching stops. The desire to scratch is analogous to the desire to cough. In both cases, the cycle of itch-scratch and tickle-cough requires control of the sensation for healing to occur.

Clinical observations suggested that stress and anxiety contribute to habit cough in some patients. A description of stress associated with habit cough was described by Papadopoulou et al. [13]. However, association does not prove etiology. The stresses described by Papadopoulou et al. are not unique and occur also in children without chronic cough.

3.5. Treatment of Habit Cough

Habit cough has been effectively treated by various forms of suggestion therapy. This was first reported in 1966 by Berman [5]. It has been extensively used at the University of Iowa since 1975 [6,11]. A successful variation includes suggesting that a sheet tied around the chest enables cessations of cough [9]. Speech therapy [21] and cognitive behavioral therapy [13] have been proposed as treatments for habit cough, but no outcome data are reported for those. Hypnosis has been successfully used [10].

Suggestion therapy has now been used to the greatest extent for the successful treatment of habit cough. Increasing numbers of physicians and some nurse practitioners have found the approach to be effective. Although the provider of the suggestion therapy can alter the wording, major elements of suggestion therapy for habit cough include:

- Establish rapport with the patient and parents.
- Be honest and forthright with patients and parents.
- Tell the parents that you want to talk to the patient and ask them to sit quietly in the background, phones turned off.
- Body temperature water should be at the patient's side or in hand to take small sips in anticipation of a cough.
- Explain the cough as a vicious cycle that started with an initial irritant that is now gone; it is now the cough itself that is causing the feeling that stimulates the coughing.
- Explain that cough is the body's natural response to feeling that something is in their airway.
- Explain that the brain can control that response, but it takes a lot of concentration.
- Instruct the patient to focus on the provider of the suggestion therapy who is to keep up a relaxed soft patter.
- The patient is instructed to be aware when a cough may be coming and take a small sip of the water and hold the cough back.
- Begin with a request to hold the cough back for a defined period of time, beginning small and progressing as successes occur.
- Tell the patient that each second the cough is delayed makes it easier to suppress further coughing.
- Repeat expressions of confidence that the patient is developing the ability to resist the urge to cough: "It's becoming easier to hold back the cough, isn't it?" (Nodding your head generally makes the child nod their head in agreement.)

- When the patient shows that he or she is able to suppress the cough (usually after about 10 min), ask in a rhetorical manner, "You're beginning to feel that you can resist the urge to cough, aren't you?" (Say with an affirmative head nod.)
- Express confidence that if the urge to cough recurs, the patient can do the same thing at home (autosuggestion).

Autosuggestion should routinely be provided for patients to continue treatment at home. Autosuggestion refers to quiet sessions at home, with or without parental guidance depending on the patient's preference, in which the patient performs their own suggestion by concentrating on holding back the cough using sips of body temperature water to "ease the irritation" causing cough. The use of online videos where suggestion therapy is successfully provided is helpful [22].

The first online video of habit cough treated by suggestion therapy was in February 2019 when one of the authors, MW, was contacted by the father of a 12-year-old girl (coauthor DB) with 3 months of a repetitive loud chronic barking cough that prevented her school attendance and disrupted the family milieu. Although the cough was absent during sleep, the cough repeated throughout all waking hours. A recording of that video was placed by her father on a website he created, www.habitcough.com (accessed on 1 November 2022), and on YouTube. That video has since become an important source of treatment (Figure 2).

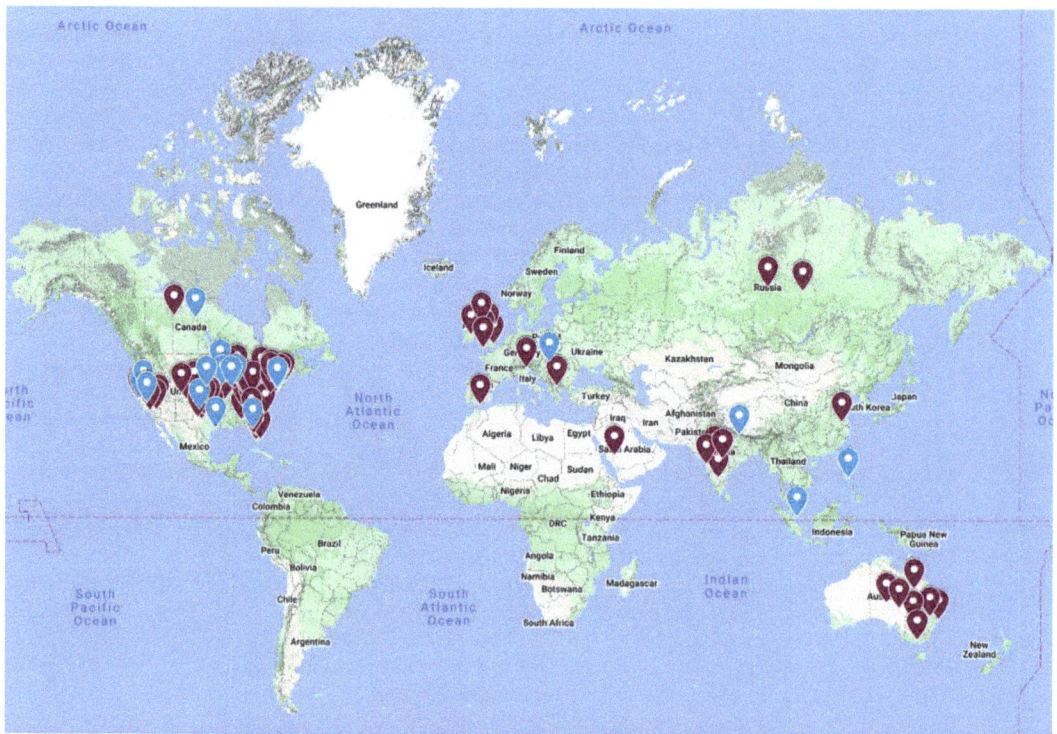

Figure 2. A map of 91 children (red dots) and 20 adults (blue dots) who informed us by email (via parents for children) of cough cessation from watching the video of a girl with chronic daily cough successfully stopped by suggestion therapy.

3.6. Outcome of Habit Cough

A 15–30 min suggestion therapy strategy was used and taught during the 40 years of the corresponding author's (MW) tenure at the University of Iowa Pediatric Allergy and

Pulmonary Division [11]. The standard of care for habit cough at the University of Iowa Pediatric Allergy and Pulmonary Clinic was suggestion therapy provided by any of the faculty assigned to the clinic.

Suggestion therapy by direct contact and autosuggestion (self-suggestion) was more effective than just providing reassurance [23]. Of 85 children who received direct suggestion therapy in the clinic, 81 stopped coughing during 15–30 min of suggestion therapy. Three of the four who did not respond to suggestion therapy had apparent psychological problems that have been described previously (the fourth was not further evaluated) [24]. Autosuggestion instructions were provided to both those who did not receive suggestion therapy in the clinic and in addition to those who received direct suggestion therapy in the clinic since the continued desire to cough might last for days or weeks.

Since the video became publicly available, 91 parents of children with habit cough and 20 adults from the U.S. and 15 other countries informed us by email that watching the video enabled cessation of coughing (Figure 2). Many found that repeated watching of the video was helpful. Eighteen of the ninety-one children additionally requested video contact with the doctor, author MW. A few requested the option of talking to the girl in the video, which was provided by video teleconference. The coughing stopped immediately in some, while sustained effort, rewatching the video, and repeated practice were described by others. The following emails illustrate these different responses:

This email was from a mother with whom we never had direct contact:

"Our daughter, Riley, is seven years old (will be eight in May). A few months back, she had a really bad cold which led to a bad cough. After a few weeks the cold symptoms went away except for that cough. There was no stop to it. Just so much coughing.

I finally decided to just pull your video up on YouTube and we all sat there and watched it. It was very emotional for all of us and at the end Riley was in tears (we all were). We hugged for a time. She said to us "I can hold the cough back. And the ... THE COUGHING STOPPED! Like turning off a switch. For four days now, I have not heard her cough except for a few random ones here and there. The cough is GONE!"

The following email is from the mother of a 14-year-old boy with a history of coughing about two times per minute during waking hours. This continued for more than a month after the clinical symptoms of a viral respiratory infection. Suggestion therapy was provided by MW via remote video conferencing:

"He is doing so much better. He went back to school this week. The first 2 days he had to really work to control the cough and had a few bouts of having a difficult time of doing so. However, the last few days he hasn't coughed at all and the urge is less and less."

These two cases demonstrate the variability in response to suggestion therapy, immediate cessation of coughing or motivated daily practice to accomplish cessation of cough.

We have no way of estimating how many others have watched the video and never contacted us. Physicians in the U.S., Ireland, Israel, and Australia have reported to us that they have referred habit cough patients to that video and received feedback from parents of chronic cough cessation, but we have only the attestation of the physician for those communications.

3.7. Clinical Course of Untreated Habit Cough

In 1991, Mayo Clinic in Rochester, Minnesota reported an 18-year follow-up of 60 children in their medical record archives with "childhood involuntary cough syndrome" consistent with habit cough [25]. The ages of the children were similar to those reported at the University of Iowa [11]. Since no treatment beyond diagnosis and counseling was given, this essentially provided the natural history for untreated habit cough. Cough spontaneously resolved only after a mean duration of 6.1 months after diagnosis in 44 (73%) of the 60. Sixteen (27%) were still coughing a mean of 5.9 years from the time of diagnosis.

At the Brompton Hospital in London, parents were provided only "simple reassurance [12]". A follow-up for 1.9 years was reported in 39 of the 55 children who they were able to contact. Spontaneous resolution of cough was reported in 59% of the 39 within 4 weeks; the others had persistent coughing for longer periods, especially if there was skepticism by the parents regarding the diagnosis.

Further evidence of the potential duration of habit cough was obtained from four adults among the remote contact patients. Their ages ranged from 23 to 32. They described 8–15 years of chronic cough that had begun when they were adolescents. Their clinical characteristics were consistent with habit cough, i.e., daily repetitive nonproductive cough that was absent when asleep. The available data, therefore, show eventual spontaneous resolution for chronic cough in many, but some continue with a persistent cough for years. Consequently, when encountering a child with habit cough, a wait-and-see approach for spontaneous resolution is not a justifiable strategy.

3.8. When Suggestion Therapy Is Not Effective

One of the authors of the article, RA, is a pediatric pulmonologist with skills in medical hypnosis that have been used to successfully treat habit cough [10]. Results of hypnosis for habit cough have found that approximately half of all patients with habit cough who use hypnosis initially resolve their cough immediately after the first application of hypnotic relaxation. Most of the others with typical habit cough who are helped with hypnosis resolve their cough within a month.

Of ten patients from the remote contact source who failed to respond to suggestion therapy, only two improved with hypnotic relaxation alone. Four of those ten patients improved after the use of hypnosis to promote interactions with the part of the mind of which one is not fully aware. Although subconscious, this can nonetheless influence actions and feelings. The use of this strategy is demonstrated in a case study described in *Changing Children's Lives with Hypnosis* [26].

An example of a patient benefiting from sessions with a medical hypnotist was Stella. Stella was a delightful 12-year-old girl from Texas whose father contacted the author MW in February 2022. Her ambition was to be an actress. She coughed about every 3–5 s continually throughout all waking hours but did not cough when sleeping. Despite several remote conversations where she was fully cooperative and highly motivated to stop, there was no progress. Local hypnosis and counseling were arranged by her father at the recommendation of author RA. Six months later her father described the successful cessation of Stella's habit cough after eight sessions with a local hypnotist selected on the basis of being skilled in medical hypnosis for children.

Interestingly, the few children resistant to suggestion therapy appeared to differ from those who responded to suggestion therapy. The "tickle," the feeling in the throat that was typically present in patients with habit cough, was not present in these children. They did not notice any precough tickle or stimulus. They also had persistent very high cough frequency, cough every few seconds, without the greater variation from distraction commonly present in others. In some, the cough seemed to occur with every exhalation.

What are we to think about these markedly different responses to suggestion therapy and hypnosis in this small minority of children diagnosed with habit cough? Are they totally different disorders or, as with many diseases, are there different phenotypes of habit cough?

4. Discussion

Chronic cough is a horribly unpleasant ailment. Coughing hundreds of times every hour of their waking lives has a profound impact on their quality of life. Muscular pain, headache, and depression are common in children and adults with this functional cough. Habit cough has been in the medical literature for over 300 years. The children from the University of Iowa and the remote contact data set we have accumulated provide evidence for a serious disorder that, while not common, is also not rare. Two major referral centers, one in the U.S. and one in England, reported an average of nine children with habit cough per year in their clinics.

4.1. What Is the Current Status of Identifying and Treating Habit Cough

Just as Dr. Berman recognized and treated habit cough in his 1966 publication [5], other physicians have recognized incessant coughing without an apparent cause as a habit disorder and used their clinical skills to provide their own approach to break the habit [9,10]. Publications over the past few years [11,22,24] and invited presentations to 12 pediatric pulmonary divisions in the U.S. and pediatric pulmonary conferences in London and Taipei have resulted in an increasing number of physicians who provide recognition and competent treatment for habit cough. A link for the recording of one of those presentations at the National Children's Hospital is available at www.milesweinberger.com (accessed on 1 November 2022).

Despite the increased awareness of some physicians, primarily pediatric pulmonologists, frustrated parents continue to contact us because their medical providers do not recognize or know how to treat the "horror" cough from which the child is suffering. The awareness of the medical community about habit cough needs to be substantially increased.

4.2. Barriers to Diagnosis and Treatment

Why the difficulty in recognizing and treating a disorder that a Boston allergist reported as responsive to "the art of suggestion" in 1966? [5]. False beliefs about habit cough have been a major barrier (Table 1).

Table 1. Popular factoids and actual facts regarding habit cough.

• **Children with habit cough exhibit *la belle indifférence*.**
It has been suggested that children with habit cough appear to not care about their cough. While children may adapt to living with a chronic cough, few if any have appeared to us content about their cough. It is life-altering for the child and their family and, if asked, the children express concern about their cough. They are not indifferent to their cough.
• **School phobia can precipitate or perpetuate habit cough.**
This claim was made in a 2020 Chest publication [27]. The reference used to support that claim was a case series of adults at a psychiatric facility [28]. While there are occasional patients with school phobia as a factor, our experience does not support the assertion that school phobia is a common concern as a cause of habit cough. We have observed that the children with habit cough are generally concerned about missing school. Those who had been out of school because of the cough are generally enthusiastic about returning.
• **Habit cough is exclusively a pediatric disorder.**
We have been contacted by 20 adults from eight countries with chronic cough who reported to us by email that their coughing was stopped by suggestion therapy from viewing the video made available by coauthor DB (see Figure 2). In addition, three adults had their chronic cough resolved by hypnosis therapy performed by coauthor RA. It is not known how many with habit cough are among the 40% of adults with idiopathic or refractory cough [29,30]. Our serendipitous experience identified 20 adults with the same clinical characteristics as the children with habit cough who described cessation of cough by suggestion therapy. Interestingly, Peter Dicpinigaitis, editor of the journal *Lung*, states in a publication that among 1000 patients he has never seen psychogenic cough (a euphemism for habit cough) [31]. However, Dr. Kefang Lai described 23 adults that he termed "somatic cough syndrome" (another euphemism for habit cough) [32]. Other case reports of psychogenic cough in adults also has been described [33,34].
• **Habit cough diagnosis requires that all other causes of cough are eliminated.**
While this has been stated without support in guidelines for chronic cough, habit cough has a sufficiently distinctive clinical presentation that major centers experienced with this disorder make the diagnosis with little testing or therapeutic trials. Efforts to examine for other causes of cough only add to the morbidity and cost [11,12]. Treating habit cough early in the course of its clinical presentation can prevent unnecessary and expensive investigations that delay resolution.

Table 1. *Cont.*

- **Habit cough is a tic disorder, a *forme fruste* of Tourette's syndrome.**

This was claimed by Dr. Alyn Morice, a prominent cough specialist, who wrote in an email, "You are describing, but failing to recognize, a *forme fruste* of Tourette's syndrome". However, cough is not supported as a usual finding in Tourette's 1884 publication [35]. Moreover, during interviews with parents of children with Tourette's, cough was readily recognized as cough and not a tic and was regarded as separate from the symptoms of Tourette's in their child.

A concerning barrier to recognition and treatment of habit cough is that the perceptions of some physicians are not consistent with the morbidity caused by this disorder. Perceptions that habit cough was not as important as physical disorders were occasionally expressed as were concerns about the time required for suggestion therapy. However, despite the absence of a physical cause, these children have serious morbidity that is readily treatable. As to having the time, that is a lame comment. When necessary, a physician makes the time to provide appropriate care for a patient in need.

A debate on the subject of terminology for this cough disorder was arranged by Richard Irwin, a cough specialist and editor of the journal *Chest*, between one of the authors of this article (MW) and a neurologist, Tamara Pringsheim, MD [36]. Skepticism regarding habit cough also was expressed by Dr. Peter Dicpinigaitis, current editor of the journal *Lung*. When provided a description of habit cough from one of the authors, he stated in an email, "I'm not a fan of science fiction".

While cough may occur in patients with Tourette's syndrome, our experience with five patients who had Tourette's syndrome found that cough was in addition to Tourette's typical symptoms of motor tics and vocalizations. One patient was Jacob, an 11-year-old boy whose father and he both had typical symptoms of Tourette's. Following symptoms of a common cold, he developed a severe repetitive cough, absent during sleep, for a month prior to contact with us. His cough responded to suggestion therapy without any effect on his tics or occasional vocalizations. Father, who had lived with his own Tourette's symptoms indicated that the 1 month of cough experienced by his son was not related to symptoms of Tourette's. Another example of the lack of association of habit cough and Tourette's was Soraya, a 10-year-old girl with typical symptoms of Tourette's since age 3. After symptoms of a cold, she had repetitive coughing, multiple times per minute, absent only during sleep, for 2 months. She responded readily to suggestion therapy by proxy. A recurrence a year later after another cold was stopped within a week after suggestion therapy was provided by remote video conferencing.

An unfortunate consequence of this diagnostic dialectic is the experience of Tom, a 16-year-old boy with 3 years of chronic cough. In 2020, a neurologist at Children's Hospital of Philadelphia attributed his cough to Tourette's syndrome, a diagnosis that stayed with him until suggestion therapy provided by remote video conferencing enabled him to control his cough more than 2 years later. Three days after the remote video conferencing, Tom reported coughing had gone from thousands per day to no more than ten. Ten days later, Tom was continuing to be free of his former daily repetitive cough with no symptoms of Tourette's.

Thus, our experience has been that motor tics were not associated with habit cough. Cough was distinct from the echophenomena of Tourette's. While there have been published case reports of chronic cough attributed to Tourette's [37,38], our experience indicates that when typical symptoms of Tourette's are present, a chronic repetitive dry cough present during most waking hours that is absent during sleep is likely a separate clinical problem and not a component of the Tourette's.

Because of the nature of habit cough and its cure by a simple behavioral technique, suggestion therapy, a degree of incredulousness has inhibited more widespread attention to this disorder. Newspaper articles hoping to educate the public have been few. The Daily Beast on 29 April 2019 was the only story about the habit cough and its cure by suggestion in the U.S. An article in the *Scotsman*, a major Scottish newspaper, on 21 March 2021 described the cure of habit cough in an 11-year-old girl who had been coughing for a year. She stopped coughing by watching the video of suggestion therapy provided to a 12-year-old girl. Further publication in the health section of major newspapers would distribute information that enables parents to seek earlier diagnosis and treatment.

4.3. Guidelines for Chronic Cough from Professional Societies

A guideline for the diagnosis and treatment of chronic cough in adults and children was published by the European Respiratory Society in 2020 with 18 authors [39]. Recommendations were for therapeutic trials of inhaled corticosteroids with and without a long-acting bronchodilator, an antileukotriene, and a macrolide. Low-dose morphine and gabapentin were suggested for adults. An antibiotic trial was recommended for children. The recommendation was indicated as conditional with the level of evidence rated low to moderate. This guideline addressed gastrointestinal reflux and postnasal drip, also known as upper airway cough syndrome, two disorders some cough specialists have regarded as contentious. Habit or tic cough was suggested to be labeled somatic cough disorder, and the guideline indicated that the diagnosis should only be made after an extensive evaluation that rules out tic disorders and uncommon causes of chronic cough. That guideline did not recognize that four major referral centers, the University of Iowa, SUNY Upstate Medical University, Rainbow Children's Hospital in Cleveland, and Brompton Hospital in London had been diagnosing habit cough for years based on the unique clinical presentation without extensive evaluation [11,12].

A guideline published in 2020 by an Expert Panel in the journal *Chest* focused on chronic cough in children [27]. The report acknowledged that many questions addressed in systematic reviews of chronic cough did not contain high-quality studies or evidence. Gastroesophageal reflux and postnasal drip were not supported as being of concern in children. Emphasis was placed on the importance of identifying various diseases that cause cough, such as tuberculosis, pertussis, and protracted bacterial bronchitis. While habit cough, also known as tic cough or somatic cough syndrome, was discussed, a major characteristic of habit cough was discounted. Specifically, the expert panel concluded that "the presence or absence of cough when sleeping should not be used to diagnose or exclude psychogenic or habit cough". This was inconsistent with virtually every publication describing absence when asleep as a characteristic of habit cough [4–11].

4.4. Strengths and Limitations of This Report

The strength of this report is the presentation of the extensive past and present experiences with habit cough of the authors, the provision of data related to the clinical course of children not treated with suggestion therapy, and the observations that suggestion therapy stops chronic cough in a substantial number of children and some adults with this disorder. Suggestion therapy is effectively provided by direct contact, indirect contact by remote video conferencing, and by proxy using a video of an effective session of suggestive therapy.

A limitation of the report is that all of our data are observational with no comparative control group. Although we serendipitously found habit cough responsive to suggestion therapy in 20 adults, we do not know what portion of the 40% of adults with idiopathic or refractory chronic cough have habit cough [29,30].

5. Conclusions and Recommendations

Habit cough is a distinctive disorder characterized by a repetitive daily nonproductive cough that generally persists during all waking hours but is absent once asleep. This description is the basis for diagnosis. Major medical centers that have routinely made the diagnosis of habit cough primarily on that clinical presentation include 140 children over 20 years at the University of Iowa, 56 children over 5 years at SUNY Upstate Medical University and Rainbow Children's Hospital in Cleveland, and 55 children over 6 years at

Brompton Hospital in London, England. Treatment by suggestion therapy is extraordinarily successful and should now be the standard of care for children with this disorder.

The provision of suggestion therapy can potentially be provided by the patient's physician that makes the diagnosis. The characteristic clinical presentation of a repetitive dry cough that is absent when asleep is generally sufficient for diagnosis. While a chest X-ray and spirometry may help provide assurance for the family of the absence of an organic cause, there is rarely an indication for more testing or therapeutic trials. Suggestion therapy should be approached with positivity. Suggestion therapy is not something to be tried, it is to be executed with confidence.

There is evidence that habit cough also can be a cause of chronic cough in adults. Medical books more than 300 years ago [2,3] described a habitual severe cough in adults, and one describes the absence once asleep, a *sine qua non* for the diagnosis of habit cough [2]. Emails to us from 20 adults describe the same clinical pattern of cough and the same response to suggestion therapy as in children with this disorder. The prevalence of habit cough in adult populations with idiopathic or refractory chronic cough warrants investigation. Those with a clinical pattern consistent with habit cough should be considered for a controlled clinical trial of suggestion therapy.

Author Contributions: Conceptualization, M.W.; Methodology, M.W., D.B. and R.D.A.; Validation, M.W., D.B. and R.D.A.; Resources, M.W. and D.B.; Writing—original draft preparation, M.W.; Writing—review and editing, M.W., D.B. and R.D.A.; Supervision, M.W. and D.B.; Project administration, M.W. and D.B.; Visualization, D.B. All authors have read and agreed to the published version of the manuscript.

Funding: This research received no external funding.

Informed Consent Statement: This publication involved no human experimentation or identification. In the few places where specific patients were mentioned, identification was not provided and all patients or parents of children who voluntarily provided clinical information signed a release permitting sharing of that information.

Data Availability Statement: Data in the form of parent of patient email communications are available for purposes of further research of habit cough.

Conflicts of Interest: The authors declare no conflict of interest.

References

1. Hurvitz, M.; Weinberger, M. Functional respiratory disorders in children. In Pulmonary Manifestations of Pediatric Diseases, Pediatr Clinics of North America. *Pediatr. Clin.* **2021**, *68*, 223–237.
2. Willis, T. *The London Practice of Physick, in the Pharmaceutic Rationalis*; 1685; p. 265.
3. Mercurius, F. *Habitual Cough, in The Spirit of Diseases*; Printed for Sarah Hawkins in George-Yard, in Lombard-Street; 1694; p. 118.
4. Creighton, C. *Illustrations of Unconscious Memory in Disease*; HK Lewis: London, UK, 1886; p. 63.
5. Berman, B.A. Habit cough in adolescent children. *Ann. Allergy* **1966**, *24*, 43–46.
6. Lokshin, B.; Lindgren, S.; Weinberger, M.; Koviach, J. Outcome of habit cough in children treated with a brief session of suggestion therapy. *Ann. Allergy* **1991**, *67*, 579–582. [PubMed]
7. Kravitz, H.; Gomberg, R.M.; Burnstine, R.C.; Hagler, S.; Korach, A. Psychogenic cough tic in children and adolescents. Nine case histories illustrate the need for re-evaluation of this common but frequently unrecognized problem. *Clin. Pediatr.* **1969**, *8*, 580–583. [CrossRef] [PubMed]
8. Weinberg, E.G. 'Honking': Psychogenic cough tic in children. *S. Afr. Med. J.* **1980**, *57*, 198–200.
9. Cohlan, S.Q.; Stone, S.M. The cough and the bedsheet. *Pediatrics* **1984**, *74*, 11–15. [CrossRef]
10. Anbar, R.D.; Hall, H. Childhood habit cough treated with self-hypnosis. *J. Pediatr.* **2004**, *144*, 213–217. [CrossRef]
11. Weinberger, M.; Hoegger, M. The cough without a cause: Habit cough syndrome. *J. Allergy Clin. Immunol.* **2015**, *137*, 930–931. [CrossRef]
12. Wright, M.F.A.; Balfour-Lynn, I.M. Habit-tic cough: Presentation and outcome with simple reassurance. *Pediatr. Pulmonol.* **2018**, *53*, 512–516. [CrossRef]
13. Papadopoulou, A.; Mermiri, D.-Z.T.; Gritzelas, G.; Tsouridi, O.; Dimara, D.; Yapijakis, C.; Chrousos, G.P. Increased incidence of stress-related tic habit cough in children during the recent Greek financial crisis. *In Vivo* **2021**, *35*, 1811–1820. [CrossRef]
14. Chang, A.B.; Robertson, C.F.; Van Asperen, E.P. A multicenter study on chronic cough in children: Buren and etiologies based on a standardized management pathway. *CHEST* **2012**, *1442*, 943–950. [CrossRef]

15. Rouadi, P.W.; Idriss, S.A.; Bousquet, J.; Laidlaw, T.M.; Azar, C.R.; Al-Ahmad, M.S.; Yañez, A.; Al-Nesf, M.A.Y.; Nsouli, T.M.; Bahna, S.L.; et al. WAO-ARIA consensus on chronic cough—Part II: Phenotypes and mechanisms of abnormal cough presentation—Updates in COVID-19. *World Allergy Organ. J.* **2021**, *14*, 24–26. [CrossRef] [PubMed]
16. Di Cicco, M.; Tozzi, M.G.; Ragazzo, V.; Peroni, D.; Kantar, A. Chronic respiratory diseases other than asthma in children: The COVID-19 tsunami. *Ital. J. Pediatr.* **2021**, *47*, 220. [CrossRef] [PubMed]
17. Doležalová, K.; Tuková, J.; Pohunek, P. The respiratory consequences of COVID-19 lasted for a median of 4 months in a cohort of children aged 2–18 years of age. *Acta Paediatr.* **2022**, *111*, 1201–1206. [CrossRef]
18. Morice, A.H.; Millqvist, E.; Belvisi, M.G.; Bieksiene, K.; Birring, S.S.; Chung, K.F.; Negro, R.W.D.; Dicpinigaitis, P.; Kantar, A.; McGarvey, L.P.; et al. Expert opinion on the cough hypersensitivity syndrome in respiratory medicine. *Eur. Respir. J.* **2014**, *44*, 1132–1148. [CrossRef] [PubMed]
19. Irwin, R.S.; Ownbey, R.; Cagle, P.T.; Stephen Baker, S.; Fraire, A.E. Interpreting the histopathology of chronic cough: A prospective, controlled, comparative study. *CHEST* **2006**, *130*, 362–370. [CrossRef] [PubMed]
20. Shapiro, C.O.; Proskocil, B.J.; Oppegard, L.J.; Blum, E.D.; Kappel, N.L.; Chang, C.H.; Fryer, A.D.; Jacoby, D.B.; Costello, R.W.; Drake, M.G. Airway sensory nerve density is increased in chronic cough. *Am. J. Respir. Crit. Care Med.* **2021**, *203*, 348–355. [CrossRef] [PubMed]
21. Slinger, C.; Mehdi, S.B.; Milan, S.J.; Dodd, S.; Matthews, J.; Vyas, A.; Marsden, P.A. Speech and language therapy for management of chronic cough. *Cochrane Database Syst Rev.* **2019**, *7*, CD013067. [CrossRef]
22. Weinberger, M.; Buettner, D. Cures of the cough without a cause. *Ann Allergy Asthma Immunol.* **2021**, *127*, 381–383. [CrossRef]
23. Weinberger, M. Commentary: The habit cough: Diagnosis and treatment. *Pediatr. Pulmonol.* **2018**, *53*, 535–537. [CrossRef]
24. Weinberger, M. The habit cough syndrome and its variations. *Lung* **2012**, *190*, 45–53. [CrossRef]
25. Rojas, A.R.; Sachs, M.I.; Yunginger, J.W.; O'Connell, E.J. Childhood involuntary cough syndrome: A long-term follow-up study. *Ann Allergy* **1991**, *66*, 106.
26. Anbar, R.D. *Changing Children's Lives with Hypnosis: A Journey to the Center*; Rowman & Littlefield: New York, NY, USA, 2021; Chapter 12.
27. Chang, A.B.; Oppenheimer, J.J.; Irwin, R.S.; CHEST Expert Cough Panel. Managing chronic cough as a symptom in children and management algorithms—CHEST guideline and expert panel report. *Chest* **2020**, *158*, 303–329. [CrossRef] [PubMed]
28. Bhatia, M.S.; Chandra, R.; Vaid, L. Psychogenic cough: A profile of 32 cases. *Int. J. Psychiatry Med.* **2002**, *32*, 353–360. [CrossRef] [PubMed]
29. Gibson, P.G. Management of cough. *J. Allergy Clin. Immunol. Pract.* **2019**, *7*, 1724–1729. [CrossRef]
30. Smith, J.A.; Woodcock, A. Chronic cough. *N. Engl. J. Med.* **2016**, *375*, 1544–1551. [CrossRef] [PubMed]
31. Dicpinigaitis, P.V. Thoughts on one thousand chronic cough patients. *Lung* **2012**, *190*, 593–596. [CrossRef]
32. Lai, K.; Peng, W.; Zhan, W.; Xie, J.-X.; Tian, J.; Zuo, X.-P.; Long, L.; Tang, J.-M.; Pan, J.-Y.; Jiang, M.; et al. Clinical characteristics in adult patients with somatic cough syndrome. *Ther. Adv. Respir. Dis.* **2022**, *16*, 17534666221092993. [CrossRef]
33. Gay, M.; Blager, F.; Bartsch, K.; Emery, C.F.; Rosenstiel-Gross, A.K.; Spears, J. Psychogenic habit cough: Review and case reports. *J. Clin. Psychiatry* **1987**, *48*, 483–486.
34. Mastrovich, J.D.; Greenberger, P.A. Psychogenic cough in adults: A report of two cases and review of the literature. *Allergy Asthma Proc.* **2003**, *23*, 27–33.
35. Lajonchere, C.; Nortz, M.; Finger, S. Gilles de la Tourette and the discovery of Tourette syndrome. Includes a translation of his 1884 article. *Arch Neurol.* **1996**, *53*, 567–574. [CrossRef]
36. Weinberger, M.; Pringsheim, T. Point-counterpoint and rebuttals: Is the term habit cough an inaccurate use of the term? *Chest* **2019**, *156*, 821–825. [CrossRef] [PubMed]
37. Duncan, K.L.; Faust, R.A. Tourette syndrome manifest as chronic cough. *Int. J. Pediatr. Otorhinolaryngol.* **2002**, *65*, 65–68. [CrossRef]
38. Tan, H.; Büyükavci, M.; Arık, A. Tourette's syndrome manifests as chronic persistent cough. *Yonsei Med. J.* **2004**, *45*, 145–149. [CrossRef] [PubMed]
39. Morice, A.H.; Millqvist, E.; Bieksiene, K.; Birring, S.S.; Dicpinigaitis, P.; Ribas, C.D.; Boon, M.H.; Kantar, A.; Lai, K.; McGarvey, L.; et al. ERS guidelines on the diagnosis and treatment of chronic cough in adults and children. *Eur. Respir. J.* **2019**, *55*, 1901136. [CrossRef] [PubMed]

Disclaimer/Publisher's Note: The statements, opinions and data contained in all publications are solely those of the individual author(s) and contributor(s) and not of MDPI and/or the editor(s). MDPI and/or the editor(s) disclaim responsibility for any injury to people or property resulting from any ideas, methods, instructions or products referred to in the content.

MDPI
St. Alban-Anlage 66
4052 Basel
Switzerland
www.mdpi.com

Journal of Clinical Medicine Editorial Office
E-mail: jcm@mdpi.com
www.mdpi.com/journal/jcm

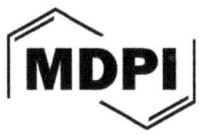

Disclaimer/Publisher's Note: The statements, opinions and data contained in all publications are solely those of the individual author(s) and contributor(s) and not of MDPI and/or the editor(s). MDPI and/or the editor(s) disclaim responsibility for any injury to people or property resulting from any ideas, methods, instructions or products referred to in the content.

www.ingramcontent.com/pod-product-compliance
Lightning Source LLC
LaVergne TN
LVHW070613100526
838202LV00012B/636